FUSION GENES AND CANCER

FUSION GENES AND CANCER

Editors

Ajaikumar B. Kunnumakkara
Ganesan Padmavathi
Nand Kishor Roy

Indian Institute of Technology (IIT) Guwahati, India

World Scientific

NEW JERSEY • LONDON • SINGAPORE • BEIJING • SHANGHAI • HONG KONG • TAIPEI • CHENNAI • TOKYO

Published by

World Scientific Publishing Co. Pte. Ltd.
5 Toh Tuck Link, Singapore 596224
USA office: 27 Warren Street, Suite 401-402, Hackensack, NJ 07601
UK office: 57 Shelton Street, Covent Garden, London WC2H 9HE

Library of Congress Cataloging-in-Publication Data
Names: Kunnumakkara, Ajaikumar B., editor. | Padmavathi, Ganesan, editor. | Roy, Nand Kishor, editor.
Title: Fusion genes and cancer / edited by Ajaikumar B. Kunnumakkara, Ganesan Padmavathi & Nand Kishor Roy.
Description: New Jersey : World Scientific, [2016] | Includes bibliographical references and index.
Identifiers: LCCN 2016039026 | ISBN 9789813200937 (hardcover : alk. paper)
Subjects: | MESH: Gene Fusion | Neoplasms--genetics
Classification: LCC RC268.4 | NLM QU 475 | DDC 616.99/4042--dc23
LC record available at https://lccn.loc.gov/2016039026

British Library Cataloguing-in-Publication Data
A catalogue record for this book is available from the British Library.

Desk Editors: Herbert Moses/Joy Quek

Typeset by Stallion Press
Email: enquiries@stallionpress.com

Printed in Singapore

Our Acharyas, Gurus and Parents whose wisdom continues to inspire and guide us!

Preface

Cancer is one of the foremost health concerns of people today affecting more than 14 million people across the globe. Both genetic and environmental factors contribute enormously to the risk of cancer occurrence. However, influence of inherited risk factors on cancer development is relatively very less compared to the 90–95% dominance of environmental factors such as poor diet, consumption of tobacco and alcohol, exposure to diverse occupational carcinogens, radiations and infections, etc. Sustained exposure to these factors increases the susceptibility to mutations (abnormal changes in DNA) ultimately leading to the development of cancer. Genome of cancer cells holds thousands of such irreparable mutations like insertion, deletion, translocation, etc. and these molecular alterations result in collective abnormality of the cell. Interestingly, some of them are being used as molecular markers and targets for cancer diagnosis and treatment. In the recent years, a distinct class of mutations known as "fusion genes" is found to be implicated in the development and maintenance of many cancers. The concept of gene fusions was seeded way back in 20th century when the Philadelphia chromosome with t(9;22) translocation was first identified in leukemic patient in 1960. Subsequent discovery of BCR-ABL fusion oncogene paved way towards a new era of cancer genomics signifying the formation of chimera of two distinct genes to produce novel fusion gene either with completely different function from the partner genes or with enhanced activity of wild-type partner genes. Further, the identification of BCR-ABL led to the discovery of more than 400 fusion genes in different cancers. Extensive research over the past several decades successfully unraveled the impact of few such fusion genes on the development of cancer and some of them are being used as diagnostic biomarkers as well as therapeutic targets to facilitate improved clinicomanagement of cancer. However, among the numerous fusion genes identified thus far, only very few have been well characterized and ascertained to possess a strong correlation with the process of carcinogenesis. Moreover, there is a lack of knowledge among the scientific community on these fusion genes and their enormous importance in cancer, which definitely demands an all-inclusive book on this topic. Therefore, this monograph is our sincere attempt to give a detailed idea about various fusion genes and their role in different cancers through exclusive compilation of available literature.

Aforementioned, certain fusion genes are found to be unique for a particular cancer thus marking them as potential diagnostic biomarkers for such cancers. Therefore, studying fusion genes would help us to unfold the knots in the development of certain cancers which are remaining elusive and also would serve as potential biomarkers for the diagnosis and treatment of cancer. Further, it is essential to have a fundamental knowledge on chromosomal rearrangements and fusion genes, formation of which is currently emerging as a significant molecular event in variety of cancers. Therefore, this monograph deals with the theories of initiation of chromosomal rearrangements, their formation as well as classification; techniques available for the identification of novel fusion genes, for the detection of known fusion genes and their importance in cancer diagnosis; function of fusion genes in the pathology of different cancers; and finally the significance of fusion gene inhibitors in successful cancer therapy. On the whole, we firmly believe that our book will help the readers to understand the science behind the formation of gene fusions and their importance in cancer development and treatment. Noteworthy to mention, this is the first book of its kind that gives a comprehensive review of available literature on fusion genes and cancer. Therefore, we anticipate that this monograph would benefit a wide range of readers working in the field of cancer biology, cancer genomics and proteomics, etc. and would help them to build a stronger foundation on this topic and to discover novel fusion genes as cancer biomarkers and therapeutic targets for better clinicomanagement of this disease.

Ajaikumar B. Kunnumakkara
Ganesan Padmavathi
Nand Kishor Roy

About the Editors

Dr. Ajaikumar B. Kunnumakkara is currently working as a faculty member in the Department of Biosciences and Bioengineering, Indian Institute of Technology (IIT) Guwahati, Assam, India. He earned his doctorate in 2006 from Amala Cancer Research Center, Thrissur, affiliated with University of Calicut, Kerala, India. Dr. Kunnumakkara did his first postdoctoral work at the University of Texas MD Anderson Cancer Center, Houston, Texas, USA (2005–2008) and his second postdoctoral work at the National Cancer Institute of National Institutes of Health (NCI/NIH), Bethesda, Maryland, USA (2008–2010); where he was subsequently employed as a NIH Scientist from 2010 to 2012. Dr. Kunnumakkara's research interests include identification of novel biomarkers for cancer diagnosis and prognosis; role of inflammatory pathways in cancer development; role of chromosomal translocations in the initiation, promotion and progression of cancer; and drug development from natural products. He is credited with the publication of more than sixty research articles. He has more than 14,000 citations with an h-index of >40. Currently, his work is cited over 1,700 times in the literature annually. Dr. Kunnumakkara has also edited two monographs entitled *Molecular Targets and Therapeutic Uses of Spices: Modern Uses for Ancient Medicine* and *Anticancer Properties of Fruits and Vegetables: A Scientific Review*.

Ms. Ganesan Padmavathi is currently working as a research scholar at Cancer Biology Laboratory, Department of Biosciences and Bioengineering, Indian Institute of Technology (IIT) Guwahati, Assam, India. She did her Bachelor of Technology (B.Tech) in Biotechnology from Bannari Amman Institute of Technology, Tamil Nadu, India. Her prime research interests include multi-step mutagenesis and cancer development and identification of novel molecular markers for the early diagnosis and treatment of cancer. Moreover, her research also involves the discovery of novel prognostic biomarkers for the prediction of treatment outcome. Apart from these, she is also interested in the development of novel, multi-targeted, safe and effective therapeutic agents from natural products such as nutraceuticals for the prevention and treatment of various cancers.

Mr. Nand Kishor Roy currently works as a research scholar in Cancer Biology Laboratory at Indian Institute of Technology (IIT) Guwahati, Assam, India. He completed his graduation (B.Sc.) in Zoology and Master of Science (M.Sc.) in Biotechnology from North East Hill University (NEHU) Shillong, India. His research interest is primarily focused on deciphering the role of different proteins involved in the process of tumorigenesis and finding their prospects as potential biomarkers for better diagnosis and prognosis. Beside this, he is also interested in understanding the various genetic aspects of cancer through the identification and characterization of different chromosomal rearrangements. He also shares his interest in discovery of novel natural products for developing cost-effective cancer therapy.

List of Contributors

Anand Anip holds a Bachelor of Technology (B.Tech) in Biotechnology from Indian Institute of Technology (IIT) Guwahati, Assam, India. His area of interest includes cancer genomics and proteomics and personalized cancer medicine.

Choudhary Harsha is currently working as a research scholar at Cancer Biology Laboratory, Department of Biosciences and Bioengineering, Indian Institute of Technology (IIT) Guwahati, Assam, India. She has completed her Masters in Biotechnology from North Eastern Hill University, Shillong, India. Her research interest involves identification of biomarkers for early diagnosis and treatment of cancer and studies related to nutraceuticals and nanoformulations for developing effective cancer therapies.

Devivasha Bordoloi is currently working as a research scholar at Cancer Biology Laboratory, Department of Biosciences and Bioengineering, Indian Institute of Technology (IIT) Guwahati, Assam, India. She holds a Bachelor of Technology (B.Tech) in Genetic Engineering. Her research interests include cancer chemosensitization, the role of diverse proteins in the development of chemoresistance and the mechanisms involved.

Javadi Monisha is currently working as a research scholar at Cancer Biology Laboratory, Department of Biosciences and Bioengineering, Indian Institute of Technology (IIT) Guwahati, Assam, India. She has done her Master of Technology (M.Tech) from Jawaharlal Technological University (JNTU) Hyderabad, India. Her research interest is to understand the role of various proteins that could serve as early diagnostic biomarkers, their involvement in chemoresistance and the possible approaches to overcome the problem.

Kishore Banik is currently working as a research scholar at Cancer Biology Laboratory, Department of Biosciences and Bioengineering, Indian Institute of Technology (IIT) Guwahati, Assam, India. He did his Masters in Biochemistry from University of Pune, India. His research interests involves role of inflammatory pathways in cancer development, identification of novel biomarkers for cancer diagnosis and prognosis and cancer drug discovery.

Krishan Kumar Thakur is currently working as a research scholar at Cancer Biology Laboratory, Department of Biosciences and Bioengineering, Indian Institute of Technology (IIT) Guwahati, Assam, India. He holds Bachelor of Pharmacy (B.Pharm) and Master of Science (M.S) in Biotechnology. His research interest includes cancer drug discovery and identification of novel biomarkers for cancer diagnosis and prognosis.

Contents

1

Cancer — An Overview and Molecular Alterations in Cancer

*Nand K. Roy, Devivasha Bordoloi, Javadi Monisha, Anand Anip, Ganesan Padmavathi and Ajaikumar B. Kunnumakkara**

INTRODUCTION

Cancer comprises more than 200 diseases that accounted for about 14.1 million new cases and 8.2 million deaths worldwide in the year 2012. It is responsible for most deaths in both economically developed and developing nations (Cavalieri *et al.*, 2002; Siegal *et al.*, 2012). Cancer is the result of accumulation of molecular alterations that change the normal characteristics of cells. These alterations lead to malfunctioning of the control system that otherwise prevent overgrowth and uncontrolled proliferation of the cells. The altered cells can attain distinctive features such as variation in cell structure, diminished property of cell adhesion, capability to synthesize

*Author for correspondence: Ajaikumar B. Kunnumakkara, Cancer Biology Laboratory, Department of Biosciences and Bioengineering, Indian Institute of Technology Guwahati, Assam 781039, India. kunnumakkara@iitg.ernet.in

new enzymes which helps their progeny to divide and sustain, even in the presence of normal nearby cells which can inhibit their growth (Varricchio, 2004). In general, tumors have been classified as benign (harmless) and malignant (harmful). Benign tumors are normally slow-growing expansive masses that remain confined to their original location and do not invade surrounding normal tissues and spread to distant body sites. Though they pose little threat, they can have malignant potential. A malignant tumor, on the other hand, has the potential to invade the neighboring normal tissues as well as spread all over the body by circulatory or lymphatic systems via a process of metastasis. Cancers are usually referred as malignant tumors by their capability to invade and metastasize different parts of the body which makes it life threatening. Although benign tumors can be usually removed by surgical intervention, malignant tumors are resistant to such localized treatments (Cooper and Sunderland, 2000; Alison, 2001).

Based on the cells of origin, cancer can be further classified into three main classes such as carcinomas, sarcomas, leukemias and lymphomas. Malignancies of epithelial cells are known as carcinomas that constitute approximately 90% of all human cancers which includes cancers of breast, colon, lung, pancreas and prostate. The cancers which initiate from the connective tissues like muscle, bone, cartilage and fibrous tissue are known as sarcomas, though they are quite rare in humans. The cancers which arise from blood-forming cells and from cells of the immune system are known as leukemia and lymphoma, respectively, and they account for approximately 8% of human malignancies. Tumors can additionally be divided according to the tissue of origin such as lung or breast carcinomas and the type of cells involved like fibrosarcomas arise from fibroblasts, erythroid leukemia from precursors of erythrocytes, etc. Compared to other cancers, cancers of soft tissues, brain, testes, bone and other organs are relatively rare. However, they can create significant health related complications in specific age groups and geographic regions (Varricchio, 2004; Cooper and Sunderland, 2000; Schulz, 2005).

ORIGIN, HISTORY AND THEORIES OF CANCER

The term cancer was coined from Greek word *carcinos* and *carcinoma,* which relates to non-ulcer forming and ulcer-forming tumors, respectively, by Greek physician Hippocrates (460–370 BC). In Greek language, these words are used for crab which might be applied due to the finger-like protrusions from a cancer, giving it the form of a crab. Later, the Roman physician, Celsus (28–50 BC) reworded it into *cancer* which is the Latin word for a crab. The Greek physician Galen (130–200 AD), described the phrase *oncos* for tumors (Greek for swelling) (The History of Cancer, 2014). The earliest evidence of cancer incidence dates back to 1600 BC in ancient manuscripts describing bone cancer of mummies in ancient Egypt. Though, the world's oldest recorded case of cancer was that of breast cancer reported in ancient Egypt in 1500 BC where lack of any treatment was indicated and only palliative treatment options was shown to be available (Sudhakar, 2009).

From the primeval, physicians are clueless over the causes of cancer and several theories have been put forth. The earliest theory came from Hippocrates in the form of Humoral theory where he proposed that the human body has four humors (body fluids) specifically blood, phlegm, yellow bile and black bile. He anticipated that the imbalance in these fluids can result in disease development and accumulation of black bile to a certain level in a particular organ site can result in cancer. This humoral theory of cancer was accepted for over 1,300 years in the middle ages. Later, it was replaced by Lymph theory where it was anticipated that cancer formation is the result of another body fluid known as lymph. It was emphasized that life consists of continuous flow of fluids like blood and lymph in the body. This theory was promoted extensively in 17th century where it was thought that tumors arise from the lymph coming out of the blood. In 1838, German pathologist Johannes Muller put forth the theory of Blastema and proved that cancer is composed of cells and not lymph. He proposed that budding elements (blastema) are responsible for the development of cancer cells developed between normal tissues. Later, his student Virchow (1821–1902) determined that all cells along with cancer cells originates from other cells and proposed chronic irritation theory where he stated that chronic irritation is responsible for cancer though he mistakenly considered that cancers "spread like a liquid". But in 1860, German surgeon, Karl Thiersch, determined that cancers can metastasize by the spreading of malignant cells and not by any means of unidentified fluid. From the late 1800s to the 1920s, trauma theory was followed which proposed trauma to be the cause of cancer. Later, parasite theory was accepted till 18th century and scientists assumed that cancer was contagious and spread by parasite infection. Identification of oncogenes and tumor suppressor genes in the 20th century has revolutionized the understanding of cancer. Oncogenes are genes that alter the normal cells to grow unregulated to become cancer cells. They are initiated by mutations of certain proto-oncogenes that normally regulate cell division and the degree of differentiation. The normal genes which control cell division, deoxyribonucleic acid (DNA) repair and apoptosis are known as tumor suppressor genes and any deregulation in these genes can cause cancer (Sudhakar, 2009).

CHARACTERISTICS OF CANCER CELLS

Cancer is the result of mutations and genetic changes that accumulate in cells. During the course of time, the normal cell acquires distinct characteristics to transform into cancerous cells (Figure 1.1) (Loeb *et al.*, 2003). Unlike the normal cells, cancer cells do not discontinue their division when come in contact with neighboring cell when they are propagated in a laboratory. It was observed that cancer cells have very less requirement for growth factors to sustain growth and proliferation. Moreover, the cancer cells show trait of anchorage independence i.e. they do not require attachment to a physical substrate to grow. Also, cancer cells are considered immortal as they do not stop dividing after a predetermined number of generations (Hejmadi, 2010; Cooper and Sunderland, 2000; Lodish *et al.*, 2000a). Hanahan and Weinberg have well defined the properties of cancer cells as "Hallmarks of Cancer" where they have discussed different biological capabilities attained at the time of human tumor development which is a multistep process. The hallmarks include sustaining proliferative signaling, evading growth suppressors, resisting cell death, facilitating replicative immortality, inducing angiogenesis, activating invasion and metastasis, genome instability, energy metabolism reprogramming and evading immune destruction (Hanahan and Weinberg, 2000, 2011).

CAUSES OF CANCER

The knowledge accumulated so far suggests that the predisposition of cancer is the outcome of environmental (carcinogens) as well as genetic

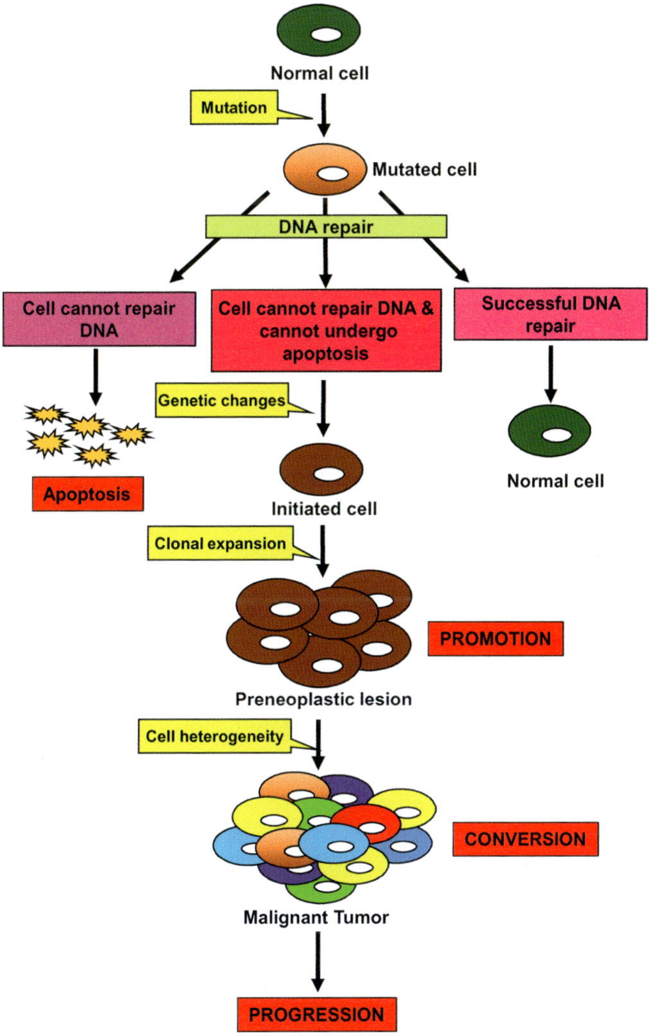

Figure 1.1: Development and progression of cancer.

factors (Clapp *et al.*, 2008). It is now well established that same extent of DNA aberrations or same mutations in oncogenes and tumor suppressor genes in various species of animals result in the development of different cancers due to numerous polymorphic tumor susceptibility genes. In the same way, recent epidemiological data have implied that susceptibility to common "sporadic" cancers in humans is attributed to multiple polymorphic host genes with relatively weak effects. This signifies that in addition to hereditary familial cancer syndromes, sporadic cancer is also under strong genetic control (Demant, 2005). The genotype difference of an individual at a particular locus can either increase or decrease their susceptibility to develop the pathology especially in response to environmental agent exposure (Migliore and Coppedè, 2002). The concept of environment is used to define all non-genetic factors such as diet, lifestyle and infectious agents which are responsible for the development of approximately 80–85% of human cancers. A substance that causes cancer is known as carcinogen. Environment can expose a person to possible carcinogens such as asbestos, outdoor and indoor air pollution, environmental tobacco smoke (ETS), indoor radon, arsenic, chlorination by-products, etc. in drinking water which have been implicated in cancer development (Boffetta and Nyberg, 2003). Lifestyle factors, such as addictive behavior of smoking and alcohol usage, obesity, diet, physical inactivity and reproductive and hormonal factors are treated as the basis of cancer and they can be mainly targeted for primary prevention. Several lines of evidence suggested that most cancer-related deaths are due to tobacco usage (25–30%) and almost 30–35% is because of diet-related anomalies, infections account for about 15–20% such as human papillomavirus (HPV), Epstein–Barr virus (EBV), etc. and the remaining percentage includes factors of radiation, stress, lack of physical activity, exposure to environmental pollutants, etc. Remarkably, it has been proved that the cancer rate can be reduced by half in economically developed societies by preventing smoking, reducing alcohol consumption, weight control and physical exercise and adapting a vegetarian diet and breast-feeding (Katzke *et al.*, 2015; Weiderpass, 2010; Anand *et al.*, 2008).

MOLECULAR ALTERATIONS IN CANCER

Cancer is a slowly developing disease and for most of the solid human tumors, it requires a 20-year interval from the time of carcinogen exposure to reach the stage of clinical detection. During this phase, cancer cells attain the capability to divide, invade and metastasize. The mutator phenotype hypothesis postulated that these phenotypes arise because of mutations in genes that maintain genetic stability in normal cells (Loeb *et al.*, 2003). The initial report for the genetic basis of cancers came through the work of Peyton Rous in 1911, which showed that sarcomas (solid tumors) in chickens could be disseminated between different animals by the help of "cell-free filtrate". Later, the active component was identified as Rous sarcoma virus. Viruses are considered as small entity having package of genes which can infect an appropriate host cell by delivering viral genes. Tumors are also thought to be induced by the addition with successive expression of viral genetic material (Gorga, 1998). It is now well established that cancer is the result of a series of molecular alterations at the genetic and epigenetic level that normally regulates cell proliferation consequently leading to uncontrolled cell growth. These alterations are mutations occurring from spontaneous and environmentally-induced DNA damage. The genes involved in tumorigenesis normally regulate cell proliferation, apoptosis and repairing of damaged DNA. Based on the processes which they affect, these genes are classified into the categories of tumor suppressor genes (growth inhibitory) and proto-oncogenes (growth promoting) (Hemminki and Hemminki, 2005). A proto-oncogene regulates cell growth and division. If any aberrations occur in these genes, it becomes an oncogene and promotes the development of cancer by typically increasing the encoded protein activity or high expression of the normal gene. Such alterations can be dominant (gain-of-function) type. Hence, only one copy of the altered gene is sufficient for cancer promotion. Different from oncogenes, tumor suppressor genes help in preventing cancer by keeping cell growth under control. Since tumor suppressor genes have the opposite effect of oncogenes, they are often referred as anti-oncogenes. The tumor suppressor genes act as recessive genes and they need to assume loss of function mutation for tumor initiation (Lodish *et al.*, 2000b; Devi, 2004; Luo *et al.,* 2009).

Aforementioned, the genetic alterations disrupt the normal pattern of gene expression, which can cause abnormal gene expression resulting in constitutively active proteins, whereas the epigenetic alterations have the potential to deregulate transcriptional control which may lead to improper silencing or activation of cancer-related genes. These alterations can be inherited at the cellular level, thus helping in clonal expansion of the cancer cells (Herceg and Hainaut, 2007). The epigenetic modifications can initiate via DNA methylation and demethylation, acetylation or phosphorylation of histones and the proteins around which DNA is intertwined to take the form of chromatin (Novak, 2004; Sharma *et al.*, 2010). The genetic alterations observed in human tumor cells can be instigated by point mutations, deletions, insertions, chromosomal rearrangements, aneuploidy, gene amplification and overexpression (Hemminki and Hemminki, 2005; Sarasin and Kauffmann, 2008).

MUTATIONS

Mutations are considered as one of the major hallmarks of cancer as they play a prominent role in the evolution of cancer cells. It is well established that cancer can be inherited at the cellular level with multiple mutations which indicates that tumor progression is a mutagenesis associated process. Moreover, now it has become evident that cancer cells are unstable which can result in cascade of mutations and some of these mutations can allow cancer cells to circumvent the normal host regulatory processes which are involved in regulating cell location, division, expression, adaptation and death. The replication errors or DNA damage can initiate mutations which are either repaired erroneously or left unrepaired. DNA damage is the consequence of exogenous factors such as chemicals, ultraviolet (UV) light, ionizing radiation (IR), endogenous factors like ROS (reactive oxygen species), aldehydes or mitotic errors and enzymes responsible for DNA repair or genome editing. Moreover, viruses and endogenous retrotransposons can also cause insertions of DNA sequence leading to mutation. Rate of different mutational processes significantly varies depending on the type of cancer. It is estimated that most cancers possess approximately 1,000–20,000 somatic point mutations and hundreds of insertions, deletions and rearrangements (Watson *et al.*, 2013; Martincorena and Campbell, 2015). The extensive heterogeneity of cancer cells present within the tumor is the result of genetic instability (Loeb and Loeb, 2000; Kim, 2015).

ANEUPLOIDY

The phenomenon of numeric alterations in chromosomes is known as aneuploidy and is one of the most common hallmarks of cancer. Almost a century ago, Theodor Boveri (a German zoologist) proposed that aneuploidy leads to cell death. But he also anticipated that some anomalous chromosomal distributions encourage uncontrolled proliferation and tumor development. Although solid tumors (90%) and hematopoietic neoplasms (85%) are aneuploids, whether they are a cause or a consequence of tumor development is still a matter of debate. However, several empirical reports strongly suggested that aneuploidy is a distinct chromosomal mutation and it helps in malignant transformation of a normal cell and its progression. Further, careful examination of various primary cancer tissues with *in situ* hybridization and comparative genomic hybridization (CGH) assays have affirmed that particular chromosome aneusomies are correlated with discrete tumor phenotypes. Besides, aneuploid tumor cell lines and *in vitro* transformed rodent cells have shown to bear highly unstable chromosomes signifying aneuploidy to be a dynamic chromosomal mutation process linked with cancerous transformation of cells. Moreover, numerous genes of mitotic process which regulate chromosomal segregation have also been found to be mutated in various human cancer cells that are responsible for initiation of aneuploidy. For instance, few of these mutations were known to cause unequal segregation of chromosomes attributed to compromised mitotic checkpoint which in turn produced aneuploidy and induced malignant transformation of cells *in vitro*. As mentioned earlier, chromosomal instability (CIN) can be a possible reason for aneuploidy as it increased the vulnerability of chromosomal gain or loss which can result in unbalanced karyotypes. The gene dosage variation arising from CIN can enable proliferative advantages by escalating the mutation rate in oncogenes, tumor suppressors or tumor susceptibility genes (Sen, 2000; Weaver and Cleveland, 2006; Manchado and Malumbres, 2011; Manchado *et al.*, 2012). By making thousands of genes unstable, aneuploidy disrupts the club of proteins which are involved in segregation, synthesis and repair of chromosomes. Aneuploidy, thus, is responsible for creating karyotypic–phenotypic variations from which, in classical Darwinian terms, cancer-specific aneuploidies are selected and support the evolution and later malignant "progressions" of cancer cells. The variation rates are directly proportional to the aneuploidy degrees, and can surpass the conventional mutation up to 4–7 orders of intensity. This transforms cancer cells into new cell "species" with discrete and uneven karyotypes, instead of mutant cells (Duesberg *et al.*, 2006).

GENE AMPLIFICATION

The phrase of gene amplification is applied to the selective increase of gene copy number and more precisely termed as DNA amplification. It is different from high gene expression, though amplification can elevate the level of encoded proteins. The cells can accomplish the exceeding demand of synthesis of specific gene products beyond the transcriptional efficiency of single copy gene by means of amplification. The gene amplification is promoted by common chromosomal fragile sites, defects in DNA replication and telomere dysfunction. Cytogenetic methods have revealed the presence of chromosomal abnormalities such as double minutes (DMs), C-bandless chromosomes or homogeneously staining chromosomal regions (HSRs) in human and animal tumor cells which act as a diagnostic tool for amplified DNA. MYCN (v-Myc avian myelocytomatosis viral oncogene neuroblastoma derived homolog) was the first oncogene reported to be amplified in solid tumors, and later various oncogenes undergoing amplification were subsequently added to the list. Drug-resistant phenotype due to gene amplification is a common phenomenon in *in vitro* cultured cells but not very prevalent in human tumors. Mostly, amplifications of proto-oncogenes occur in any of the three families (erbB, ras, myc) or they belong to the 11q13 locus. The amplification of gene is suggested to be selected during tumor growth as it is found to be tumor specific and is absent in constitutional DNA of the cancer patient. At present, amplification and overexpression of many genes have been identified and recognized as a major player in the tumor progression in humans and have been correlated with clinical behavior (Jandrig, 1990; Brison, 1993; Schwab, 1999; Albertson, 2006; Santarius *et al.,* 2010). Defining oncogene amplification can prove to be very advantageous because it can help as a prognostic marker in clinic, for instance, *HER2* targeted agents are administered in breast cancer patients having high level of *HER2* overexpression as a therapeutic target. Moreover, it can also find its relevance in diagnostics and in understanding the mechanism of acquired drug resistance (Albertson, 2006; Bagci and Kurtgöz, 2015).

CHROMOSOMAL TRANSLOCATION

Chromosomal translocations can be defined as the structural anomaly formed as a result of reciprocal exchange of the segments of two different chromosomes following DNA double-strand breakages (DSBs) (Oliveira and Fletcher, 2002). These DSBs can be formed by internal or external causes. Endogenously, translocations can result from incorrect recombination activating gene (RAG) or activation-induced deaminase (AID) function in the course of immune receptor maturation. Non-canonical DNA structures or collapsed replication forks can cause endogenous DSBs. External sources such as IR and cancer chemotherapy can serve for exogenous DSBs. The spatial immediacy of the heterologous chromosomes is one of the essential requirements for translocations. Ample amount of evidence suggests that most of the translocations occur through alternative non-homologous end joining (aNHEJ). The poly ADP-ribose polymerase 1 (PARP1) assists in the initiation of the process and it serves as an important molecular mediator for chromosomal translocations (Byrne *et al.*, 2014). In the recent period, various haematological and solid tumors have been shown to possess the oncogenic fusion genes suggesting the importance of translocations in malignancy. The applications of sequencing methods have established that the cancer cells have distinctive characteristic of non-clonal translocations. The chromosome rearrangements are fairly complicated and include DNA segments from different genomic sites. The chromosomal translocations that advance towards cancer can occur through two ways, either by oncogenic fusion protein creation or by oncogene activation through new fused promoter or enhancer. The translocation that displaces the coding sequence of a gene into proximity of the regulatory sequence of other gene can result in the development of cancer. This type of translocation was first reported in translocation of chromosomes 8 and 14 of a patient suffering from Burkitt's lymphoma. In this translocation event, the MYC proto-oncogene from chromosome 8 becomes placed under the regulation of powerful immunoglobulin heavy (IGH) chain gene promoter of the chromosome 14. In normal condition, MYC protein controls cell proliferation and translocation, thereby resulting in excessive amount of MYC overexpression in lymphoid cells under the influence IGH promoter. In some other cancers, translocations result in the production of fusion genes that can potentially act as oncogenes. For instance, in chronic myelogenous leukemia (CML), Philadelphia chromosome is involved which is the product of reciprocal translocation of 9 and 22 chromosomes. Subsequent molecular analyses have confirmed that the translocation resulted in the fusion of the coding sequence of the breakpoint cluster region (BCR) gene (chromosome 22) and the coding sequence of the Abelson murine leukemia viral oncogene homolog 1 (ABL) gene (chromosome 9). The result is the formation of a chimeric protein tyrosine kinase that becomes constitutively active, causing over activation of signaling pathways of cell growth and proliferation. Information of this particular translocation has revolutionized the treatment of CML as investigators could use the available sequence information to overexpress and crystallize the BCR-ABL protein, which subsequently helped in drug development that could inhibit the activity of this protein (Zheng, 2013; Bunting and Nussenzweig, 2013; O'Connor, 2008; Wang, 2012).

CONCLUSION

Cancer is a multistage process that involves aggregation of multiple genetic alterations regulated through different genetic pre-disposition as well as external factors. These endogenous and exogenous sources can result in various genetic and molecular aberrations that can be detected by means of molecular studies. In majority of the cases, these aberrations affect the two different subsets of genes: oncogenes and tumor suppressor genes. Oncogenes are activated by point mutation, overexpression, amplification, translocation, oxidative stress, epigenetic modifications (micro RNA, CpG island methylation, histone modification, chromatin remodeling), chromosomal changes such as terminal deletion, deletion, insertion, duplication, inversion, reciprocal translocation, Robertsonian translocation, ring chromosome, isochromosome. Nucleotide changes such as nucleotide deletion, nucleotide insertion and nucleotide substitution also contribute to the process of tumorigenesis.

CONFLICT OF INTEREST

The authors express no conflict of interest.

REFERENCES

Albertson, D.G., Gene amplification in cancer, *Trends Genet* **22**(8): 447–455 (2006).

Alison. M.R., Cancer, *Encyclopedia of Life Sciences*, Nature Publishing Group, (2001), www.els.net.

Anand, P., A.B. Kunnumakkara, C. Sundaram, K.B. Harikumar, S.T. Tharakan, O.S. Lai, B. Sung, and B.B. Aggarwal, Cancer is a preventable disease that requires major lifestyle changes, *Pharm Res* **25**(9): 2097–2116 (2008).

Bagci, O. and S. Kurtgöz, Amplification of cellular oncogenes in solid tumors, *N Am J Med Sci* **7**(8): 341–346 (2015).

Boffetta, P. and F. Nyberg, Contribution of environmental factors to cancer risk, *Br Med Bull* **68**: 71–94 (2003)

Brison, O., Gene amplification and tumor progression, *Biochim Biophys Acta* **1155**(1): 25–41 (1993).

Bunting, S.F. and A. Nussenzweig, End-joining, translocations and cancer, *Nat Rev Cancer* **13**(7): 443–454 (2013).

Byrne, M., J. Wray, B. Reinert, Y. Wu, J. Nickoloff, S.H. Lee, R. Hromas, and E. Williamson, Mechanisms of oncogenic chromosomal translocations, *Ann N Y Acad Sci* **1310**: 89–97 (2014).

Cavalieri, E.L., E.G. Rogan, and D. Chakravarti, Initiation of cancer and other diseases by catechol ortho-quinones: a unifying mechanism, *Cell Mol Life Sci* **59**(4): 665–681 (2002).

Cell Biology and Cancer. *Rediscovering Biology.*

Clapp, R.W., M.M. Jacobs, and E.L. Loechler, Environmental and occupational causes of cancer: new evidence 2005–2007, *Rev Environ Health* **23**(1): 1–37 (2008).

Cooper, G.M. and M.A. Sunderland, *The Development and Causes of Cancer, The Cell: A Molecular Approach*, 2nd edition. Sinauer Associates (2000).

Demant, P., The genetic factors in cancer development and their implications for cancer prevention and detection, *Radiat Res* **164**(4 Pt 2): 462–466 (2005).

Devi, P.U., Basics of carcinogenesis, *Health Administrator* **17**(1): 16–24 (2004).

Duesberg, P., R. Li, A. Fabarius, and R. Hehlmann, Aneuploidy and cancer: from correlation to causation, *Contrib Microbiol* **13**: 16–44 (2006).

Gorga, F., The molecular basis of cancer, *Bridgewater Review* **17**(2), 3–6 (1998).

Hanahan, D. and R.A. Weinberg, The hallmarks of cancer, *Cell* **100**(1): 57–70 (2000).

Hanahan, D. and R.A. Weinberg, Hallmarks of cancer: the next generation, *Cell* **144**(5): 646–674 (2011).

Hemminki, A. and K. Hemminki, The genetic basis of cancer, *Cancer Gene Therapy*, Humana Press (2005), pp. 9–18.

Herceg, Z. and P. Hainaut, Genetic and epigenetic alterations as biomarkers for cancer detection, diagnosis and prognosis, *Mol Oncol* **1**(1): 26–41 (2007).

Jandrig, B., Amplification of oncogenes and disease prognosis, *Arch Geschwulstforsch* **60**(2): 141–148 (1990).

Katzke, V.A., R. Kaaks, and T. Kühn, Lifestyle and cancer risk, *Cancer J* **21**(2): 104–110 (2015).

Kim, S., New and emerging factors in tumorigenesis: an overview, *Cancer Manag Res* **7**: 225–239 (2015).

Lodish, H., A. Berk, S.L. Zipursky, P. Matsudaira, D. Baltimore, and J. Darnell, Tumor cells and the onset of cancer, *Molecular Cell Biology*, 4th edition. W.H. Freeman and Company, New York (2000a), Section 24.1.

Lodish, H., A. Berk, S.L. Zipursky, P. Matsudaira, D. Baltimore, and J. Darnell, Proto-oncogenes and tumor-suppressor genes, *Molecular Cell Biology*, 4th edition. W.H. Freeman and Company, New York (2000b), Section 24.2.

Loeb, K.R. and L.A. Loeb, Significance of multiple mutations in cancer, *Carcinogenesis* **21**(3): 379–385 (2000).

Loeb, L.A., K.R. Loeb, and J.P. Anderson, Multiple mutations and cancer, *Proc Natl Acad Sci USA* **100**(3): 776–781 (2003).

Luo, J., N.L. Solimini and S.J. Elledge, Principles of cancer therapy: oncogene and non-oncogene addiction, *Cell* **136**(5): 823–837 (2009).

Manchado, E., M. Guillamot and M. Malumbres, Killing cells by targeting mitosis, *Cell Death Differ* **19**(3): 369–377 (2012).

Manchado, E. and M. Malumbres, Targeting aneuploidy for cancer therapy, *Cell.* **144**(4): 465–466 (2011).

Martincorena, I. and P.J. Campbell, Somatic mutation in cancer and normal cells, *Science* **349**(6255): 1483–1489 (2015).

Migliore, L. and F. Coppedè, Genetic and environmental factors in cancer and neurodegenerative diseases, *Mutat Res* **512**(2–3): 135–153 (2002).

Hejmadi, M., *Introduction to Cancer Biology*, Book BooN.com (2010).

Novak, K., Epigenetics Changes in Cancer Cells: Highlights of the American Association for Cancer Research Special Conference on Chromatin, Chromosomes, and Cancer Epigenetics, *Medscape General Medicine* **6**(4), 17 (2004).

O'Connor, C., Human chromosome translocations and cancer, *Nature Education* **1**(1): 56 (2008).

Oliveira, A.M. and J.A. Fletcher, Translocation breakpoints in cancer, *eLS* (2002).

Santarius, T., J. Shipley, D. Brewer, M.R. Stratton, and C.S. Cooper, A census of amplified and overexpressed human cancer genes, *Nat Rev Cancer* **10**(1): 59–64 (2010).

Sarasin, A. and A. Kauffmann, Overexpression of DNA repair genes is associated with metastasis: a new hypothesis, *Mutat Res* **659**(1–2): 49–55 (2008).

Schwab, M., Oncogene amplification in solid tumors, *Semin Cancer Biol* **9**(4): 319–325 (1999).

Sen, S., Aneuploidy and cancer, *Curr Opin Oncol* **12**(1): 82–88 (2000).

Sharma, S., T.K. Kelly, and P.A. Jones, Epigenetics in cancer, *Carcinogenesis.* **31**(1): 27–36 (2010).

Siegel, R., D. Naishadham, and A. Jemal, Cancer statistics, 2012, *CA Cancer J Clin* **62**(1): 10–29 (2012).

Sudhakar, A., History of cancer, ancient and modern treatment methods, *J Cancer Sci Ther* **1**(2): 1–4 (2009).

The History of Cancer, American cancer society, Retrieved from http://www.cancer.org/cancer/cancerbasics/thehistoryofcancer/the-history-of-cancer-what-is-cancer (2014).

Varricchio G. Claudette, *A cancer source book for nurses*, Eighth edition. Jones & Bartlett Learning, American Cancer Society (2004).

Wang, J.H., Mechanisms and impacts of chromosomal translocations in cancers, *Front Med* **6**(3): 263–274 (2012).

Watson, I.R., K. Takahashi, P.A. Futreal, and L. Chin, Emerging patterns of somatic mutations in cancer, *Nat Rev Genet* **14**(10): 703–718 (2013).

Weaver, B.A. and D.W. Cleveland, Does aneuploidy cause cancer? *Curr Opin Cell Biol* **18**(6): 658–667 (2006).

Weiderpass, E., Lifestyle and cancer risk, *J Prev Med Public Health* **43**(6): 459–471 (2010).

Schulz, W., *Molecular Biology of Human Cancers: An Advanced Student's Textbook*, Springer Science & Business Media (2005).

Zheng, J., Oncogenic chromosomal translocations and human cancer (review), *Oncol Rep* **30**(5): 2011–2019 (2013).

2

Basic Concepts of Fusion Genes and Their Classification

*Ganesan Padmavathi, Nand K. Roy, Devivasha Bordoloi, Javadi Monisha and Ajaikumar B. Kunnumakkara**

INTRODUCTION

The concept of genomic instability and rearrangements are considered as hallmarks of cancer. Genomic rearrangements can result in novel chimeric genes which are formed from the linkage of two physically separated genes. These chimeric genes are the result of chromosomal structural rearrangements such as inversion, deletion, amplification and inter-chromosomal/intra-chromosomal translocation which in turn are the consequence of improper transcription or DNA DSBs (Annala *et al.*, 2013; Engreitz *et al.*, 2012; Wang *et al.*, 2015; White *et al.*, 2013; Leow *et al.*, 2012). Generally, transcriptional coactivators, tyrosine kinase receptors and transcription

*Author for correspondence: Ajaikumar B. Kunnumakkara, Cancer Biology Laboratory, Department of Biosciences and Bioengineering, Indian Institute of Technology Guwahati, Assam 781039, India. kunnumakkara@iitg.ernet.in

factors involved in growth factor signaling and cell cycle regulation are susceptible for the gene rearrangements and fusions (Stenman, 2013). The term "fusion gene" gained much attention of the researchers when the Philadelphia chromosome with t(9;22) translocation was first identified in 1960 (Nowell and Hungerford, 1960; Groffen *et al.*, 1984). Consequently, fabrication of such fusion genes being a distinct class of "mutations" was considered as one of the key events responsible for the initiation and progression of various tumors accounting for approximately 20% of total cancer morbidity. The rate of occurrence of fusion genes varies considerably, from 0% to 100%, among different cancer types and the extent of gene fusion-positive cases is similar between both solid and liquid tumors (Wang *et al.*, 2015; Mitelman *et al.*, 2007; Nicorici *et al.*, 2014). Gene fusions are mostly gain of function mutations in cancer, acting either by creation of chimeric proteins with new or altered activities of their wild-type gene partners as in case of BCR-ABL, or by overexpression of any one of the partner oncogenes or by down-regulation of a tumor suppressor gene. Moreover, in general, the chromosomal rearrangements position the 5′-component of a proto-oncogene in proximal to the 3′-end of a strong promoter, thereby causing an aberrant regulation of the former and most often the resultant fusion products are either tyrosine kinases or transcription factors (Pierotti *et al.*, 1998; Soda *et al.*, 2007; Charest *et al.*, 2003; Leow *et al.*, 2012).

MODELS AND THEORIES OF GENE FUSION

Different models have been proposed to explain the gene fusion. However, the exact mechanism of gene fusion is poorly understood. Initially, recombinase enzymes of immune system were thought to be the driving factor for the translocation (Gu *et al.*, 1992a). However, there is an uncertainty as the participation of recombinases was not proved evidently (Reichel *et al.*, 1998). Next, two more hypotheses, namely, "contact first" and "breakage first" were proposed for DSBs induced translocations. According to the "contact first" hypothesis, gene fusion was favored by the chromosomal breakpoints co-localization in the nucleus (Engreitz *et al.*, 2012; Aten *et al.*, 2004). Co-transcription of genes may facilitate this co-localization (Wright *et al.*, 2014). However, this theory is questionable since some studies showed contradictory results i.e. close proximity gene partners exhibited lesser rate of chromosomal rearrangements (Gué *et al.*, 2006). Therefore, the "breakage first" hypothesis was proposed which predicts that the DSBs are first created in distal chromosomes and the broken pairs are diffused in the nucleus to find their counter partners for fusion (Aten *et al.*, 2004). Further in general, the rearrangements are believed to be driven by two pathways first being "breakage and re-joining" and second being "crossing-over between repetitive DNA". As per the "breakage and re-joining" theory, first step in the creation of gene fusion is the formation of DSBs in the chromosome. These DSBs have to be repaired by joining the broken parts of the genome which otherwise are detrimental to the cell. During the repair mechanism, assembly of the two ends of same breaks results in the normal parent DNA. But, if joined, ends of two different breaks result in the chromosomal rearrangements producing novel chimeric genes. However, these rearrangements, to become inherited to the progenies, should possess one centromere and two telomeres which are essential for proper anaphase separation and DNA replication. According to "crossing-over between repetitive DNA" theory, homologous repetitive sequences present in either same or different chromosomes serve as the sites for improper crossing-over producing significant chromosomal rearrangements (Griffiths *et al.*, 1999).

CLASSIFICATION OF FUSION GENES

Chromosomal rearrangements are broadly classified as balanced and imbalanced rearrangements, the former including inversions and translocations with no change in dosage of genetic materials; and the latter including deletions and duplications that alter the gene dosage (Griffiths *et al.*, 1999). Further, inversions are subclassified into paracentric and pericentric inversions depending on the involvement of centromere; and translocations are subclassified into reciprocal and non-reciprocal depending on the involvement of homologous and non-homologous chromosomes (Griffiths *et al.*, 1999). Based on this, in this section of the chapter, we attempt to classify the various fusion genes identified thus far into subgroups (Figure 2.1 and Tables 2.1–2.3).

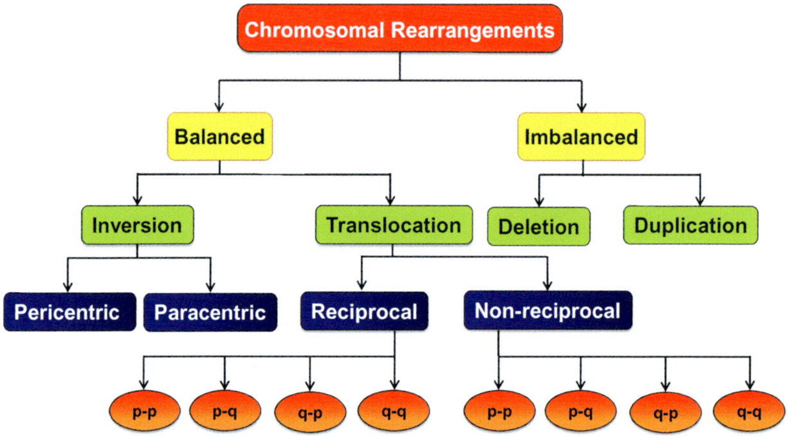

Figure 2.1: Classification of chromosomal rearrangements.

Deletions

Removal of a part of chromosome resulting in the loss of genetic material due to errors in chromosomal crossover is termed as deletion mutation. It is further classified as: (i) terminal deletions taking place near the end of a chromosome; (ii) intercalary deletion occurring from the interior of a chromosome; and (iii) microdeletion, which is the deletion of very small segment upto 5 Mb (*World Heritage Encyclopedia*). The deletion mutations producing fusion of certain genes with altered functions are listed in Table 2.1.

Duplications

It is one of the major genetic events responsible for the evolution of new genes creating unique genetic makeup of every organism in which duplicate copies of a chromosomal segment have been generated as a result of unequal crossing over, retrotransposition and replication slippage, etc. (Magadum *et al.*, 2013).

Table 2.1: Classification of fusion genes based on deletions.

Sl. no.	Deletion	Gene product	Cancer(s)	References
1.	del(1p/19q)		Glioma	Jenkins *et al.* (2006)
2.	del(1)(p36p36)	RERE-PIK3CD	Prostate cancer and lymphoma	McPherson *et al.* (2011) and Le Baccon *et al.* (2001)
3.	del(1)(q44q44)	ZNF695-TFB2M	Lung cancer	Rudin *et al.* (2012)
4.	del(2)(p21p23)		Soft tissue tumors	Walther *et al.* (2011) and Bassett *et al.* (2005)
5.	del(4)(p16p16)	FGFR3-TACC3	Cervical cancer, lung cancer	Carneiro *et al.* (2015) and Capelletti *et al.* (2014)

Table 2.2: Classification of fusion genes based on inversion.

Sl. no.	Inversion	Type of inversion	Fusion gene	Cancer(s)	References
			p–p		
1.	inv(1)(p34p34)	Paracentric inversion	RLF-MYCL	Lung cancer	Rudin *et al.* (2012) and Iwakawa *et al.* (2013)
2.	inv(2)(p21p23)	Paracentric inversion	EML4-ALK	Lung cancer	Perner *et al.* (2008) and Soda *et al.* (2007)
3.	inv(9)(p13p24)	Paracentric inversion	PAX5-JAK2	Leukemia	Nebral *et al.* (2009) and Schinnerl *et al.* (2015)
4.	inv(X)(p11.4p11.22)	Paracentric inversion	BCOR-CCNB3	Bone cancer	Pierron *et al.* (2012)
			q–q		
5.	inv(1)(q21q23)	Paracentric inversion	TPM3-NTRK1	Thyroid cancer	Beimfohr *et al.* (1999) and Butti *et al.* (1995)
6.	inv(1)(q23q31)	Paracentric inversion	TPR-NTRK1	Thyroid cancer	Greco *et al.* (1997) and Beimfohr *et al.* (1999)
7.	inv(3)(q21q26)	Paracentric inversion	RPN1-MECOM	Leukemia	Medeiros *et al.* (2010)

8.	inv(6)(q22q25)	Paracentric inversion	EZR-ROS1	Lung cancer	Takeuchi *et al.* (2012), Li *et al.* (2015) and Matsuura *et al.* (2013)
9.	inv(7)(q21q34)	Paracentric inversion	AKAP9-BRAF	Thyroid cancer	Ciampi *et al.* (2005) and Fusco *et al.* (2005)
10.	inv(8)(q12q12)	Paracentric inversion	CHCHD7-PLAG1	Head and neck cancer	Asp *et al.* (2006)
11.	inv(10)(q11q11)	Paracentric inversion	RET-NCOA4	Thyroid cancer	Santoro *et al.* (1994)
12.	inv(11)(q13q23)	Paracentric inversion	KMT2A-BTBD18	Leukemia	Alonso *et al.* (2010)
13.	inv(11)(q21q23)	Paracentric inversion	KMT2A-MAML2	Leukemia	Nemoto *et al.* (2007), Takei *et al.* (2006) and Obama *et al.* (1998)
14.	inv(12)(q13q13)	Paracentric inversion	NAB2-STAT6	Solitary fibrous tumor	Robinson *et al.* (2013) and Chmielecki *et al.* (2013)
15.	inv(14)(q11q32.1)	Paracentric inversion	TRA/TCL1A	Leukemia	Chervinsky *et al.* (1995)

(Continued)

Table 2.2: (*Continued*)

Sl. no.	Inversion	Type of inversion	Fusion gene	Cancer(s)	References
16.	inv(14)(q11q32)	Paracentric inversion	CEBPE-IGH	Leukemia	Akasaka *et al.* (2007)
p–q					
17.	inv(2)(p23q13)	Pericentric inversion	RANBP2-ALK	Leukemia and inflammatory myofibroblastic tumor	Maesako *et al.* (2014), Takeoka *et al.* (2015), Lim *et al.* (2014), Chen *et al.* (2008) and Ma *et al.* (2003)
18.	inv(2)(p23q35)	Pericentric inversion	ATIC-ALK	Anaplastic large cell lymphoma (ALCL) and inflammatory myofibroblastic tumor	Ma *et al.* (2000), Wlodarska *et al.* (1998), Trinei *et al.* (2000), Colleoni *et al.* (2000) and Debiec-Rychter *et al.* (2003)
19.	inv(7)(p15q34)	Pericentric inversion	TRB-HOXA10	Leukemia	Speleman *et al.* (2005) and Yasukawa *et al.* (1987)
20.	inv(8)(p11q13)	Pericentric inversion	KAT6A-NCOA2 (or) MOZ-TIF2	Leukemia	Deguchi *et al.* (2003), Carapeti *et al.* (1998) and Aguiar *et al.* (1997)
21.	inv(10)(p12.1q11.2)	Pericentric inversion	ACBD5-RET	Thyroid cancer	Hamatani *et al.* (2014)

22.	inv(10)(p11q11)	Pericentric inversion	CCDC6-RET	Thyroid cancer and lung cancer	Zhang *et al.* (2015), Matsubara *et al.* (2012), Takeuchi *et al.* (2012) and Wang *et al.* (2012)
23.	inv(10)(p11q11)	Pericentric inversion	KIF5B-RET	Lung cancer	Cai *et al.* (2013)
24.	inv(11)(p15q22)	Pericentric inversion	NUP98-DDX10	Leukemia	Arai *et al.* (1997), Ikeda *et al.* (1999), Yamamoto *et al.* (2005) and Morerio *et al.* (2006)
25.	inv(12)(p13q15)	Pericentric inversion	ETV6-PTPRR	Leukemia	Setoyama *et al.* (1998) and Welborn *et al.* (2004)
26.	inv(16)(p13q22)	Pericentric inversion	CBFB-MYH11	Leukemia	Shurtleff *et al.* (1995) and van der Reijden *et al.* (1995, 1999)
27.	inv(16)(p13q24)	Pericentric inversion	CBFA2T3-GLIS2	Leukemia	Gruber *et al.* (2012)
28.	inv(19)(p13q13)	Pericentric inversion	TCF3-TFPT (or) E2A-FB1	Leukemia	Brambillasca *et al.* (1999)
29.	inv(X)(p11q12)	Pericentric inversion	NonO-TFE3	Papillary renal cell carcinoma	Clark *et al.* (1997) and Shav-Tal *et al.* (2002)

Table 2.3: Classification of fusion genes based on translocations

Sl. no.	Translocation	Type of Translocation (inter-intra)	Sub-type	Fusion gene	Cancer(s)	References
				p–p		
1.	t(2;10)(p23;p11)	Reciprocal/inter	p–p	KIF5B-ALK	Lung cancer	Takeuchi *et al.* (2009)
2.	t(8;9)(p22;p24)	Reciprocal/inter	p–p	PCM1-JAK2	Leukemia	Bousquet *et al.* (2005), Reiter *et al.* (2005) and Murati *et al.* (2005)
3.	t(9;12)(p24;p13)	Reciprocal/inter	p–p	ETV6-JAK2	Leukemia	Peeters *et al.* (1997) and Zhou *et al.* (2012)
4.	t(11;16)(p11;p11)	Reciprocal/inter	p–p	FUS-CREB3L1	Low-grade fibromyxoid sarcoma	Mertens *et al.* (2005), Prieto-Granada *et al.* (2015) and Hisaoka *et al.* (2012)
				q–q		
5.	t(1;21)(q32;q22)	Reciprocal/inter	q–q	SLC45A3-ERG	Prostate cancer	Perner *et al.* (2013) and Esgueva *et al.* (2010)

6.	t(1;3)(q23;q12)	Reciprocal/inter	q–q	TFG-NTRK1	Papillary thyroid carcinoma	Roccato *et al*. (2003)
7.	t(1;6)(q21;q22)	Reciprocal/inter	q–q	TPM3-ROS1	Lung adenocarcinoma	Cheng *et al*. (2014)
8.	t(2;11)(q11;q23)	Reciprocal/inter	q–q	KMT2A-AFF3	Leukemia	Hiwatari *et al*. (2003)
9.	t(2;13)(q35;q14)	Reciprocal/inter	q–q	PAX3-FOXO1	Rhabdomyosarcoma	Biegel *et al*. (1995) and Douglass *et al*. (1987)
10.	t(3;12)(q27;q15)	Reciprocal/inter	q–q	HMGA2-LPP	Mesenchymal tumors	Hess (1998), Petit *et al*. (1996) and Rogalla *et al*. (1998)
11.	t(3;11)(q21;q23)	Reciprocal/inter	q–q	KMT2A-EEFSEC	Leukemia	http://cancer.sanger.ac.uk/cosmic/fusion
12.	t(4;11)(q21;q23)	Reciprocal/inter	q–q	KMT2A-AFF1	Leukemia	Blütters-Sawatzki *et al*. (1995) and Gu *et al*. (1992b)
13.	t(5;6)(q33;q22)	Reciprocal/inter	q–q	CD74-ROS1	Lung cancer	Davies *et al*. (2012) and Rimkunas *et al*. (2012)

(*Continued*)

Table 2.3: *(Continued)*

Sl. no.	Translocation	Type of Translocation (inter/intra)	Sub-type	Fusion gene	Cancer(s)	References
14.	t(6;12)(q22;q14.1)	Reciprocal/inter	q–q	LRIG3-ROS1	Lung cancer	Takeuchi *et al.* (2012)
15.	t(6;20)(q22;q12)	Reciprocal/inter	q–q	SDC4-ROS1	Lung cancer	Davies *et al.* (2012) and Takeuchi *et al.* (2012)
16.	t(8;21)(q22;q22)	Reciprocal/inter	q–q	RUNX1-RUNX1T1	Leukemia	Ohki (1993) and Maseki *et al.* (1993)
17.	t(8;14)(q24;q32)	Reciprocal/inter	q–q	IGH-MYC	Lymphoma and leukemia	Busch *et al.* (2004) and Kuriakose *et al.* (2004)
18.	t(9;22)(q34;q11)	Reciprocal/inter	q–q	BCR-ABL	Leukemia	Kurzrock *et al.* (1991) and Heisterkamp *et al.* (1991)
19.	t(9;22)(q22-31; q11-12)	Reciprocal/inter	q–q	EWSR1-NR4A3	Bone cancer	Hinrichs *et al.* (1985), Clark *et al.* (1996) and Labelle *et al.* (1999)
20.	t(10;17)(q11.2;q23)	Reciprocal/inter	q–q	PRKAR1A-RET (or) RET-PTC2	Thyroid cancer	Santoro *et al.* (2013) and Sozzi *et al.* (1994)

21.	t(11;22)(q24;q12)	Reciprocal/inter	q–q	EWS-FLI1	Ewing's sarcoma, pancreatic cancer, neuroectodermal tumor	Delattre *et al*. (1994), Scotlandi *et al*. (2000), Maitra *et al*. (2000) and Thorner *et al*. (1996)
22.	t(11;17)(q23;q25)	Reciprocal/inter	q–q	KMT2A-SEPT9	Leukemia	Osaka *et al*. (1999)
23.	t(11;17)(q23;q21)	Reciprocal/inter	q–q	ZBTB16-RARA (or) PLZF-RARA	Leukemia	Chen *et al*. (1993) and Chen *et al*. (1994)
24.	t(12;22)(q13;q12)	Reciprocal/inter	q–q	EWSR1-ATF1	Soft tissue tumors	Hallor *et al*. (2005) and Zucman *et al*. (1993)
25.	t(12;22)(q13;q12)	Reciprocal/inter	q–q	EWS-CHOP	Liposarcoma	Panagopoulos *et al*. (1996)
26.	t(15;17)(q22;q21)	Reciprocal/inter	q–q	PML-RARA	Leukemia	Bennour *et al*. (2013)
27.	t(17;22)(q22;q13)	Reciprocal/inter	q–q	COL1A1-PDGFB	Dermatofibrosarcomas and giant-cell fibroblastomas	O'Brien *et al*. (1998), Segura *et al*. (2011) and Ha *et al*. (2013)

(Continued)

Table 2.3: (*Continued*)

Sl. no.	Translocation	Type of Translocation (inter/intra)	Sub-type	Fusion gene	Cancer(s)	References
28.	t(17;21)(q21;q22)	Reciprocal/inter	q–q	TMPRSS2-ETV4	Prostate cancer	Tomlins *et al*. (2006)
29.	t(21;22)(q22;q12)	Reciprocal/inter	q–q	EWSR1-ERG	Ewing's sarcoma and Wilms tumor	Tarazona *et al*. (2015), Maesawa *et al*. (2002) and Stewénius *et al*. (2008)
				p–q		
30.	t(1;11)(p32;q23)	Reciprocal/inter	p–q	MLL-EPS15	Leukemia	So *et al*. (2003) and Bernard *et a*l. (1994)
31.	t(1;13)(p36;q14)	Reciprocal/inter	p–q	PAX7-FOXO1	Alveolar rhabdomyosarcoma	Davis *et al*. (1997), and Barr (2001)
32.	t(X;1)(p11;q21)	Reciprocal/inter	p–q	PRCC-TFE3	Renal cell carcinoma	Ohe *et al*. (2012), Sidhar *et al*. (1996) and Weterman *et al*. (1996)
33.	t(2;17)(p23;q23)	Reciprocal/inter	p–q	CLTC-ALK	ALK+ diffuse large B-cell lymphomas	Momose *et al*. (2009), Li *et al*. (2009) and Choung *et al*. (2008)

34.	t(2;14)(p23;q32)	Reciprocal/inter	p–q	KLC1-ALK	Lung cancer	Togashi *et al.* (2012)
35.	t(2;5)(p23;q35)	Reciprocal/inter	p–q	NPM1-ALK	Lymphomas and leukemias	Falini *et al.* (2007), Wellmann *et al.* (1995), and Morris *et al.* (1994)
36.	t(2;3)(p23;q21)	Reciprocal/inter	p–q	TFG-ALK	ALCL	Rosenwald *et al.* (1999) and Hernández *et al.* (1999)
37.	t(4;6)(p15;q22)	Reciprocal/inter	p–q	SLC34A2-ROS1	Lung cancer	Davies *et al.* (2012), and Rimkunas *et al.* (2012)
38.	t(7;21)(p21;q22)	Reciprocal/inter	p–q	TMPRSS2-ETV1	Prostate cancer	Dai *et al.* (2008) and Tomlins *et al.* (2005)
39.	t(9;12)(p22;q14)	Reciprocal/inter	p–q	HMGA2-NFIB	Lipoma	Nilsson *et al.* (2005)
40.	t(9;11)(p22;q23)	Reciprocal/inter	p–q	KMT2A-MLLT3	Leukemia	Joh *et al.* (1996) and Ney Garcia *et al.* (2015)

(*Continued*)

Table 2.3: (*Continued*)

Sl. no.	Translocation	Type of Translocation (inter/intra)	Sub-type	Fusion gene	Cancer(s)	References
41.	t(10;11)(p12;q23)	Reciprocal/inter	p–q	KMT2A-MLLT10 (or) KMT2A-NEBL	Leukemia	Chaplin *et al.* (1995), Cóser *et al.* (2010) and Emerenciano *et al.* (2013)
42.	t(11;22)(p13;q12)	Reciprocal/inter	p–q	EWS-WT1	Desmoplastic small round cell tumor	Kim *et al.* (1998), Gerald *et al.* (1998) and Benjamin *et al.* (1996)
43.	t(12;15)(p13;q25)	Reciprocal/inter	p–q	ETV6-NTRK3	Leukemia, fibrosarcoma	Eguchi *et al.* (1999) and Lannon *et al.* (2005)
44.	t(12;21)(p13;q22)	Reciprocal/inter	p–q	ETV6-RUNX1 (or) TEL-AML1	Leukemia	Raynaud *et al.* (1996) and Romana *et al.* (1995)
45.	t(X;17)(p11;q25)	Reciprocal/inter	p–q	ASPSCR1-TFE3	Renal cancers	Aulmann *et al.* (2007), Uppal *et al.* (2003), Hernandez-Martí *et al.* (1995) and Argani *et al.* (2001)

46.	t(X;18)(p11;q11)	Reciprocal/inter	p–q	SS18-SSX (or) SS18-SSX1 (or) SS18-SSX2 (or) SS18-SSX4	Synovial sarcoma	Lubieniecka *et al.* (2008) and Törnkvist *et al.* (2004)
q-p						
47.	t(1;7)(q32;p21)	Reciprocal/inter	q–p	SLC45A3-ETV1	Prostate cancer	Miyagi *et al.* (2010) and Tomlins *et al.* (2007)
48.	t(1;19)(q23;p13)	Reciprocal/inter	q–p	TCF3-PBX1 (or) E2A-PBX1	Lung cancer, Leukemia	Mo *et al.* (2013) and Fu *et al.* (1997)
49.	t(1;2)(q25;p23)	Reciprocal/inter	q–p	TPM3-ALK	Inflammatory myofibroblastic tumors (IMTs) and ALCL	Lamant *et al.* (1999), Lawrence *et al.* (2000) and Ladanyi (2000)
50.	t(5;9)(q14.1;p24.1)	Reciprocal/inter	q–p	SSBP2-JAK2	Leukemia	Poitras *et al.* (2008)
51.	t(6;9)(q22-23;p23-24)	Reciprocal/inter	q–p	MYB-NFIB	Adenoid cystic carcinomas (ACC) of the breast and head and neck	Fehr *et al.* (2011) and Persson *et al.* (2009)

(*Continued*)

Table 2.3: (*Continued*)

Sl. no.	Translocation	Type of Translocation (inter/intra)	Sub-type	Fusion gene	Cancer(s)	References
52.	t(7;16)(q33;p11)	Reciprocal/inter	q–p	FUS-CREB3L2	Low grade fibromyxoid sarcoma	Storlazzi *et al.* (2003)
53.	t(11;19)(q21;p13.1)	Reciprocal/inter	q–p	CRTC1-MAML2	Skin cancer, head and neck cancer	El-Naggar *et al.* (1996) and Behboudi *et al.* (2005)
54.	t(11;19)(q23;p13.3)	Reciprocal/inter	q–p	KMT2A-MLLT1	Leukemia	Rubnitz *et al.* (1999)
55.	t(12;16)(q13;p11)	Reciprocal/inter	q–p	FUS-ATF-1	Fibrous histiocytoma	Waters *et al.* (2000) and Raddaoui *et al.* (2002)
56.	t(12;16)(q13;p11)	Reciprocal/inter	q–p	FUS-DDIT3	Liposarcoma	Panagopoulos *et al.* (1997) and Pérez-Mancera *et al.* (2005)
57.	t(15;19)(q14;p13)	Reciprocal/inter	q–p	BRD4-NUTM1	NUT midline carcinoma	French *et al.* (2003), Engleson *et al.* (2006) and Kubonishi *et al.* (1991)

58.	t(16;17)(q22;p13)	Reciprocal/inter	q–p	CDH11-USP6	Bone cancer	Herens *et al.* (2001) and Wyatt-Ashmead *et al.* (2001)
			Non-reciprocal translocations			
59.	t(2;2)(p23;p22)	Non-reciprocal/intra	p–p	STRN-ALK	Lung cancer and thyroid carcinoma	Majewski *et al.* (2013) and Pérot *et al.* (2014)
60.	t(6;6)(q21;q22)	Non-reciprocal/intra	q–q	GOPC-ROS1	Lung cancer	Rimkunas *et al.* (2012) and Suehara *et al.* (2012)
61.	t(21;21)(q22;q22)	Non-reciprocal/intra	q–q	TMPRSS2-ERG	Prostate cancer	Soller *et al.* (2006), Dai *et al.* (2008), Swanson *et al.* (2011) and Polson *et al.* (2013)
62.	t(16;16)(p13;q22)	Non-reciprocal/intra	p–q	CBFB-MYH11	Leukemia	van der Reijden *et al.* (1995, 1999) and Shurtleff *et al.* (1995)

Inversions

Inversion is an intrachromosomal rearrangement i.e. reversed end to end rearrangement of a chromosomal segment within the same chromosome. It is of two types: (i) paracentric inversion not involving centromere where the breakpoint occurs in the same arm of the chromosome; and (ii) pericentric inversion involving centromere where the breakpoint occurs in both the arms of the chromosome. In certain cases of inversion, functional fusion proteins are produced which are implicated in different cancers (Griffiths *et al.*, 1999; Pierotti *et al.*, 2003). Such fusion products are listed in Table 2.2.

Translocations

Exchange of genetic materials between two non-homologous chromosomes resulting in relocation of genes is termed as translocation. Reciprocal translocation is the rearrangement of genetic materials between two non-homologous chromosomes where two chromosomal segments are exchanged and non-reciprocal translocation is most commonly the rearrangement of genetic material within the same chromosome, however, only relocation of one segment occurs i.e. one-way transfer of a chromosomal segment occurs (Griffiths *et al.*, 1999). Table 2.3 comprises the various reciprocal and non-reciprocal translocations identified to be associated with different cancers.

CONCLUSION

Chromosomal alterations such as deletions, duplications, inversions and translocations are characteristic feature of cancers. At present, it becomes evident that these chromosomal aberrations can result in the formation of fusion genes which can have tumorigenic action either by gene overexpression in one of the breakpoints or through the formation of a hybrid gene during the fusion of two genes, one in each breakpoint. As a consequence of this, the cell starts functioning in an unregulated manner and develops into a cancer cell.

CONFLICT OF INTEREST

The authors express no conflict of interest.

REFERENCES

Aguiar, R.C., A. Chase, S. Coulthard, D.H. Macdonald, M. Carapeti, A. Reiter, J. Sohal, A. Lennard, J.M. Goldman, and N.C. Cross, Abnormalities of chromosome band 8p11 in leukemia: two clinical syndromes can be distinguished on the basis of MOZ involvement, *Blood* **90**(8): 3130–3135 (1997).

Akasaka, T., T. Balasas, L.J. Russell, K.J. Sugimoto, A. Majid, R. Walewska, E.L. Karran, D.G. Brown, K. Cain, L. Harder, S. Gesk, J.I. Martin-subero Subero, M.G. Atherton, M. Brüggemann, M.J. Calasanz, T. Davies, O.A. Haas, A. Hagemeijer, H. Kempski, M. Lessard, D.M. Lillington, S. Moore, F. Nguyen-Khac, I. Radford-Weiss, C. Schoch, S. Struski, P. Talley, M.J. Welham, H. Worley, J.C. Strefford, C.J. Harrison, R. Siebert, and M.J. Dyer, Five members of the CEBP transcription factor family are targeted by recurrent IGH translocations in B-cell precursor acute lymphoblastic leukemia (BCP-ALL), *Blood* **109**(8): 3451–3461 (2007).

Alonso, C.N., C. Meyer, M.S. Gallego, J.G. Rossi, A.P. Mansini, P.L. Rubio, A. Medina, R. Marschalek, and M.S. Felice, BTBD18: A novel MLL partner gene in an infant with acute lymphoblastic leukemia and inv(11)(q13;q23), *Leuk Res* **34**(11): e294–6 (2010).

Annala, M.J., B.C. Parker, W. Zhang, and M. Nykter, Fusion genes and their discovery using high throughput sequencing, *Cancer Lett* **340**(2): 192–200 (2013).

Arai, Y., F. Hosoda, H. Kobayashi, K. Arai, Y. Hayashi, N. Kamada, Y. Kaneko, and M. Ohki, The inv(11)(p15q22) chromosome translocation of de novo and therapy-related myeloid malignancies results in fusion of the nucleoporin gene, NUP98, with the putative RNA helicase gene, DDX10, *Blood* **89**(11): 3936–3944 (1997).

Argani, P,. C.R. Antonescu, P.B. Illei, M.Y. Lui, C.F. Timmons, R. Newbury, V.E. Reuter, A.J. Garvin, A.R. Perez-Atayde, J.A. Fletcher, J.B. Beckwith, J.A. Bridge, and M. Ladanyi, Primary renal neoplasms with the ASPL-TFE3 gene fusion of alveolar soft part sarcoma: a distinctive tumor entity previously included among renal cell carcinomas of children and adolescents, *Am J Pathol* **159**(1): 179–192 (2001).

Asp, J., F. Persson, M. Kost-Alimova, and G. Stenman, CHCHD7-PLAG1 and TCEA1-PLAG1 gene fusions resulting from cryptic, intrachromosomal 8q rearrangements in pleomorphic salivary gland adenomas, *Genes Chromosomes Cancer* **45**(9): 820–828 (2006).

Aten, J.A., J. Stap, P.M. Krawczyk, C.H. van Oven, R.A. Hoebe, J. Essers, and R. Kanaar, Dynamics of DNA double-strand breaks revealed by clustering of damaged chromosome domains, *Science* **303**(5654): 92–95 (2004).

Aulmann, S., T. Longerich, P. Schirmacher, G. Mechtersheimer, and R. Penzel, Detection of the ASPSCR1-TFE3 gene fusion in paraffin-embedded alveolar soft part sarcomas, *Histopathology* **50**(7): 881–886. (2007).

Barr F.G. Gene fusions involving PAX and FOX family members in alveolar rhabdomyosarcoma, *Oncogene* **20**(40): 5736–5746 (2001).

Bassett, M.D., S.M. Schuetze, C. Disteche, T.H. Norwood, K. Swisshelm, X. Chen, J. Bruckner, and E.U. Conrad, 3rd, B.P. Rubin. Deep-seated, well differentiated lipomatous tumors of the chest wall and extremities: the role of cytogenetics in classification and prognostication, *Cancer* **103**(2): 409–416 (2005).

Behboudi, A., M. Winnes, L. Gorunova, J.J. van den Oord, F. Mertens, F. Enlund, and G. Stenman, Clear cell hidradenoma of the skin-a third tumor type with a t(11;19) — associated TORC1-MAML2 gene fusion, *Genes Chromosomes Cancer* **43**(2): 202–205 (2005).

Beimfohr, C., S. Klugbauer, E.P. Demidchik, E. Lengfelder, and H.M. Rabes, NTRK1 re-arrangement in papillary thyroid carcinomas of children after the Chernobyl reactor accident, *Int J Cancer* **80**(6): 842–847 (1999).

Beimfohr, C., S. Klugbauer, E.P. Demidchik, E. Lengfelder, and H.M. Rabes, NTRK1 re-arrangement in papillary thyroid carcinomas of children after the Chernobyl reactor accident, *Int J Cancer* **80**(6): 842–847 (1999).

Benjamin, L.E., W.J. Fredericks, F.G. Barr, and F.J. Rauscher, 3rd., Fusion of the EWS1 and WT1 genes as a result of the t(11;22)(p13;q12) translocation in desmoplastic small round cell tumors, *Med Pediatr Oncol* **27**(5): 434–439 (1996).

Biegel, J.A., L.M. Nycum, V. Valentine, F.G. Barr, and D.N. Shapiro, Detection of the t(2;13)(q35;q14) and PAX3-FKHR fusion in alveolar rhabdomyosarcoma by fluorescence *in situ* hybridization, *Genes Chromosomes Cancer* **12**(3): 186–192 (1995).

Blütters-Sawatzki, R., A. Borkhardt, J. Grathwohl, R. Repp, I. Rheinisch-Becker, R.M. Bohle and F. Lampert, Secondary acute myeloid leukemia with translocation (4;11) and MLL/AF4 rearrangement in a 15-year-old boy treated for common acute lymphoblastic leukemia 11 years earlier, *Ann Hematol* **70**(1): 31–35 (1995).

Bousquet, M., C. Quelen, V. De Mas, E. Duchayne, B. Roquefeuil, G. Delsol, G. Laurent, N. Dastugue, and P. Brousset, The t(8;9)(p22;p24) translocation in atypical chronic myeloid Leukemia yields a new PCM1-JAK2 fusion gene, *Oncogene* **24**(48): 7248–7252 (2005).

Brambillasca, F., G. Mosna, M. Colombo, A. Rivolta, C. Caslini, M. Minuzzo, G. Giudici, L. Mizzi, A. Biondi, and E. Privitera, Identification of a novel molecular partner of the E2A gene in childhood leukemia, *Leukemia* **13**(3): 369–375 (1999).

Busch, K., A. Borkhardt, W. Wössmann, A. Reiter, and J. Harbott, Combined polymerase chain reaction methods to detect c-myc/IgH rearrangement in childhood Burkitt's lymphoma for minimal residual disease analysis, *Haematologica* **89**(7): 818–825 (2004).

Butti, M.G., I. Bongarzone, G. Ferraresi, P. Mondellini, M.G. Borrello, and M.A. Pierotti, A sequence analysis of the genomic regions involved in the rearrangements between TPM3 and NTRK1 genes producing TRK oncogenes in papillary thyroid carcinomas, *Genomics* **28**(1): 15–24 (1995).

Cai, W., C. Su, X. Li, L. Fan, L. Zheng, K. Fei, and C. Zhou, KIF5B-RET fusions in Chinese patients with non-small cell lung cancer, *Cancer* **119**(8): 1486–1494 (2013).

Capelletti, M., M.E. Dodge, D. Ercan, P.S. Hammerman, S.I. Park, J. Kim, H. Sasaki, D.M. Jablons, D. Lipson, L. Young, P.J. Stephens, V.A. Miller, N.I. Lindeman, K.J. Munir, W.G. Richards, and P.A. Jänne, Identification of recurrent FGFR3-TACC3 fusion oncogenes from lung adenocarcinoma, *Clin Cancer Res* **20**(24): 6551–6558 (2014).

Carapeti, M., R.C. Aguiar, J.M. Goldman, and N.C. Cross, A novel fusion between MOZ and the nuclear receptor coactivator TIF2 in acute myeloid leukemia, *Blood* **91**(9): 3127–3133 (1998).

Carneiro, B.A., J.A. Elvin, S.D. Kamath, S.M. Ali, A.S. Paintal, A. Restrepo, E. Berry, F.J. Giles, and M.L. Johnson, FGFR3-TACC3: A novel gene fusion in cervical cancer, *Gynecol Oncol Rep* **13**: 53–56 (2015).

Catalogue of somatic mutations in cancer (COSMIC): http://cancer.sanger.ac.uk/cosmic/fusion

Chaplin, T., O. Bernard, H.B. Beverloo, V. Saha, A. Hagemeijer, R. Berger, and B.D. Young, The t(10;11) translocation in acute myeloid leukemia (M5) consistently fuses the leucine zipper motif of AF10 onto the HRX gene, *Blood* **86**(6): 2073–2076 (1995).

Charest, A., K. Lane, K. McMahon, J. Park, E. Preisinger, H. Conroy, and D. Housman, Fusion of FIG to the receptor tyrosine kinase ROS in a glioblastoma with an interstitial del (6)(q21q21), *Genes Chromosomes Cancer* **37**(1): 58–71 (2003).

Chen, S.J., A. Zelent, J.H. Tong, H.Q. Yu, Z.Y. Wang, J. Derré, R. Berger, S. Waxman, and Z. Chen, Rearrangements of the retinoic acid receptor alpha and promyelocytic leukemia zinc finger genes resulting from t(11;17)(q23;q21) in a patient with acute promyelocytic leukemia, *J Clin Invest* **91**(5): 2260–2267 (1993).

Chen, S.T., and J.C. Lee, An inflammatory myofibroblastic tumor in liver with ALK and RANBP2 gene rearrangement: combination of distinct morphologic, immunohistochemical, and genetic features, *Hum Pathol* **39**(12): 1854–1858 (2008).

Chen, Z., F. Guidez, P. Rousselot, A. Agadir, S.J. Chen, Z.Y. Wang, L. Degos, A. Zelent, S. Waxman, and C. Chomienne, PLZF-RAR alpha fusion proteins generated from the variant t(11;17)(q23;q21) translocation in acute promyelocytic leukemia inhibit ligand-dependent transactivation of wild-type retinoic acid receptors, *Proc Natl Acad Sci USA* **91**(3): 1178–1182 (1994).

Cheng, H. L. Ye, and L. Xue, [Detection of ROS1 gene rearrangement by FISH and analysis of its clinical features in non-small cell lung cancer patients], *Zhonghua Zhong Liu Za Zhi* **36**(10): 751–754 (2014).

Chervinsky, D.S., M. Grossi, S. Kakati, A.W. Block, and P.D. Aplan, Concurrent presence of inv(14)(q11q32) and t(4;11)(q21;q23) in pre-B acute lymphoblastic leukemia, *Genes Chromosomes Cancer* **12**(3): 229–236 (1995).

Chmielecki, J., A.M. Crago, M. Rosenberg, O'R. Connor, S.R. Walker, L. Ambrogio, D. Auclair, A. McKenna, M.C. Heinrich, D.A. Frank, and M. Meyerson, Whole-exome sequencing identifies a recurrent NAB2-STAT6 fusion in solitary fibrous tumors, *Nat Genet* **45**(2): 131–132 (2013).

Choung, H.S., H.J. Kim, W.S. Kim, K. Kim, and S.H. Kim, [Cytomorphology and molecular characterization of CLTC-ALK rearrangement in 2 cases of ALK-positive diffuse large B-cell lymphoma with extensive bone marrow involvement], *Korean J Lab Med* **28**(2): 89–94 (2008).

Ciampi, R., J.A. Knauf, R. Kerler, M. Gandhi, Z. Zhu, M.N. Nikiforova, H.M. Rabes, J.A. Fagin, and Y.E. Nikiforov, Oncogenic AKAP9-BRAF fusion is a novel mechanism of MAPK pathway activation in thyroid cancer, *J Clin Invest* **115**(1): 94–101 (2005).

Clark, J., H. Benjamin, S. Gill, S. Sidhar, G. Goodwin, J. Crew, B.A. Gusterson, J. Shipley, and C.S. Cooper, Fusion of the EWS gene to CHN, a member of the steroid/thyroid receptor gene superfamily, in a human myxoid chondrosarcoma, *Oncogene* **12**(2): 229–235 (1996).

Clark, J., Y.J. Lu, S.K. Sidhar, C. Parker, S. Gill, D. Smedley, R. Hamoudi, W.M. Linehan, J. Shipley, and C.S. Cooper, Fusion of splicing factor genes PSF and NonO (p54nrb) to the TFE3 gene in papillary renal cell carcinoma, *Oncogene* **15**(18): 2233–2239 (1997).

Colleoni, G.W., J.A. Bridge, B. Garicochea, J. Liu, D.A. Filippa, and M. Ladanyi, ATIC-ALK: A novel variant ALK gene fusion in anaplastic large cell lymphoma resulting from the recurrent cryptic chromosomal inversion, inv(2)(p23q35), *Am J Pathol* **156**(3): 781–789 (2000).

Cóser, V.M., C. Meyer, R. Basegio, J. Menezes, R. Marschalek, and M.S. Pombo-de-Oliveira, Nebulette is the second member of the nebulin family fused to the MLL gene in infant leukemia, *Cancer Genet Cytogenet* **198**(2): 151–154 (2010).

Dai, M.J., L.L. Chen, Y.B. Zheng, W. Chen, Z.H. Tao, Z.L. Weng, X.L. Wu, C.D. Li, Z.G. Chen, X.D. Chen, and S.B. Shi, Frequency and transcript variant analysis of gene fusions between TMPRSS2 and ETS transcription factor genes in prostate cancer, *Zhonghua Yi Xue Za Zhi* **88**(10): 669–673 (2008).

Davies, K.D., A.T. Le, M.F. Theodoro, M.C. Skokan, D.L. Aisner, E.M. Berge, L.M. Terracciano, F. Cappuzzo, M. Incarbone, M. Roncalli, M. Alloisio, A. Santoro, D.R. Camidge, M. Varella-Garcia, and R.C. Doebele, Identifying and targeting ROS1 gene fusions in non-small cell lung cancer, *Clin Cancer Res* **18**(17): 4570–4579 (2012).

Davis, R.J. and F.G. Barr, Fusion genes resulting from alternative chromosomal translocations are overexpressed by gene-specific mechanisms in alveolar rhabdomyosarcoma, *Proc Natl Acad Sci USA* **94**(15): 8047–8051 (1997).

Rychter, D.-M., P. Marynen, A. Hagemeijer, and P. Pauwels, ALK-ATIC fusion in urinary bladder inflammatory myofibroblastic tumor, *Genes Chromosomes Cancer* **38**(2): 187–190 (2003).

Deguchi, K., P.M. Ayton, M. Carapeti, J.L. Kutok, C.S. Snyder, I.R. Williams, N.C. Cross, C.K. Glass, M.L. Cleary, and D.G. Gilliland, MOZ-TIF2-induced acute myeloid leukemia requires the MOZ nucleosome binding motif and TIF2-mediated recruitment of CBP, *Cancer Cell* **3**(3): 259–271 (2003).

Delattre, O., J. Zucman, T. Melot, X.S. Garau, J.M. Zucker, G.M. Lenoir, P.F. Ambros, D. Sheer, C. Turc-Carel, T.J. Triche, *et al.*, The Ewing family of tumors — a subgroup of small-round-cell tumors defined by specific chimeric transcripts, *N Engl J Med* **331**(5): 294–299 (1994).

Douglass, E.C., M. Valentine, E. Etcubanas, D. Parham, B.L. Webber, P.J. Houghton, J.A. Houghton, and A.A. Green, A specific chromosomal abnormality in rhabdomyosarcoma, *Cytogenet Cell Genet* **45**(3–4): 148–155 (1987).

Eguchi, M., M. E-Ishimae, A. Tojo, K. Morishita, K. Suzuki, Y. Sato, S. Kudoh, K. Tanaka, M. Setoyama, F. Nagamura, S. Asano, and N. Kamada, Fusion of ETV6 to neurotrophin-3 receptor TRKC in acute myeloid leukemia with t(12;15)(p13;q25), *Blood* **93**(4): 1355–1363 (1999).

El-Naggar, A.K., M. Lovell, A.M. Killary, G.L. Clayman, and J.G. Batsakis, A mucoepidermoid carcinoma of minor salivary gland with t(11;19)(q21;p13.1) as the only karyotypic abnormality, *Cancer Genet Cytogenet* **87**(1): 29–33 (1996).

Emerenciano, M., E. Kowarz, K. Karl, de Almeida B. Lopes, B. Scholz, S. Bracharz, C. Meyer, Pombo-de-MS. Oliveira, and R. Marschalek, Functional analysis of the two reciprocal fusion genes MLL-NEBL and NEBL-MLL reveal their oncogenic potential, *Cancer Lett* **332**(1): 30–34 (2013).

Engleson, J., M. Soller, I. Panagopoulos, A. Dahlén, M. Dictor, and M. Jerkeman, Midline carcinoma with t(15;19) and BRD4-NUT fusion oncogene in a 30-year-old female with response to docetaxel and radiotherapy, *BMC Cancer* **6**: 69 (2006).

Engreitz, J.M., V. Agarwala, and L.A. Mirny, Three-dimensional genome architecture influences partner selection for chromosomal translocations in human disease, *PLoS One* 7(9): e44196 (2012).

Esgueva, R., S. Perner, J C. LaFargue, V. Scheble, C. Stephan, M. Lein, F.R. Fritzsche, M. Dietel, G. Kristiansen, and M.A. Rubin, Prevalence of TMPRSS2-ERG and SLC45A3-ERG gene fusions in a large prostatectomy cohort, *Mod Pathol* **23**(4): 539–546 (2010).

Falini, B., I. Nicoletti, N. Bolli, M.P. Martelli, A. Liso, P. Gorello, F. Mandelli, C. Mecucci, and M.F. Martelli, Translocations and mutations involving the nucleophosmin (NPM1) gene in lymphomas and leukemias, *Haematologica* **92**(4): 519–532 (2007).

Fehr, A., A. Kovács, T. Löning, H. Jr Frierson, van den J. Oord, and G. Stenman, The MYB-NFIB gene fusion-a novel genetic link between adenoid cystic carcinoma and dermal cylindroma, *J Pathol* **224**(3): 322–327 (2011).

French, C.A., I. Miyoshi, I. Kubonishi, H.E. Grier, A.R. Perez-Atayde, and J.A. Fletcher, BRD4-NUT fusion oncogene: a novel mechanism in aggressive carcinoma, *Cancer Res* **63**(2): 304–307 (2003).

Fu, X., and M.P. Kamps, E2a-Pbx1 induces aberrant expression of tissue-specific and developmentally regulated genes when expressed in NIH 3T3 fibroblasts, *Mol Cell Biol* **17**(3): 1503–1512 (1997).

Fusco, A., G. Viglietto, and M. Santoro, A new mechanism of BRAF activation in human thyroid papillary carcinomas, *J Clin Invest* **115**(1): 20–23 (2005).

Genetic deletion, *World Heritage Encyclopedia; WHEBN0011099118* available at http://www.ebooklibrary.org/articles/eng/genetic_deletion.

Gerald, W.L., M. Ladanyi, E. de Alava, M. Cuatrecasas, B.H. Kushner, M.P. LaQuaglia, and J. Rosai, Clinical, pathologic, and molecular spectrum of tumors associated with t(11;22)(p13;q12): desmoplastic small round-cell tumor and its variants, *J ClinOncol* **16**(9): 3028–3036 (1998).

Greco, A., C. Miranda, S. Pagliardini, L. Fusetti, I. Bongarzone, and M.A. Pierotti, Chromosome 1 rearrangements involving the genes TPR and NTRK1 produce structurally different thyroid-specific TRK oncogenes, *Genes Chromosomes Cancer* **19**(2): 112–123 (1997).

Griffiths, A.J.F., W.M. Gelbart, J.H. Miller, *et al.*, *Modern Genetic Analysis*, New York: W. H. Freeman (1999). Chromosomal Rearrangements. Available from: http://www.ncbi.nlm.nih.gov/books/NBK21367/.

Groffen, J., J.R. Stephenson, N. Heisterkamp, de A. Klein, C.R. Bartram, and G. Grosveld, Philadelphia chromosomal breakpoints are clustered within a limited region, bcr, on chromosome 22, *Cell* **36**(1): 93–99 (1984).

Gruber, T.A., Larson A. Gedman, J. Zhang, C.S. Koss, S. Marada, H.Q. Ta, S.C. Chen, X. Su, S.K. Ogden, J. Dang, G. Wu, V. Gupta, A.K. Andersson, S. Pounds, L. Shi, J. Easton, M.I. Barbato, H.L. Mulder, J. Manne, J. Wang, M. Rusch, S. Ranade, R. Ganti, M. Parker, J. Ma, I. Radtke, L. Ding, G. Cazzaniga, A. Biondi, S.M. Kornblau, F. Ravandi, H. Kantarjian, S.D. Nimer, K. Döhner, H. Döhner, T.J. Ley, P. Ballerini, S. Shurtleff, D. Tomizawa, S. Adachi, Y. Hayashi, A. Tawa, L.Y. Shih, D.C. Liang, J.E. Rubnitz, C.H. Pui, E.R. Mardis, R.K. Wilson, and J.R. Downing, An Inv(16)(p13.3q24.3)-encoded CBFA2T3-GLIS2 fusion protein defines an aggressive subtype of pediatric acute megakaryoblastic leukemia, *Cancer Cell* **22**(5): 683–697 (2012).

Gu, Y., G. Cimino, H. Alder, T. Nakamura, R. Prasad, O. Canaani, D.T. Moir, C. Jones, P.C. Nowell, C.M. Croce, *et al.*, The (4;11)(q21;q23) chromosome translocations in acute leukemias involve the VDJ recombinase, *Proc Natl Acad Sci USA* **89**(21): 10464–101046 (1992a).

Gu, Y., T. Nakamura, H. Alder, R. Prasad, O. Canaani, G. Cimino, C.M. Croce and E. Canaani, The t(4;11) chromosome translocation of human acute leukemias fuses the ALL-1 gene, related to Drosophila trithorax, to the AF-4 gene, *Cell* **71**(4): 701–708 (1992b).

Gué, M., J.S. Sun, and T. Boudier, Simultaneous localization MLL. of, AF4 and ENL genes in interphase nuclei by 3D-FISH: MLL translocation revisited, *BMC Cancer* **6**: 20 (2006).

Ha, S.Y., S.E. Lee, M.J. Kwon, Y.J. Kim, E.H. Lee, J. Seo, K.T. Jang, J. Lee, and Y.L. Choi, PDGFB rearrangement in dermatofibrosarcoma protuberans: correlation with clinicopathologic characteristics and clinical implications, *Hum Pathol* **44**(7): 1300–1309 (2013).

Hallor, K.H., F. Mertens, Y. Jin, J.M. Meis-Kindblom, L.G. Kindblom, M. Behrendtz, A. Kalén, N. Mandahl, and I. Panagopoulos, Fusion of the EWSR1 and ATF1 genes without expression of the MITF-M transcript in angiomatoid fibrous histiocytoma, *Genes Chromosomes Cancer* **44**(1): 97–102 (2005).

Hamatani, K., H. Eguchi, K. Koyama, M. Mukai, K. Nakachi, and Y. Kusunoki, A novel RET rearrangement (ACBD5/RET) by pericentric inversion, inv(10)(p12.1;q11.2), in papillary thyroid cancer from an atomic bomb survivor exposed to high-dose radiation, *Oncol Rep* **32**(5): 1809–1814 (2014).

Heisterkamp, N., and J. Groffen, Molecular insights into the Philadelphia translocation, *Hematol Pathol* **5**(1): 1–10 (1991).

Herens, C., A. Thiry, M.F. Dresse, J. Born, C. Flagothier, G. Vanstraelen, N. Allington, and V. Bex, Translocation (16;17)(q22;p13) is a recurrent anomaly of aneurysmal bone cysts, *Cancer Genet Cytogenet* **127**(1): 83–84 (2001).

Hernández, L., M. Pinyol, S. Hernández, S. Beà, K. Pulford, A. Rosenwald, L. Lamant, B. Falini, G. Ott, D.Y. Mason, G. Delsol, and E. Campo, TRK-fused gene (TFG) is a new partner of ALK in anaplastic large cell lymphoma producing two structurally different TFG-ALK translocations, *Blood* **94**(9): 3265–3268 (1999).

Hernandez-Martí, M.J., Orellana-C. Alonso, Badía-L. Garrabou, A. Verdeguer Miralles, and A. Paradís-Alós, Renal adenocarcinoma in an 8-year-old child, with a t(X;17)(p11.2;q25), *Cancer Genet Cytogenet* **83**(1): 82–83 (1995).

Hess, J.L, Chromosomal translocations in benign tumors: the HMGI proteins, *Am J Clin Pathol* **109**(3): 251–261 (1998).

Hinrichs, S.H., M.A. Jaramillo, P.H. Gumerlock, M.B. Gardner, J.P. Lewis, and A.E. Freeman, Myxoid chondrosarcoma with a translocation involving chromosomes 9 and 22, *Cancer Genet Cytogenet* **14**(3–4): 219–226 (1985).

Hisaoka, M., A. Matsuyama, T. Aoki, A. Sakamoto, and K. Yokoyama, Low-grade fibromyxoid sarcoma with prominent giant rosettes and heterotopic ossification, *Pathol Res Pract* **208**(9): 557–560 (2012).

Hiwatari, M., T. Taki, T. Taketani, M. Taniwaki, K. Sugita, M. Okuya, M. Eguchi, K. Ida and Y. Hayashi, Fusion of an AF4-related gene, LAF4, to MLL in childhood acute lymphoblastic leukemia with t(2;11)(q11;q23), *Oncogene* **22**(18): 2851–2855 (2003).

Ikeda, T., K. Ikeda, K. Sasaki, K. Kawakami, and J. Takahara, The inv(11)(p15q22) chromosome translocation of therapy-related myelodysplasia with NUP98-DDX10 and DDX10-NUP98 fusion transcripts, *Int J Hematol* **69**(3): 160–164 (1999).

Iwakawa, R., M. Takenaka, T. Kohno, Y. Shimada, Y. Totoki, T. Shibata, K. Tsuta, R. Nishikawa, M. Noguchi, A. Sato-Otsubo, S. Ogawa and J. Yokota, Genome-wide identification of genes with amplification and/or fusion in small cell lung cancer, *Genes Chromosomes Cancer* **52**(9): 802–816 (2013).

Jenkins, R.B., H. Blair, K.V. Ballman, C. Giannini, R.M. Arusell, M. Law, H. Flynn, S. Passe, S. Felten, P.D. Brown, E.G. Shaw, and J.C. Buckner, A t(1;19)(q10;p10) mediates the combined deletions of 1p and 19q and predicts a better prognosis of patients with oligodendroglioma, *Cancer Res* **66**(20): 9852–9861 (2006).

Joh, T., Y. Kagami, K. Yamamoto, T. Segawa, J. Takizawa, T. Takahashi, R. Ueda, and M. Seto, Identification of MLL and chimeric MLL gene products involved in 11q23 translocation and possible mechanisms of leukemogenesis by MLL truncation, *Oncogene* **13**(9): 1945–1953 (1996).

Kim, J., K. Lee, and J. Pelletier, The desmoplastic small round cell tumor t(11;22) translocation produces EWS/WT1 isoforms with differing oncogenic properties, *Oncogene* **16**(15): 1973–1979 (1998).

Kubonishi, I., N. Takehara, J. Iwata, H. Sonobe, Y. Ohtsuki, T. Abe, and I. Miyoshi, Novel t(15;19)(q15;p13) chromosome abnormality in a thymic carcinoma, *Cancer Res* **51**(12): 3327–3328 (1991).

Kuriakose, P. N. Perveen, K. Maeda, A. Wiktor, and D.L. Van Dyke, Translocation (8;14)(q24;q32) as the sole cytogenetic abnormality in B-cell prolymphocytic leukemia, *Cancer Genet Cytogenet* **150**(2): 156–158 (2004).

Kurzrock, R., and M. Talpaz, The molecular pathology of chronic myelogenous Leukemia, *Br J Haematol* 79 Suppl **1**: 34–37 (1991).

Labelle, Y., J. Bussières, F. Courjal, and M.B. Goldring, The EWS/TEC fusion protein encoded by the t(9;22) chromosomal translocation in human chondrosarcomas is a highly potent transcriptional activator, *Oncogene* **18**(21): 3303–3308. PubMed PMID: 10359536 (1999).

Ladanyi, M, Aberrant ALK tyrosine kinase signaling. Different cellular lineages, common oncogenic mechanisms, *Am J Pathol* **157**(2): 341–345 (2000).

Lamant, L., N. Dastugue, K. Pulford, G. Delsol, and B. Mariamé, A new fusion gene TPM3-ALK in anaplastic large cell lymphoma created by a (1;2) (q25;p23) translocation, *Blood* **93**(9): 3088–3095 (1999).

Lannon, C.L., and P.H. Sorensen, ETV6-NTRK3: a chimeric protein tyrosine kinase with transformation activity in multiple cell lineages, *Semin Cancer Biol* **15**(3): 215–223 (2005).

Lawrence, B., Perez-A. Atayde, M.K. Hibbard, B.P. Rubin, Dal P. Cin, J.L. Pinkus, G.S. Pinkus, S. Xiao, E.S. Yi, C.D. Fletcher, and J.A. Fletcher, TPM3-ALK and TPM4-ALK oncogenes in inflammatory myofibroblastic tumors, *Am J Pathol* **157**(2): 377–384 (2000).

Le Baccon, P., D. Leroux, C. Dascalescu, S. Duley, D. Marais, E. Esmenjaud, J.J. Sotto, and M. Callanan, Novel evidence of a role for chromosome 1 pericentric heterochromatin in the pathogenesis of B-cell lymphoma and multiple myeloma, *Genes Chromosomes Cancer* **32**(3): 250–264 (2001).

Leow, P.C., C.S. Ku, R. Soo, and R. Soong, Technological advances in the detection of novel fusion genes, *eLS* (2012).

Li, H., Y. Pan, R. Wang, Y. Li, Y. Sun, and H. Chen, Response to crizotinib observed in metastatic mediastinum lymph node from a non-small cell lung cancer patient harboring EZR-ROS1 fusion, *J Cancer Res Clin Oncol* **141**(1): 185–187 (2015).

Li, S, Anaplastic lymphoma kinase-positive large B-cell lymphoma: a distinct clinicopathological entity, *Int J Clin Exp Pathol* **2**(6): 508–518 (2009).

Lim, J.H., S. Jang, C.J. Park, Y.U. Cho, J.H. Lee, K.H. Lee, J.O. Lee, J.Y. Shin, J.I. Kim, J. Huh, and E.J. Seo, RANBP2-ALK fusion combined with monosomy 7 in acute myelomonocytic leukemia, *Cancer Genet* **207**(1–2): 40–45 (2014).

Lubieniecka, J.M., D.R. de Bruijn, L. Su, A.H. van Dijk, S. Subramanian, van de M. Rijn, N. Poulin, A.G. van Kessel, and T.O. Nielsen, Histone deacetylase inhibitors reverse SS18-SSX-mediated polycomb silencing of the tumor suppressor early growth response 1 in synovial sarcoma, *Cancer Res* **68**(11): 4303–4310 (2008).

Ma, Z., J. Cools, P. Marynen, X. Cui, R. Siebert, S. Gesk, B. Schlegelberger, B. Peeters, De Wolf-C. Peeters, I. Wlodarska, and S.W. Morris, Inv(2) (p23q35) in anaplastic large-cell lymphoma induces constitutive anaplastic lymphoma kinase (ALK) tyrosine kinase activation by fusion ATIC. to, an enzyme involved in purine nucleotide biosynthesis, *Blood* **95**(6): 2144–2149 (2000).

Ma, Z., D.A. Hill, M.H. Collins, S.W. Morris, J. Sumegi, M. Zhou, C. Zuppan, and J.A. Bridge, Fusion of ALK to the Ran-binding protein 2 (RANBP2) gene in inflammatory myofibroblastic tumor, *Genes Chromosomes Cancer* **37**(1): 98–105 (2003).

Maesako, Y., K. Izumi, S. Okamori, K. Takeoka, C. Kishimori, A. Okumura, G. Honjo, T. Akasaka, and H. Ohno, inv(2)(p23q13)/RAN-binding protein 2 (RANBP2)-ALK fusion gene in myeloid leukemia that developed in an elderly woman, *Int J Hematol* **99**(2): 202–207 (2014).

Maesawa, C., S. Iijima, N. Sato, N. Yoshinori, M. Suzuki, M. Tarusawa, K. Ishida, G. Tamura, K. Saito, and T. Masuda, Esophageal extraskeletal Ewing's sarcoma, *HumPathol* **33**(1): 130–132 (2002).

Magadum, S., U. Banerjee, P. Murugan, D. Gangapur, and R. Ravikesavan, Gene duplication as a major force in evolution, *J Genet* **92**(1): 155–161 (2013).

Maitra, A., A.G. Weinberg, N. Schneider, and K. Patterson, Detection of t(11;22)(q24;q12) translocation and EWS-FLI-1 fusion transcript in a case of solid pseudopapillary tumor of the pancreas, *Pediatr Dev Pathol* **3**(6): 603–605 (2000).

Majewski, I.J., L. Mittempergher, N.M. Davidson, A. Bosma, S.M. Willems, H.M. Horlings, I. de Rink, L. Greger, G.K. Hooijer, D. Peters, P.M. Nederlof, I. Hofland, J. de Jong, J. Wesseling, R.J. Kluin, W. Brugman, R. Kerkhoven, F. Nieboer, P. Roepman, A. Broeks, T.R. Muley, J. Jassem, J. Niklinski, N. van Zandwijk, A. Brazma, A. Oshlack, M. van den Heuvel, and R. Bernards, Identification of recurrent FGFR3 fusion genes in lung cancer through kinome-centred RNA sequencing, *J Pathol* **230**(3): 270–276 (2013).

Maseki, N., H. Miyoshi, K. Shimizu, C. Homma, M. Ohki, M. Sakurai, and Y. Kaneko, The 8;21 chromosome translocation in acute myeloid leukemia is always detecTable by molecular analysis using AML1, *Blood* **81**(6): 1573–1579 (1993).

Matsubara, D., Y. Kanai, S. Ishikawa, S. Ohara, T. Yoshimoto, T. Sakatani, S. Oguni, T. Tamura, H. Kataoka, S. Endo, Y. Murakami, H. Aburatani, M. Fukayama, and T. Niki, Identification of CCDC6-RET fusion in the human lung adenocarcinoma cell line, LC-2/ad, *J Thorac Oncol* **7**(12): 1872–1876 (2012).

Matsuura, S., K. Shinmura, T. Kamo, H. Igarashi, K. Maruyama, M. Tajima, H. Ogawa, M. Tanahashi, H. Niwa, K. Funai, T. Kohno, T. Suda, and H. Sugimura, CD74-ROS1 fusion transcripts in resected non-small cell lung carcinoma, *Oncol Rep* **30**(4): 1675–1680 (2013).

McPherson, A., C. Wu, I. Hajirasouliha, F. Hormozdiari, F. Hach, A. Lapuk, S. Volik, S. Shah, C. Collins and S.C. Sahinalp, Comrad: detection of expressed rearrangements by integrated analysis of RNA-Seq and low coverage genome sequence data, *Bioinformatics* **27**(11): 1481–1488 (2011).

Medeiros, B.C., H.E. Kohrt, D.A. Arber, C.D. Bangs, A.M. Cherry, R. Majeti, K.E. Kogel, C.A. Azar, S. Patel, and A.A. Alizadeh, Immunophenotypic features of acute myeloid leukemia with inv(3)(q21q26.2)/t(3;3)(q21;q26.2), *Leuk Res* **34**(5): 594–597 (2010).

Mertens, F., C.D. Fletcher, C.R. Antonescu, J.M. Coindre, M. Colecchia, H.A. Domanski, Downs-E. Kelly, C. Fisher, J.R. Goldblum, L. Guillou, R. Reid, J. Rosai, R. Sciot, N. Mandahl, and I. Panagopoulos, Clinicopathologic and molecular genetic characterization of low-grade fibromyxoid sarcoma, and cloning of a novel FUS/CREB3L1 fusion gene, *Lab Invest* **85**(3): 408–415 (2005).

Mitelman, F., B. Johansson, and F. Mertens, The impact of translocations and gene fusions on cancer causation, *Nat Rev Cancer* **7**(4): 233–245 (2007).

Miyagi, Y., T. Sasaki, K. Fujinami, J. Sano, Y. Senga, T. Miura, Y. Kameda, Y. Sakuma, Y. Nakamura, M. Harada, and E. Tsuchiya, ETS family-associated gene fusions in Japanese prostate cancer: analysis of 194 radical prostatectomy samples, *Mod Pathol* **23**(11): 1492–1498 (2010).

Mo, M.L., Z. Chen, H.M. Zhou, H. Li, T. Hirata, D.M. Jablons, and B. He, Detection of E2A-PBX1 fusion transcripts in human non-small-cell lung cancer, *J Exp Clin Cancer Res* **32**: 29 (2013).

Momose, S., J. Tamaru, H. Kishi, I. Mikata, M. Mori, Y. Toyozumi, and S. Itoyama, Hyperactivated STAT3 in ALK-positive diffuse large B-cell lymphoma with clathrin-ALK fusion, *Hum Pathol* **40**(1): 75–82 (2009).

Morerio, C., M. Acquila, A. Rapella, E. Tassano, C. Rosanda, and C. Panarello, Inversion (11)(p15q22) with NUP98-DDX10 fusion gene in pediatric acute myeloid leukemia, *Cancer Genet Cytogenet* **171**(2): 122–125 (2006).

Morris, S.W., M.N. Kirstein, M.B. Valentine, K.G. Dittmer, D.N. Shapiro, D.L. Saltman, and A.T. Look, Fusion of a kinase gene, ALK, to a nucleolar protein gene, NPM, in non-Hodgkin's lymphoma, *Science* **263**(5151): 1281–1284. Erratum in: *Science* **267**(5196): 316–317 (1995).

Murati, A., Gelsi-V. Boyer, J. Adélaïde, C. Perot, P. Talmant, S. Giraudier, L. Lodé, A. Letessier, B. Delaval, V. Brunel, M. Imbert, R. Garand, L. Xerri, D. Birnbaum, M.J. Mozziconacci, and M. Chaffanet, PCM1-JAK2 fusion in myeloproliferative disorders and acute erythroid leukemia with t(8;9) translocation, *Leukemia* **19**(9): 1692–1696 (2005).

Nebral, K., D. Denk, A. Attarbaschi, M. König, G. Mann, O.A. Haas, and S. Strehl, Incidence and diversity of PAX5 fusion genes in childhood acute lymphoblastic leukemia, *Leukemia* **23**(1): 134–143 (2009).

Nemoto, N., K. Suzukawa, S. Shimizu, A. Shinagawa, N. Takei, T. Taki, Y. Hayashi, H. Kojima, Y. Kawakami, and T. Nagasawa, Identification of a novel fusion gene MLL-MAML2 in secondary acute myelogenous leukemia and myelodysplastic syndrome with inv(11)(q21q23), *Genes Chromosomes Cancer* **46**(9): 813–819 (2007).

Ney Garcia, D.R., T. Liehr, M. Emerenciano, C. Meyer, R. Marschalek, S. Pombo-de-Oliveira Mdo, R.C. Ribeiro, M.G. Poirot Land and M.L. Macedo Silva, Molecular studies reveal a MLL-MLLT3 gene fusion displaced in a case of childhood acute lymphoblastic leukemia with complex karyotype, *Cancer Genet* **208**(4): 143–147 (2015).

Nicorici, D., M. Satalan, H. Edgren, S. Kangaspeska, A. Murumagi, O. Kallioniemi, S. Virtanen, and O. Kilkku, FusionCatcher-a tool for finding somatic fusion genes in paired-end RNA-sequencing data, *bioRxiv* 011650 (2014).

Nilsson, M., I. Panagopoulos, F. Mertens, and N. Mandahl, Fusion of the HMGA2 and NFIB genes in lipoma, *Virchows Arch* **447**(5): 855–858 (2005).

Nowell, P.C., and D.A. Hungerford, A minute chromosome in human chronic granulocytic leukemia [abstract], *Science* **132**: 1497 (1960).

Obama, K., Y. Furukawa, M. Tara, and K. Niina, Secondary monocytic leukemia with rearrangement of the MLL gene occurring during the course of adult T-cell leukemia, *Int J Hematol* **68**(3): 323–326 (1998).

O' Brien, K.P., E. Seroussi, P. Dal Cin, R. Sciot, N. Mandahl, J.A. Fletcher, C. Turc-Carel, and J.P. Dumanski, Various regions within the alpha-helical domain of the COL1A1 gene are fused to the second exon of the PDGFB gene in dermatofibrosarcomas and giant-cell fibroblastomas, *Genes Chromosomes Cancer* **23**(2): 187–193 (1998).

Ohe, C., N. Kuroda, O. Hes, M. Michal, T. Vanecek, P. Grossmann, Y. Tanaka, M. Tanaka, H. Inui, Y. Komai, T. Matsuda, and Y. Uemura, A renal epithelioid angiomyolipoma/perivascular epithelioid cell tumor with TFE3 gene break visualized by FISH, *Med Mol Morphol* **45**(4): 234–237 (2012).

Ohki, M, Molecular basis of the t(8;21) translocation in acute myeloid Leukemia, *Semin Cancer Biol* **4**(6): 369–375 (1993).

Osaka, M., J.D. Rowley, and N.J. Zeleznik-Le, MSF (MLL septin-like fusion), a fusion partner gene MLL. of, in a therapy-related acute myeloid leukemia with a t(11;17)(q23;q25), *Proc Natl Acad Sci USA* **96**(11): 6428–6433 (1999).

Panagopoulos, I., M. Höglund, F. Mertens, N. Mandahl, F. Mitelman, and P. Aman, Fusion of the EWS and CHOP genes in myxoid liposarcoma, *Oncogene* **12**(3): 489–494 (1996).

Panagopoulos, I., C. Lassen, M. Isaksson, F. Mitelman, N. Mandahl, and P. Aman, Characteristic sequence motifs at the breakpoints of the hybrid genes FUS/CHOP, EWS/CHOP and FUS/ERG in myxoid liposarcoma and acute myeloid leukemia, *Oncogene* **15**(11): 1357–1362 (1997).

Peeters, P., S.D. Raynaud, J. Cools, I. Wlodarska, J. Grosgeorge, P. Philip, F. Monpoux, Van L. Rompaey, M. Baens, H. Van den Berghe, and P. Marynen, Fusion TEL. of, the ETS-variant gene 6 (ETV6), to the receptor-associated kinase JAK2 as a result of t(9;12) in a lymphoid and t(9;15;12) in a myeloid leukemia, *Blood* **90**(7): 2535–2540 (1997).

Pérez-Mancera, P.A., and I. Sánchez-García, Understanding mesenchymal cancer: theliposarcoma-associated FUS-DDIT3 fusion gene as a model, *Semin Cancer Biol* **15**(3): 206–214 (2005).

Perner, S., N.J. Rupp, M. Braun, M.A. Rubin, H. Moch, M. Dietel, N. Wernert, K. Jung, C. Stephan, and G. Kristiansen, Loss of SLC45A3 protein (prostein) expression in prostate cancer is associated with SLC45A3-ERG gene rearrangement and an unfavorable clinical course, *Int J Cancer* **132**(4): 807–812 (2013).

Perner, S., P.L. Wagner, F. Demichelis, R. Mehra, C.J. Lafargue, B.J. Moss, S. Arbogast, A. Soltermann, W. Weder, T.J. Giordano, D.G. Beer, D.S. Rickman, A.M. Chinnaiyan, H. Moch, and M.A. Rubin, EML4-ALK fusion lung cancer: a rare acquired event, *Neoplasia* **10**(3): 298–302 (2008).

Pérot, G., I. Soubeyran, A. Ribeiro, B. Bonhomme, F. Savagner, Boutet-N. Bouzamondo, I. Hostein, F. Bonichon, Y. Godbert, and F. Chibon, Identification of a recurrent STRN/ALK fusion in thyroid carcinomas, *PLoS One* **9**(1): e87170 (2014).

Persson, M., Y. Andrén, J. Mark, H.M. Horlings, F. Persson, and G. Stenman, Recurrent fusion of MYB and NFIB transcription factor genes in carcinomas of the breast and head and neck, *Proc Natl Acad Sci USA* **106**(44): 18740–18744 (2009).

Petit, M.M., R. Mols, E.F. Schoenmakers, N. Mandahl, and W.J. Van de Ven, LPP, thepreferred fusion partner gene of HMGIC in lipomas, is a novel member of the LIM protein gene family, *Genomics* **36**(1): 118–129 (1996).

Pierotti, M.A., G. Sozzi, and C.M. Croce, Mechanisms of oncogene activation. In: D.W. Kufe, R.E. Pollock, R.R. Weichselbaum, *et al.* (eds.). *Holland-Frei Cancer Medicine*, 6th edition. Hamilton (ON): BC Decker; 2003. Available from: http://www.ncbi.nlm.nih.gov/books/NBK12538/.

Pierron, G., F. Tirode, C. Lucchesi, S. Reynaud, S. Ballet, S. Cohen-Gogo, V. Perrin, J.M. Coindre, and O. Delattre, A new subtype of bone sarcoma defined by BCOR-CCNB3 gene fusion, *Nat Genet* **44**(4): 461–466 (2012).

Pierotti, M.A., P. Vigneri, and I. Bongarzone, Rearrangements of RET and NTRK1 tyrosinekinase receptors in papillary thyroid carcinomas, *Recent Results Cancer Res* **154**: 237–247 (1998).

Poitras, J.L., Dal P. Cin, J.C. Aster, D.J. Deangelo, and C.C. Morton, Novel SSBP2-JAK2 fusion gene resulting from a t(5;9)(q14.1;p24.1) in pre-B acute lymphocytic leukemia, *Genes Chromosomes Cancer* **47**(10): 884–889 (2008).

Polson, E.S., J.L. Lewis, H. Celik, V.M. Mann, M.J. Stower, M.S. Simms, G. Rodrigues, A.T. Collins, and N.J. Maitland, Monoallelic expression of TMPRSS2/ERG in prostate cancer stem cells, *Nat Commun* **4**: 1623 (2013).

Prieto-Granada, C., L. Zhang, H.W. Chen, Y.S. Sung, N.P. Agaram, A.A. Jungbluth, and C.R. Antonescu, A genetic dichotomy between pure sclerosing epithelioid fibrosarcoma (SEF) and hybrid SEF/low-grade fibromyxoid sarcoma: a pathologic and molecular study of 18 cases, *Genes Chromosomes Cance*r **54**(1): 28–38 (2015).

Raddaoui, E., L.R. Donner, and I. Panagopoulos, Fusion of the FUS and ATF1 genes in a large, deep-seated angiomatoid fibrous histiocytoma, *Diagn Mol Pathol* **11**(3): 157–162 (2002).

Raynaud, S., H. Cave, M. Baens, C. Bastard, V. Cacheux, J. Grosgeorge, Guidal-C. Giroux, C. Guo, E. Vilmer, P. Marynen, and B. Grandchamp, The 12;21 translocation involving TEL and deletion of the other TEL allele: two frequently associated alterations found in childhood acute lymphoblastic leukemia, *Blood* **87**(7): 2891–2899 (1996).

Reichel, M., E. Gillert, I. Nilson, G. Siegler, J. Greil, G.H. Fey, and R. Marschalek, Fine structure of translocation breakpoints in leukemic blasts with chromosomal translocation t(4;11): the DNA damage-repair model of translocation, *Oncogene* **17**(23): 3035–3044 (1998).

Reiter, A., C. Walz, A. Watmore, C. Schoch, I. Blau, B. Schlegelberger, U. Berger, N. Telford, S. Aruliah, J.A. Yin, D. Vanstraelen, H.F. Barker, P.C. Taylor, O'A. Driscoll, F. Benedetti, C. Rudolph, H.J. Kolb, A. Hochhaus, R. Hehlmann, A. Chase, and N.C. Cross, The t(8;9)(p22;p24) is a recurrent abnormality in chronic and acute leukemia that fuses PCM1 to JAK2, *Cancer Res* **65**(7): 2662–2667 (2005).

Rimkunas, V.M., K.E. Crosby, D. Li, Y. Hu, M.E. Kelly, T.L. Gu, J.S. Mack, M.R. Silver, X. Zhou, and H. Haack, Analysis of receptor tyrosine kinase ROS1-positive tumors in non-small cell lung cancer: identification of a FIG-ROS1 fusion, *Clin Cancer Res* **18**(16): 4449–4457 (2012).

Rimkunas, V.M., K.E. Crosby, D. Li, Y. Hu, M.E. Kelly, T.L. Gu, J.S. Mack, M.R. Silver, X. Zhou, and H. Haack, Analysis of receptor tyrosine kinase ROS1-positive tumors in non-small cell lung cancer: identification of a FIG-ROS1 fusion, *Clin Cancer Res* **18**(16): 4449–4457 (2012).

Robinson, D.R., Y.M. Wu, S. Kalyana-Sundaram, X. Cao, R.J. Lonigro, Y.S. Sung, C.L. Chen, L. Zhang, R. Wang, F. Su, M.K. Iyer, S. Roychowdhury,

J. Siddiqui, K.J. Pienta, L.P. Kunju, M. Talpaz, J.M. Mosquera, S. Singer, S.M. Schuetze, C.R. Antonescu, and A.M. Chinnaiyan, Identification of recurrent NAB2-STAT6 gene fusions in solitary fibrous tumor by integrative sequencing, *Nat Genet* **45**(2): 180–185 (2013).

Roccato, E., S. Pagliardini, L. Cleris, S. Canevari, F. Formelli, M.A. Pierotti, and A. Greco, Role of TFG sequences outside the coiled-coil domain in TRK-T3 oncogenic activation, *Oncogene* **22**(6): 807–818 (2003).

Rogalla, P., B. Kazmierczak, K. Meyer-Bolte, K.H. Tran, and J. Bullerdiek, The t(3;12)(q27;q14-q15) with underlying HMGIC-LPP fusion is not determining an adipocytic phenotype, *Genes Chromosomes Cancer* **22**(2): 100–104 (1998).

Romana, S.P., H. Poirel, M. Leconiat, M.A. Flexor, M. Mauchauffé, P. Jonveaux, E.A. Macintyre, R. Berger, and O.A. Bernard, High frequency of t(12;21) in childhood B-lineage acute lymphoblastic leukemia, *Blood* **86**(11): 4263–4269 (1995).

Rosenwald, A., G. Ott, K. Pulford, T. Katzenberger, J. Kühl, J. Kalla, M.M. Ott, D.Y. Mason, and H.K. Müller-Hermelink, t(1;2)(q21;p23) and t(2;3)(p23;q21): two novel variant translocations of the t(2;5)(p23;q35) in anaplastic large cell lymphoma, *Blood* **94**(1): 362–364 (1999).

Rubnitz, J.E., B.M. Camitta, H. Mahmoud, S.C. Raimondi, A.J. Carroll, M.J. Borowitz, J.J. Shuster, M.P. Link, D.J. Pullen, J.R. Downing, F.G. Behm, and C.H. Pui, Childhood acute lymphoblastic leukemia with the MLL-ENL fusion and t(11;19)(q23;p13.3)translocation, *J Clin Oncol* **17**(1): 191–196 (1999).

Rudin, C.M., S. Durinck, E.W. Stawiski, J.T. Poirier, Z. Modrusan, D.S. Shames, E.A. Bergbower, Y. Guan, J. Shin, J. Guillory, C.S. Rivers, C.K. Foo, D. Bhatt, J. Stinson, F. Gnad, P.M. Haverty, R. Gentleman, S. Chaudhuri, V. Janakiraman, B.S. Jaiswal, C. Parikh, W. Yuan, Z. Zhang, H. Koeppen, T.D. Wu, H.M. Stern, R.L. Yauch, K.E. Huffman, D.D. Paskulin, P.B. Illei, M. Varella-Garcia, A.F. Gazdar, F.J. de Sauvage, R. Bourgon, J.D. Minna, M.V. Brock, and S. Seshagiri, Comprehensive genomic analysis identifies SOX2 as a frequently amplified gene in small-cell lung cancer, *Nat Genet* **44**(10): 1111–1116 (2012).

Santoro, M., N.A. Dathan, M.T. Berlingieri, I. Bongarzone, C. Paulin, M. Grieco, M.A. Pierotti, G. Vecchio and A. Fusco, Molecular characterization of RET-PTC3; a novel rearranged version of the RET proto-oncogene in a human thyroid papillary carcinoma, *Oncogene* **9**(2): 509–516 (1994).

Santoro, M., and F. Carlomagno, Central role of RET in thyroid cancer, *Cold Spring Harb Perspect Biol* **5**(12): a009233 (2013).

Schinnerl, D., K. Fortschegger, M. Kauer, J.R. Marchante, R. Kofler, M.L. Den Boer, and Strehl S, The role of the Janus-faced transcription factor PAX5-JAK2 in acute lymphoblastic leukemia, *Blood* **125**(8): 1282–1291 (2015).

Scotlandi, K., T. Chano, S. Benini, M. Serra, M.C. Manara, V. Cerisano, P. Picci, and N. Baldini, Identification of EWS/FLI-1 transcripts in giant-cell tumor of bone, *Int J Cancer* **87**(3): 328–335 (2000).

Segura, S., R. Salgado, A. Toll, G. Martín-Ezquerra, M. Yébenes, A. Sáez, F. Solé, C. Barranco, P. Umbert, B. Espinet, and R.M. Pujol, Identification of t(17;22)(q22;q13) (COL1A1/PDGFB) in dermatofibrosarcoma protuberans by fluorescence *in situ* hybridization in paraffin-embedded tissue microarrays, *Hum Pathol* **42**(2): 176–184 (2011).

Setoyama, M., A. Tojo, F. Nagamura, S. Asano, M. Ishimae, M. Eguchi and N. Kamada, A unique translocation of the TEL gene in a case of acute myelogenous leukemia with inv(12)(p13q15), *Blood* **92**(4): 1454–1455 (1998).

Shav-Tal, Y., and D. Zipori, PSF and p54(nrb)/NonO — multi-functional nuclear proteins, *FEBS Lett* **531**(2): 109–114 (2002).

Shurtleff, S.A., S. Meyers, S.W. Hiebert, S.C. Raimondi, D.R. Head, C.L. Willman, S. Wolman, M.L. Slovak, A.J. Carroll, and F. Behm, Heterogeneity in CBF beta/MYH11 fusion messages encoded by the inv(16)(p13q22) and the t(16;16)(p13;q22) in acute myelogenous leukemia, *Blood* **85**(12): 3695–3703 (1995).

Sidhar, S.K., J. Clark, S. Gill, R. Hamoudi, A.J. Crew, R. Gwilliam, M. Ross, W.M.S. Linehan Birdsall, J. Shipley, and C.S. Cooper, The t(X;1)(p11.2;q21.2) translocation in papillary renal cell carcinoma fuses a novel gene PRCC to the TFE3 transcription factor gene, *Hum Mol Genet* **5**(9): 1333–1338 (1996).

So, C.W., M. Lin, P.M. Ayton, E.H. Chen, and M.L. Cleary, Dimerization contributes to oncogenic activation of MLL chimeras in acute leukemias, *Cancer Cell* **4**(2): 99–110 (2003).

Soda, M., Y.L. Choi, M. Enomoto, S. Takada, Y. Yamashita, S. Ishikawa, S.I. Fujiwara, H. Watanabe, K. Kurashina, H. Hatanaka, and M. Bando, Identification of the transforming EML4–ALK fusion gene in non-small-cell lung cancer, *Nature* **448**(7153): 561–566 (2007).

Soller, M.J., M. Isaksson, P. Elfving, W. Soller, R. Lundgren, and I. Panagopoulos, Confirmation of the high frequency of the TMPRSS2/ERG fusion gene in prostate cancer, *Genes Chromosomes Cancer* **45**(7): 717–719 (2006).

Sozzi, G., I. Bongarzone, M. Miozzo, M.G. Borrello, M.G. Blutti, S. Pilotti, G. Della Porta, and M.A. Pierotti, A t(10;17) translocation creates the RET/

PTC2 chimeric transforming sequence in papillary thyroid carcinoma, *Genes Chromosomes Cancer* **9**(4): 244–250 (1994).

Speleman, F., B. Cauwelier, N. Dastugue, J. Cools, B. Verhasselt, B. Poppe, N. Van Roy, J. Vandesompele, C. Graux, A. Uyttebroeck, M. Boogaerts, B. De Moerloose, Y. Benoit, D. Selleslag, J. Billiet, A. Robert, F. Huguet, P. Vandenberghe, A. De Paepe, P. Marynen, and A. Hagemeijer, A new recurrent inversion, inv(7)(p15q34), leads to transcriptional activation of HOXA10 and HOXA11 in a subset of T-cell acute lymphoblastic leukemias, *Leukemia* **19**(3): 358–366 (2005).

Stenman, G., Fusion oncogenes in salivary gland tumors: molecular and clinical consequences, *Head Neck Pathol* **7**(Suppl 1): S12–19. doi: 10.1007/s12105-013–0462-z. Epub 2013 Jul 3. Review. PubMed PMID:

Stewénius, Y., Y. Jin, I. Ora, I. Panagopoulos, E. Möller, F. Mertens, B. Sandstedt, J. Alumets, M. Akerman, J.H. Merks, J. de Kraker, and D. Gisselsson, High-resolution molecular cytogenetic analysis of Wilms tumors highlights diagnostic difficulties among small round cell kidney tumors, *Genes Chromosomes Cancer* **47**(10): 845–852 (2008).

Storlazzi, C.T., F. Mertens, A. Nascimento, M. Isaksson, J. Wejde, O. Brosjo, N. Mandahl, and I. Panagopoulos, Fusion of the FUS and BBF2H7 genes in low grade fibromyxoid sarcoma, *Hum Mol Genet* **12**(18): 2349–2358 (2003).

Suehara, Y., M. Arcila, L. Wang, A. Hasanovic, D. Ang, T. Ito, Y. Kimura, A. Drilon, U. Guha, V. Rusch, M.G. Kris, M.F. Zakowski, N. Rizvi, R. Khanin, and M. Ladanyi, Identification of KIF5B-RET and GOPC-ROS1 fusions in lung adenocarcinomas through a comprehensive mRNA-based screen for tyrosine kinase fusions, *Clin Cancer Res* **18**(24): 6599–6608 (2012).

Swanson, T.A., S.A. Krueger, S. Galoforo, B.J. Thibodeau, A.A. Martinez, G.D. Wilson, and B. Marples, TMPRSS2/ERG fusion gene expression alters chemo- and radio-responsiveness in cell culture models of androgen independent prostate cancer, *Prostate* **71**(14): 1548–1558 (2011).

Takei, N., K. Suzukawa, H.Y. Mukai, T. Itoh, Y. Okoshi, Y. Yoda, and T. Nagasawa, Therapy-related acute myeloid leukemia 6 years after clonal detection of inv(11)(q21q23) and MLL gene rearrangement, *Int J Hematol* **83**(3): 247–251 (2006).

Takeoka, K., A. Okumura, Y. Maesako, T. Akasaka, and H. Ohno, Crizotinib resistance in acute myeloid leukemia with inv(2)(p23q13)/RAN binding protein 2 (RANBP2) anaplastic lymphoma kinase (ALK) fusion and monosomy 7, *Cancer Genet* **208**(3): 85–90 (2015).

Takeuchi, K., Y.L. Choi, Y. Togashi, M. Soda, S. Hatano, K. Inamura, S. Takada, T. Ueno, Y. Yamashita, Y. Satoh, S. Okumura, K. Nakagawa, Y. Ishikawa, and H. Mano, KIF5B-ALK, a novel fusion oncokinase identified by an immunohistochemistry-based diagnostic system for ALK-positive lung cancer, *Clin Cancer Res* **15**(9): 3143–3149 (2009).

Takeuchi, K., M. Soda, Y. Togashi, R. Suzuki, S. Sakata, S. Hatano, R. Asaka, W. Hamanaka, H. Ninomiya, H. Uehara, Y. Lim Choi, Y. Satoh, S. Okumura, K. Nakagawa, H. Mano, and Y. Ishikawa, RET, ROS1 and ALK fusions in lung cancer, *Nat Med* **18**(3): 378–381 (2012).

Tarazona, N., L. Navarro, J.M. Cejalvo, V. Gambardella, J.A. Pérez-Fidalgo, A. Sempere, S. Navarro, and A. Cervantes, Primary paraesophageal Ewing's sarcoma: an uncommon case report and literature review, *Onco Targets Ther* **8**: 1053–1059 (2015).

Testoni, N., G. Borsaru, G. Martinelli, C. Carboni, D. Ruggeri, E. Ottaviani, S. Pelliconi, P. Ricci, R. Pastano, G. Visani, A. Zaccaria, and S. Tura, 3q21 and 3q26 cytogenetic abnormalities in acute myeloblastic leukemia: biological and clinical features, *Haematologica* **84**(8): 690–694 (1999).

Thorner, P., J. Squire, Chilton-S. MacNeil, P. Marrano, J. Bayani, D. Malkin, M. Greenberg, A. Lorenzana, and M. Zielenska, Is the EWS/FLI-1 fusion transcriptspecific for Ewing sarcoma and peripheral primitive neuroectodermal tumor? Areport of four cases showing this transcript in a wider range of tumor types, *Am J Pathol* **148**(4): 1125–1138 (1996).

Togashi, Y., M. Soda, S. Sakata, E. Sugawara, S. Hatano, R. Asaka, T. Nakajima, H. Mano, and K. Takeuchi, KLC1-ALK: a novel fusion in lung cancer identified using a formalin-fixed paraffin-embedded tissue only, *PLoS One* **7**(2): e31323 (2012).

Tomlins, S.A., B. Laxman, S.M. Dhanasekaran, B.E. Helgeson, X. Cao, D.S. Morris, A. Menon, X. Jing, Q. Cao, B. Han, J. Yu, L. Wang, J.E. Montie, M.A. Rubin, K.J. Pienta, D. Roulston, R.B. Shah, S. Varambally, R. Mehra and A.M. Chinnaiyan, Distinct classes of chromosomal rearrangements create oncogenic ETS gene fusions in prostate cancer, *Nature* **448**(7153): 595–599 (2007).

Tomlins, S.A., R. Mehra, D.R. Rhodes, L.R. Smith, D. Roulston, B.E. Helgeson, X. Cao, J.T. Wei, M.A. Rubin, R.B. Shah, and A.M. Chinnaiyan, TMPRSS2:ETV4 gene fusions define a third molecular subtype of prostate cancer, *Cancer Res* **66**(7): 3396–3400 (2006).

Tomlins, S.A., D.R. Rhodes, S. Perner, S.M. Dhanasekaran, R. Mehra, X.W. Sun, S. Varambally, X. Cao, J. Tchinda, R. Kuefer, C. Lee, J.E. Montie, R.B. Shah, K.J. Pienta, M.A. Rubin, and A.M. Chinnaiyan, Recurrent fusion of

TMPRSS2 and ETS transcription factor genes in prostate cancer, *Science* **310**(5748): 644–648 (2005).

Törnkvist, M., J. Wejde, J. Ahlén, B. Brodin, and O. Larsson, A novel case of synovial sarcoma of the kidney: impact of SS18/SSX analysis of renal hemangiopericytoma-like tumors, *Diagn Mol Pathol* **13**(1): 47–51 (2004).

Trinei, M., L. Lanfrancone, E. Campo, K. Pulford, D.Y. Mason, P.G. Pelicci, and B. Falini, A new variant anaplastic lymphoma kinase (ALK)-fusion protein (ATIC-ALK) in a case of ALK-positive anaplastic large cell lymphoma, *Cancer Res.* **60**(4): 793–798 (2000).

Uppal, S., H. Aviv, F. Patterson, S. Cohen, J. Benevenia, S. Aisner, and M. Hameed, Alveolar soft part sarcoma — reciprocal translocation between chromosome 17q25 and Xp11. Report of a case with metastases at presentation and review of the literature, *Acta Orthop Belg* **69**(2): 182–187 (2003).

van der Reijden, B.A., H.G. Dauwerse, R.H. Giles, S. Jagmohan-Changur, C. Wijmenga, P.P. Liu, B. Smit, H.W. Wessels, G.C. Beverstock, M. Jotterand-Bellomo, D. Martinet, D. Mühlematter, M. Lafage-Pochitaloff, J. Gabert, J. Reiffers, C. Bilhou-Nabera, G.J. van Ommen, A. Hagemeijer, and M.H. Breuning, Genomic acute myeloid leukemia-associated inv(16)(p13q22) breakpoints are tightly clustered, *Oncogene* **18**(2): 543–550 (1999).

van der Reijden, B.A., H.G. Dauwerse, R.H. Giles, S. Jagmohan-Changur, C. Wijmenga, P.P. Liu, B. Smit, H.W. Wessels, G.C. Beverstock, M. Jotterand-Bellomo, D. Martinet, D. Mühlematter, M. Lafage-Pochitaloff, J. Gabert, J. Reiffers, C. Bilhou-Nabera, G.J. van Ommen, A. Hagemeijer, and M.H. Breuning, Genomic acute myeloid leukemia-associated inv(16)(p13q22) breakpoints are tightly clustered, *Oncogene* **18**(2): 543–550 (1999).

van der Reijden, B.A., M. Lombardo, H.G. Dauwerse, R.H. Giles, D. Mühlematter, M.J. Bellomo, H.W. Wessels, G.C. Beverstock, G.J. van Ommen, A. Hagemeijer, *et al.*, RT-PCR diagnosis of patients with acute nonlymphocytic leukemia and inv(16)(p13q22) and identification of new alternative splicing in CBFB-MYH11 transcripts, *Blood* **86**(1): 277–282 (1995).

van der Reijden, B.A., M. Lombardo, H.G. Dauwerse, R.H. Giles, D. Mühlematter, M.J. Bellomo, H.W. Wessels, G.C. Beverstock, G.J. van Ommen, A. Hagemeijer, *et al.*, RT-PCR diagnosis of patients with acute nonlymphocytic leukemia and inv(16)(p13q22) and identification of new alternative splicing in CBFB-MYH11 transcripts, *Blood* **86**(1): 277–282 (1995).

von Bergh, A.R., H.B. Beverloo, P. Rombout, E.R. van Wering, M.H. van Weel, G.C. Beverstock, P.M. Kluin, R.M. Slater, and E. Schuuring, LAF4, an AF4-related gene, is fused to MLL in infant acute lymphoblastic leukemia, *Genes Chromosomes Cancer* **35**(1): 92–96 (2002).

Walther, C., H.A. Domanski, F.V. von Steyern, N. Mandahl, and F. Mertens, Chromosome banding analysis of cells from fine-needle aspiration biopsy samples from soft tissue and bone tumors: is it clinically meaningful? *Cancer Genet* **204**(4): 203–206 (2011).

Wang, R., H. Hu, Y. Pan, Y. Li, T. Ye, C. Li, X. Luo, L. Wang, H. Li, Y. Zhang, F. Li, Y. Lu, Q. Lu, J. Xu, D. Garfield, L. Shen, H. Ji, W. Pao, Y. Sun, and H. Chen, RET fusions define a unique molecular and clinicopathologic subtype of non-small-cell lung cancer, *J Clin Oncol* **30**(35): 4352–4359 (2012).

Wang, Y., N. Wu, J. Liu, Z. Wu, and D. Dong, FusionCancer: a database of cancer fusion genes derived from RNA-seq data, *Diagnostic pathology* **10**(1): 131 (2015).

Waters, B.L., I. Panagopoulos, and E.F. Allen, Genetic characterization of angiomatoid fibrous histiocytoma identifies fusion of the FUS and ATF-1 genes induced by a chromosomal translocation involving bands 12q13 and 16p11, *Cancer Genet Cytogenet* **121**(2): 109–116 (2000).

Welborn, J., H. Jenks, J. Taplett, and P. Walling, Inversion of chromosome 12 and lineage promiscuity in hematologic malignancies, *Cancer Genet Cytogenet* **148**(2): 91–103 (2004).

Wellmann, A., T. Otsuki, M. Vogelbruch, H.M. Clark, E.S. Jaffe and M. Raffeld, Analysis of the t(2;5)(p23;q35) translocation by reverse transcription-polymerase chain reaction in CD30+ anaplastic large-cell lymphomas, in other non-Hodgkin's lymphomas of T-cell phenotype, and in Hodgkin's disease, *Blood* **86**(6): 2321–2328 (1995).

Weterman, M.A., M. Wilbrink, and A. Geurts van Kessel, Fusion of the transcription factor TFE3 gene to a novel gene, PRCC, in t(X;1)(p11;q21)-positive papillary renal cell carcinomas, *Proc Natl Acad Sci USA* **93**(26): 15294–15298 (1996).

White, N.M., F.Y. Feng, and C.A. Maher, Recurrent rearrangements in prostate cancer: causes and therapeutic potential, *Current Drug Targets* **14**(4): 450–459 (2013).

Wlodarska, I., C. De Wolf-Peeters, B. Falini, G. Verhoef, S.W. Morris, A. Hagemeijer, and H. Van den Berghe, The cryptic inv(2)(p23q35) defines a new molecular genetic subtype of ALK-positive anaplastic large-cell lymphoma, *Blood* **92**(8): 2688–2695 (1998).

Wright, R.L., and A.T. Vaughan, A systematic description of MLL fusion gene formation, *Crit Rev Oncol Hematol* **91**(3): 283–291 (2014).

Wyatt-Ashmead, J., L. Bao, R.E. Eilert, P. Gibbs, G. Glancy, and L. McGavran, Primary aneurysmal bone cysts: 16q22 and/or 17p13 chromosome abnormalities, *Pediatr Dev Pathol* **4**(4): 418–419 (2001).

Yamamoto, M., K. Kakihana, T. Kurosu, N. Murakami, and O. Miura, Clonal evolution with inv(11)(p15q22) and NUP98/DDX10 fusion gene in imatinib-resistant chronic myelogenous leukemia, *Cancer Genet Cytogenet* **157**(2): 104–108 (2005).

Yasukawa, M., K. Iwamasa, S. Kawamura, S. Murakami, K. Takada, T. Hato, T. Shiosaka, T. Tamai, T. Fukuoka, S. Fujita, *et al.*, Phenotypic and genotypic analysis of chronic myelogenous Leukemia with T lymphoblastic and megakaryoblastic mixed crisis, *Br J Haematol* **66**(3): 331–336 (1987).

Zhang, T., Y. Lu, Q. Ye, M. Zhang, L. Zheng, X. Yin, P. Gavine, Z. Sun, Q. Ji, G. Zhu, and X. Su, An evaluation and recommendation of the optimal methodologies to detect RET gene rearrangements in papillary thyroid carcinoma, *Genes Chromosomes Cancer* **54**(3): 168–176 (2015).

Zhou, M.H., L. Gao, Y. Jing, Y.Y. Xu, Y. Ding, N. Wang, W. Wang, M.Y. Li, X.P. Han, J.Z. Sun, L.L. Wang, and L. Yu, Detection of ETV6 gene rearrangements in adult acute lymphoblasticleukemia, *Ann Hematol* **91**(8): 1235–1243 (2012).

Zucman, J., O. Delattre, C. Desmaze, A.L. Epstein, G. Stenman, F. Speleman, C.D. Fletchers, A. Aurias, and G. Thomas, EWS and ATF-1 gene fusion induced by t(12;22) translocation in malignant melanoma of soft parts, *Nat Genet* **4**(4): 341–345 (1993).

3

Techniques to Identify Novel Fusion Genes and to Detect Known Fusion Genes

*Nand K. Roy, Ganesan Padmavathi, Devivasha Bordoloi and Ajaikumar B. Kunnumakkara**

INTRODUCTION

Cancer is driven by genes which often have recurring tumor specific DNA aberrations. According to the Cancer Gene Census of the Welcome Trust Sanger Institute, there are around 384 validated cancer genes which are beyond 1.5% of all transcribed human genes. Fusion oncogenes are frequent events of somatic DNA alteration detected in 282 from 384 validated cancer genes (Kaye, 2009). A fusion gene can be defined as chimeric gene formed by amalgamation of two different genes at transcript or

*Author for correspondence: Ajaikumar B. Kunnumakkara, Cancer Biology Laboratory, Department of Biosciences and Bioengineering, Indian Institute of Technology Guwahati, Assam 781039, India. kunnumakkara@iitg.ernet.in

genomic level. From the time of detection of the recurrent BCR-ABL1 fusion gene in CML and TMPRSS2-ETS related gene (ERG) fusion gene in solid tumor, it has been widely accepted that fusion genes play significant roles in cancer development. To date, more than 800 different fusion genes have been discovered in human cancer (Ge *et al.*, 2011; Leow *et al.*, 2012). More than 80% of the entire known fusion genes are reported in hematological cancers though it represents for only 10% of all human malignancies whereas in solid tumors which accounts for 80% of cancer-related mortalities, approximately 10% of the gene fusions are only known till date. This highlights the narrow degree of understanding of fusion genes in solid tumors and emphasizes the need of further advancing the research avenues in this field. In the present time interval, discovery of various recurrent gene fusions in solid tumors like prostate and lung cancers have revitalized the research in identification of novel fusions (Leow *et al.*, 2012).

The identification of an ever increasing number of fusion genes can serve as a clinical mean to diagnose, stage, classify, prognoses and treat the cancer. One of the significant characteristics of gene fusions as biomarkers is their absence in normal tissues. Thus, targeting fusion transcripts can help in providing a very specific biomarker. Moreover, gene fusions are known to have a direct functional influence on the molecular processes in the cell. For instance, TMPRSS2-ERG gene fusion is responsible for overexpression of ERG and hence develops androgen independence in several prostate cancer cases. In addition, the limited expression of these hybrid genes only in cancer cells can provide an opportunity to target them specifically through therapeutics such as Gleevec™ (imatinib), a small molecule TKI that specifically targets the BCR-ABL1 fusion protein in CML (Supper *et al.*, 2013; Leow *et al.*, 2012). Therefore, identification of fusion genes helps in better treatment of these malignancies.

For identification of fusion genes, many methodologies are available which can be mainly categorized into traditional cytogenetic-based and non-cytogenetic-based methods. Traditionally, chromosomal alterations were identified by fluorescence *in situ* hybridization (FISH) or CGH techniques. In the subsequent period, high-throughput array-CGH and SNP array were established to identify genomic copy number shift at 1 Kb resolution level. The development of next-generation sequencing (NGS) has radically revolutionized the area by generating the data up to base-pair resolution that allowed the discovery and characterization of genomic variation with added detail. With the help of NGS fusion genes were identified by the means of genomic DNA sequencing (gDNA-seq) and transcriptome sequencing (RNA-seq) as well (Ge *et al.*, 2011).

CONVENTIONAL METHODS FOR THE DETECTION OF FUSION GENES

In the earlier days, fusion genes were microscopically detected with the help of conventional cytogenetic banding techniques. Later in the coming years, molecular assays like FISH, polymerase chain reaction (PCR)-based methods and phosphoproteomic approach have been introduced for more sensitive identification and characterization of the fusion genes with more emphasis on its precise location (Leow *et al.*, 2012).

CHROMOSOME BANDING METHODS

Chromosome banding pattern was initially used for the identification of fusion genes. In this process, the chromosomes are stained with a dye or assayed for a particular function. The dye-based banding of chromosome includes G-(Giemsa), R-(reverse), C-(centromere) and Q-(quinacrine) banding. Bands which develop intense staining are taken as positive bands while faint stained bands are considered as negative bands. Although the staining pattern is not totally black and white, it can have varied intensities. G-positive bands are known as G-bands and similarly for R positive R-bands. Constitutive heterochromatins are represented by positive C-bands. Q-bands are similar to G-bands. With the help of these methods, each and every chromosome and chromosomal site could be detected depending on their distinctive banding pattern (Francke, 1994; Bickmore, 2001). In the year 1980, the first fusion gene was reported, almost 10 years after the discovery of various chromosomal rearrangements related to different diseases with the aid of banding analyses. Banding pattern analyses have remarkably helped in the identification of different structural chromosomal alterations, like inversions or reciprocal translocations in metaphase spreads obtained from cultured tumor cells, and also enabled the assignment of these rearranged breakpoints to the specific chromosomes as well as chromosome bands. The first report of balanced rearrangements in neoplasia came in 1973, where the Ph chromosome in CML was found to be associated with translocation of chromosomes 9, and 22 t(9;22(q34;q11), and t(8;21)(q22;q22) in case of acute myeloid leukemia (AML) (Mertens and Tayebwa, 2014; Mertens *et al.*, 2015; Rowley, 1973a, 1973b). Presently, there is an increasing attention in cytogenetic analysis of other hematological neoplasms and various translocations have been reported such as t(8;14)(q24;q32), t(2;8)(p11;q24), and t(8;22)(q24;q11) in Burkitt lymphoma (BL), t(4;11)(q21;q23) in acute lymphoblastic leukemia (ALL), t(15;17)(q22;q21) in acute promyelocytic leukemia (APL), and t(14;18)(q32;q21) in follicular lymphoma (Fukuhara *et al.*, 1979). The first evidence of specific translocations in neoplasms in animal models was discovered through mouse plasmacytoma (MPC) that is similar to BL having equivalent characteristic rearrangements present in human BL. Similarly in other cancers also, several translocations such as t(2;13)(q36;q14) in alveolar rhabdomyosarcoma (ARMS); t(X;1)(p11;q21) in kidney cancer; t(6;9)(q23;p23) in adenoid cystic carcinoma (ACC) of the salivary glands; t(11;22)(q24;q12) in Ewing sarcoma; t(3;8)(p21;q12) in salivary gland adenoma (SGA) and t(3;12)(q27;q13) in lipoma have been identified using this technique (Ohno *et al.*, 1979; Mark *et al.*, 1980; Seidal *et al.*, 1982; Aurias *et al.*, 1983, 1986; Turc-Carel *et al.*, 1983, 1986; de Jong *et al.*, 1986; Stenman *et al.*, 1986; Heim *et al.*, 1986).

FLUORESCENCE *IN SITU* HYBRIDIZATION (FISH)

FISH is a well-known molecular cytogenetic method applied in diagnostic pathology. Interphase FISH is most commonly used to detect gene amplification, gene rearrangements, microdeletions and chromosomal duplication. The process of FISH requires hybridization of a DNA probe labeled either directly with a fluorochrome (rhodamine or fluorscein-5-thiocyanate) or indirectly by means of haptens (biotin or digoxigenin). The DNA probes used in FISH can have three classes such as full chromosome painting probes used for identification of entire sequence of a particular chromosome for discovering the structural rearrangements, centromeric probes, applied to locate repetitive probes present in the centromere which targets the tandem repeat sequences of α-satellite DNA; locus specific probes for identification of chromosome site or specific gene bearing structural rearrangements and varied copy number. Different variations of FISH such as multiplex FISH, spectral karyotyping (SKY), combined binary ratio labeling (COBRA) FISH, high resolution multicolor-banding (mBAND), etc., are applied in cancer research (Langer-Safer *et al.*, 1982; Speicher *et al.*, 1996; Schrock *et al.*, 1996; Tanke *et al.*, 1999; Das and Tan, 2013). FISH techniques have enabled the cytogeneticists to increase the resolution level of breakpoint sites up to a few hundred Kb in comparison to 5–10 Mb resolution level of chromosome band alone (Gisselsson, 2009; Mertens and Tayebwa, 2014). The two most admired FISH assay methods used are "Break-apart probe" and "fusion probe" which frequently are used in combination. In case of "break-apart probe" assay, two differentially labeled fluorescent probes are hybridized with target gene sequences located within 1Mb distance to establish overlapping or co-localization of the probes in gene fusion deficient cells. The event of translocation is indicated by single color signal, while signal loss represents a deletion. In "fusion probe" method, two different probes are used targeting the two different chromosomes. Co-localized signals represent chromosomal translocation, but normal diploid nucleus indicates two separated signals. The "Break-apart probe" assay offers more advantages as it enables identification of fusion variants with many associate genes. FISH probes used for specific genes can help in the recognition of new variants of previously known fusion genes and it indicates that a number of genes like *mixed lineage leukemia* (*MLL*) gene, which are more susceptible to recombine with multiple partners (Leow *et al.*, 2012; Mertens *et al.*, 2015).

PHOSPHOPROTEOMICS

Phosphorylation is a frequently occurring post-translational modification that regulates diverse cellular processes in a cell and its aberrations are usually linked with several cancers (Hanahan and Weinberg, 2000). Mutations, overexpression of kinases or faults in negative regulated mechanism can lead to aberrant regulation (Harsha and Pandey, 2010). Also, the activation can occur as a result of fusion of genes encoding for different kinases. Phoshoproteomics approaches such as biochemical, peptide arrays, reverse-phase protein arrays, anti-body arrays and mass spectrometry may find their relevance in detection of kinase associated fusion gene. For instance, with the help of tyrosine phosphopeptide enrichment and LC-MS/MS method, Walters *et al.* (2006) have verified the presence of TEL-ARG and BCR-ABL fusion protein in HT-93 and KNM-3 cells respectively, as upstream enzymes of STAT5 (Walters *et al.*, 2006; Harsha and Pandey, 2010). The method of phosphoproteomics however can only be applied for detection or confirmation of those fusion genes where kinase activity is involved.

HIGH-THROUGHPUT ARRAY-BASED ANALYSES

Despite the enormous contributions offered by cytogenetic-based methods for detection of fusion genes, it has some limitations such as requirement of live cells for chromosome banding analysis which makes it essential for rapid delivery of tumor samples to the laboratory. In addition, difficulty in culturing of cells and preparation of metaphase spreads of high quality and low visibility of gene fusions under microscope limits the usage of cytogenetic based methods. Furthermore, even the high-quality preparations of chromosomes cannot detect the gene fusions resulting from small interstitial deletions or inversions or translocations that only affect the ends of chromosomes (Mitelman *et al.*, 2007; Watson *et al.*, 2013; Mertens and Tayebwa, 2014; Mertens *et al.*, 2015). The emergence of high- throughput methods for global genetic analyses like array-based platforms for gene expression and copy number profiling have opened new opportunities to overcome these limitations. This method presents a genome-wide view and grants much depth in the resolution as compared to chromosome banding analysis without prior culturing of cells. The principle lies in the analysis of genomic DNA by which gene fusions resulting from either unbalanced chromosomal rearrangements (small gains or losses) or balanced translocations (extensive deletions and/or duplications) in the breakpoint sites can be detected (Sinclair *et al.*, 2000; Pinkel and Albertson, 2005; Mertens and Tayebwa, 2014). By utilizing this approach the first novel gene fusion to be identified was the gene for transcription factor PAX3 and nuclear receptor co-activator 1 (NCOA1), PAX3-NCOA1, in ARMS (Wachtel *et al.*, 2004). This method has made possible to detect the fusion of genes' occurring within the same chromosome band. For instance, gene fusion of the transmembrane protease serine 2 gene (TMPRSS2) and gene E26 oncogene homologue (ERG) resulting in the TMPRSS2-ERG fusion gene was discovered through this analysis (Tomlins *et al.*, 2005). Variation of this method involves utilization of expression data at exon level instead of the entire gene. The expression data for gene is taken either as mean expression levels of different exons of a gene or single exon individually. As a result of this modification, it is possible to find a hint of rearrangements of two parts based on the difference in the expression levels of the 5′- and 3′-parts of the affected gene. With the help of this method, several fusion genes have been identified in several cancers such as tenosynovial giant cell tumor, lung cancer and chondrosarcoma. In addition, this method has also been endeavored for different clinical and diagnostic purposes. However, this method can be applied for the analysis of known fusion genes only (West *et al.*, 2006; Rikova *et al.*, 2007; Soda *et al.*, 2007; Wang *et al.*, 2012a; Løvf *et al.*, 2011; Mertens and Tayebwa, 2014).

RT-PCR IN FUSION GENE DETECTION

Real-time or reverse transcription PCR (qRT-PCR) is a commonly used tool for the detection and quantification of mRNA samples. This technique has immense prospective for high-throughput advancements. With the help of continuous introduction of improved or novel chemistries, high-end equipment and better protocols, qRT-PCR is emerged as standard clinical diagnostic assay (Bustin *et al.*, 2005). RT-PCR being a very sensitive technique can detect even a single molecule of RNA and it makes diagnostics possible with even lower amounts of complex biological materials in comparison to traditional methods. Till date, ample reports are available where their contribution in cancer research has been documented (Deepak *et al.*, 2007). Many studies are also available where application of RT-PCR in detection of fusion genes in different cancers such as acute myloid leukemia, Ewing tumors (ET), alveolar rhabdomyosarcoma (ARMS), synovial sarcoma (SS), small round cell desmoplastic tumors (SRCDT), extraskeletal myxoid chondrosarcoma, malignant melanoma of soft parts, congenital fibrosarcoma, ALCL, non-small cell lung cancers (NSCLC) have been explored (Panagopoulos *et al.*, 2014, Van Dongen *et al.*, 1999, Peter *et al.*, 2001, Wang *et al.*, 2012b, Robesova *et al.*, 2014).

RECENT METHODS FOR THE IDENTIFICATION OF FUSION GENES

Though conventional methods of molecular and cytogenetic approaches have some limitations, their contribution in identification of fusion genes are enormous. In the recent period, the rapid advancement in present technologies like genome-wide high-throughput comprehensive profiling has further improved the detection of novel fusion genes. In addition, introduction of bioinformatics and computational approach has further improvised the existing technologies and endowed significantly in the promotion of this area of research.

TRANSCRIPTOME SEQUENCING

Transcriptome or RNA sequencing is a high-throughput assay for the characterization of RNA transcribed from genome and it has emerged as the prime technique for the detection of fusion genes. It offers the advantage of direct identification of chimeric transcripts which can have functional influence on the activity of fusion gene. As compared to DNA sequencing, RNA sequencing is less tedious and more efficient as most of the genomic regions are non-coding. Moreover, in contrast to hybridization-based approaches such as tilling microarrays, CGH and FISH, RNA-sequencing (RNA-seq) does not find its limitation to identification of known transcripts only. Additionally, the process of transcriptome-sequencing can predict the specific rearrangement site up to single-base resolution making it feasible to study complex chimeric transcriptomes. Also, RNA-seq has advantages of precise quantification of gene expression levels, reproducibility, and requirement of very less quantity of sample and it needs less operational cost. By using this method and its modifications such as paired-end sequencing, many oncogenic fusion genes have been discovered in different cancers like breast, lung, prostate and uterus carcinomas (Maher *et al.*, 2009a, 2009b; Wang *et al.*, 2009, 2013; Harbers and Carninci, 2005; Leow *et al.*, 2012; Campbell *et al.*, 2008; Stephens *et al.*, 2009; Ha *et al.*, 2011; Kim *et al.*, 2015).

NEXT GENERATION SEQUENCING

Fusion genes have been the major interest amid the mostly studied variations, due to their relations with tumorigenesis (Wang *et al.*, 2013; Arsenijevic and Daus-Dusenbery, 2016). The fusion gene is also known as a "*hybrid gene*" or a "*chimeric gene*". These are neoplasia-based mutations, which are occurring from structural chromosome mutations, such as chromosomal deletion, small insertions, single-base substitutions, inversion or translocation that juxtaposes two otherwise separated genes (Liu *et al.*, 2016; Kalyana-Sundaram *et al.*, 2012; Grossmann *et al.*, 2011; Wang *et al.*, 2015; Edwards *et al.*, 2010). As a consequence of accumulation of hereditary variations, cancer can also be the outcome of fusion gene, particularly the fusions related to transcription or kinases controllers (Shyr and Liv, 2013). Moreover, owing to their prevalence and common characteristics among various cancer types, fusion genes are always considered as a distinctive mutation (Wang *et al.*, 2015). Recently, it has been revealed that emergence of wide applications of NGS aided a lot in the study of fusions genes. NGS-based technologies for the detection of cancer cell genomes, such as RNA-seq or transcriptome sequencing and whole genome sequencing (WGS) have become extremely valuable tools to identify the mechanisms of tumorigenesis (Liu *et al.*, 2016; Rizzo and Buck, 2012; Urakami *et al.*, 2016; Mertens *et al.*, 2015). NGS stimulates nucleotide acquisition by sequencing 10–100 millions of sequence targets simultaneously and thus permits a low cost comprehensive genome-wide analysis. Indeed, gene fusions that are responsible for tumorigenesis may be emerging targets for identifying diagnostic markers and the development of new drugs (Urakami *et al.*, 2016). Moreover, NGS produces output in digital format, for instance, each transcript in transcriptome sequencing data appear as counts relative to the quantitative estimate of signals obtained from data of microarray gene expression. NGS being of digital nature allows the data to be of higher resolution which in turn increases the mutation analysis resolution level to the base-pair. Additionally, NGS supported different range of applications related to human genetic research (Qingguo *et al.*, 2012; Glenn *et al.*, 2011). Depending on the nature of input resources, the gross functions of NGS could be categorized into: WGS, whole RNA-seq and whole exome sequencing (WES). WGS is a powerful sequencing technology, which provides unbiased and comprehensive categorization of genomic variations in genomes, particularly in cancer genomes. However, WGS suffers the drawback of requirement of huge quantity of sequencing and extensive analysis through computational methods. Moreover, it has been observed that the cost of NGS has decreased significantly, but is yet costly in comparison to RNA-seq (Qingguo *et al.*, 2012; Desai *et al.*, 2012). Apart from WGS and RNA-seq, NGS also has the features of targeted sequencing. The RNA-seq approach in addition to quantification of gene expression profiles can also detect RNA editing, fusion transcripts, and alternative splicing. Additionally, DNA methylation alterations, epigenetic alterations and histone modifications can be analyzed with the help of new sequencing techniques such as ChIP-seq and Bisulfite-seq. These NGS techniques in combination can enable a high-resolution as well as cancer genome's global view (Shyr and Liv, 2013). In the present days, the sequencing expenditure has significantly reduced due to the fast advancement in the NGS technologies which avail centers and core facilities in the institutes to sequence the human genomes quite regularly. The process of software development has also attained pace due to recent advances in sequencing approaches. Numerous novel software have been rapidly materialized which can detect structural variants (SVs). The gene fusions can result from various SVs like insertions, inversions, deletions and translocations (Qingguo *et al.*, 2012). Fusion genes and NGS-based studies are used presently to improve the understanding towards molecular understanding of cancers, to recognize new genetic variations responsible for tumorigenesis, cancer origins, progression and metastasis and to analyze tumor complexity and heterogeneity. These contributions have resulted in great success for different cancers including ovarian cancer, breast cancer, colorectal cancer, liver cancer, lung cancer, kidney cancer, head and neck cancer, acute myeloid leukemia, melanoma (Shyr and Liv, 2013). In the recent years, a variety of fusion genes have been predicted as vital prognostic markers or key therapeutic targets in anti-cancer therapy and treatment. For example, a new urine test was developed which could indicate the risk of prostate cancer by the detection of TMPRSS2-ERG (Tomlins *et al.*, 2011). NGS has provided great success to the researchers to identify different mutations in cancer; it has been applied to numerous clinical areas such as prenatal diagnostics, genetic mutations and pathogen detection, etc. (Desai *et al.*, 2012). Although genetic alterations have been identified with PCR, microarrays and Sanger sequencing, clinically, these techniques have certain limitations which NGS is devoid of. Hence, NGS approaches serve as excellent prognostic and diagnostic techniques and help the clinicians to recognize specific characteristics in patients which generate a new path towards personalized medicine (Shyr and Liu, 2013).

CHROMOGENIC *IN SITU* HYBRIDIZATION (CISH)

Chromogenic *in situ* hybridization (CISH) is a practical, cost-effective and promising alternative to FISH for analyzing gene alteration (Madrid and Lo, 2004). This technique may overcome the limitations of FISH because of their ability to quantify the signals acquired from conventional bright field light microscopy. Also, CISH is a completely automated bright field ISH assay and implements steady and lasting archival slides that can be analyzed through conventional bright field light microscopy (Nitta *et al.*, 2010; Bartlett *et al.*, 2009; Penault-Llorca *et al.*, 2009; Kim *et al.*, 2011). In addition, CISH has an edge over RT-PCR as DNA is found to be more stable than mRNA in sample tissues and it allows identification of fusion genes to single-cells resolution. Moreover, CISH is well suited for formalin-fixed paraffin-embedded tissue samples which otherwise has trouble if evaluated through RT-PCR (Leow *et al.*, 2012). CISH is quite similar to FISH which uses specific probes against corresponding nucleic acid in the tissue samples. It implements peroxidase enzyme-labeled probes as a replacement for fluorescent-labeled probes that permit simultaneous chromogenic visualization of both chromosomal aberrations and tissue histological characteristics of a specimen by bright-field microscope (Leow *et al.*, 2012). In an evaluation of the ALK gene rearrangement between FISH and CISH methods, it has shown great similarity and ALK FISH–CISH status was associated with ALK protein expression in lung cancer (Kim *et al.*, 2011). Similarly, CISH is taken as a reliable assay for the identification of ALK rearrangements in adenocarcinomas of the lung (Schildhaus *et al.*, 2013). In a modified CISH, use of combined dual-color chromogenic and silver *in situ* hybridization has significantly improved the identification of ERG gene rearrangement in prostate cancer (Braun *et al.*, 2012). However, bright-field ISH methods are quite new and have not yet been generally recognized in pathology/research laboratories. CISH is certainly one of the most powerful tools for the identification in addition to diagnosis of pathological gene rearrangements present in cancers (Leow *et al.*, 2012).

COMPUTATIONAL AND BIOINFORMATICS APPROACHES

Computational biology and bioinformatics have become an essential discipline of modern biological science. Generally, in computational biology, genes are identified, translated and compared within the databases, protein functions are predicted and sequences are aligned into families of similar proteins and assign their functional roles (Tsoka and Ouzounis, 2000). In the recent period, different computational approaches have been developed to detect fusion by taking advantage of the significant throughput of the new RNA-seq technologies (Ozsolak and Milos, 2011). There are different computational tools such as Bellerophontes, ChimeraScan, deFuse, FusionFinder, FusionHunter, FusionMap, MapSplice and TopHat-fusion, etc. which are used for chimeras detection (Abate *et al.*, 2012; Iyer *et al.*, 2011; McPherson *et al.*, 2011; Francis *et al.*, 2012; Li *et al.*, 2011; Ge *et al.*, 2011; Wang *et al.*, 2010; Kim and Salzberg, 2011; Carrara *et al.*, 2013). The techniques can be clumped into several subtypes depending on the chosen alignment strategies. According to Carrara and co-workers, these tools can be classified into whole paired-end, paired-end + fragmentation and direct fragmentation groups. In case of whole paired-end method, tools align the full-length paired-end reads based on reference and utilize discordant alignments for producing a set of putative fusion events that are ultimately elected by means of numerous supplementary pieces of information or filtering steps. In case of paired-end + fragmentation approach, the putative fusion events are obtained in two steps. Initially, the full-length paired-end reads are aligned on a reference, and the discordant alignments are utilized for the generation of new pseudoreference which comprises identified putative fusion events. This step is followed by fragmentation of the unaligned reads and realignment on the pseudoreference to recognize junction-spanning reads. Only the putative fusion events related to junction-spanning reads are preferred as input for filtration step. For direct fragmentation, direct exploitation of paired-end information is not required; instead, they fragment every read prior to the first alignment and identify fusion candidates aligning those fragments to a genomic reference (Carrara *et al.*, 2013). The main drawback of computational approach is the generation of false positive results which contaminate the outcome and present a prime challenge in validation (Beccuti *et al.*, 2013). Moreover, the computational gene fusion literature is discrete. For instance, many fusion landscape studies use negligible reference to bioinformatics surveys of gene fusion molecular biology, which otherwise could help in the elucidation of the function of novel fusions and order them in the context of other identified oncogenic fusions. Similarly, an elevated level of attentiveness of fusion prioritization algorithms can help the investigators in narrowing down putative fusion lists to only the occurrences that have possibility to be biologically functional (Latysheva and Babu, 2016).

CONCLUSION

Fusion genes function primarily in tumor growth of several types of cancer and thus are potential pathological tool for the diagnosis, staging, classification, prognosis and treatment of cancer. Conventionally, identifying fusion genes have been a tedious job based on FISH to sense chromosomal alterations. Moreover, identification of gene fusions in solid tumors is technically challenging. However, recent advancements obtained in genomics from NGS along with numerous emerging fields of bioinformatics and molecular tools have deciphered several novel oncogenic gene fusions in solid tumors which formerly were unrecognizable by conventional methods of cytogenetics. Also, transcriptome sequencing which is a high-throughput method of characterizing RNA transcribed from the genome is rapidly developing as a novel approach in the identification of fusion genes. Nevertheless, several challenges still persist in the detection of novel fusion genes for the diagnosis and prognosis of cancers.

CONFLICT OF INTEREST

The authors express no conflict of interest.

REFERENCES

Abate, F., A. Acquaviva, G. Paciello, C. Foti, E. Ficarra, A. Ferrarini, M. Delledonne, I. Iacobucci, S. Soverini, G. Martinelli, and E. Macii, Bellerophontes: an RNA-seq data analysis framework for chimeric transcripts discovery based on accurate fusion model, *Bioinformatics* **28**(16): 2114–2121 (2012).

Arsenijevic, V. and B.N. Davis-Dusenbery, Reproducible, scalable fusion gene detection from RNA-seq, *Cancer Gene Profiling: Methods and Protocols* **2016**: 223–237 (2016).

Aurias, A., C. Rimbaut, D. Buffe, J. Dubousset, and A. Mazabraud, Chromosomal translocations in Ewing's sarcoma, *N Engl J Med* **309**: 496–497 (1983).

Bartlett, J.M., F.M. Campbell, M. Ibrahim, P. Wencyk, I. Ellis, E. Kay, Y. Connolly, A. O'Grady, S. Di Palma, J. Starczynski, and J.M. Morgan, Chromogenic *in situ* hybridization, *Am J Clin Pathol* **132**(4): 514–520 (2009).

Beccuti, M., M. Carrara, F. Cordero, S. Donatelli, and R.A. Calogero, The structure of state-of-art gene fusion-finder algorithms, *Genome Bioinformatics* **1**: 1(2) (2013).

Bickmore, W.A., Karyotype analysis and chromosome banding. eLS (2001).

Braun, M., J. Stomper, D. Boehm, W. Vogel, V.J. Scheble, N. Wernert, Z. Shaikhibrahim, F. Fend, G. Kristiansen, and S. Perner, Improved method of detecting the ERG gene rearrangement in prostate cancer using combined dual-color chromogenic and silver *in situ* hybridization, *The Journal of Molecular Diagnostics* **14**(4): 322–327 (2012).

Bustin, S.A. and R. Mueller, Real-time reverse transcription PCR (qRT-PCR) and its potential use in clinical diagnosis, *Clin Sci* **109**(4): 365–379 (2005).

Campbell, P.J., P.J. Stephens, E.D. Pleasance, S. O'Meara, H. Li, T. Santarius, L.A. Stebbings, C. Leroy, S. Edkins, C. Hardy, and J.W. Teague, Identification of somatically acquired rearrangements in cancer using genome-wide massively parallel paired-end sequencing, *Nat Genet* **40**(6): 722–729 (2008).

Cancer Genome Atlas Research Network. Comprehensive genomic characterization of squamous cell lung cancers, *Nature* **489**(7417): 519–525 (2012).

Cancer Genome Atlas Research Network. Integrated genomic characterization of endometrial carcinoma, *Nature* **497**(7447): 67–73 (2013).

Carrara, M., M. Beccuti, F. Lazzarato, F. Cavallo, F. Cordero, S. Donatelli, and RA. Calogero, State-of-the-art fusion-finder algorithms sensitivity and specificity, *BioMed Research International* (2013).

Das, K. and P. Tan, Molecular cytogenetics: recent developments and applications in cancer, *Clin Genet* **84**(4): 315–325 (2013).

de Jong, B., I.M. Molenaar, J.A. Leeuw, V.J. Idenberg, and J.W. Oosterhuis, Cytogenetics of a renal adenocarcinoma in a 2-year-old child, *Can Genet Cytogenet* **21**(2): 165–169 (1986).

Deepak, S., K. Kottapalli, R. Rakwal *et al.*, Real-Time PCR: revolutionizing detection and expression analysis of genes. *Curr Genom* **8**(4): 234–251 (2007).

Desai, A.N. and A. Jere, Next generation sequencing: ready for the clinics? *Clin Genet* **81**(6): 503–510.

Edwards, P.A., Fusion genes and chromosome translocations in the common epithelial cancers, *The J Pathol* **220**(2): 244–254 (2012).

Francis, R.W., K. Thompson-Wicking, K.W. Carter, D. Anderson, U.R. Kees, and A.H. Beesley, FusionFinder: a software tool to identify expressed gene fusion candidates from RNA-Seq data, *PloS One* **7**(6): e39987 (2012).

Francke, U., Digitized and differentially shaded human chromosome ideograms for genomic applications, *Cytogenet Cell Genet* **65**(3): 206–218 (1994).

Fukuhara, S., J.D. Rowley, D. Variakojis, and H.M. Golomb, Chromosome abnormalities in poorly differentiated lymphocytic lymphoma, *Cancer Res* **39**(8): 3119–3128 (1979).

Ge, H., K. Liu, T. Juan, F. Fang, M. Newman, and W. Hoeck, FusionMap: detecting fusion genes from next-generation sequencing data at base-pair resolution. *Bioinformatics* **27**(14): 1922–1928 (2011).

Gisselsson, D., Cytogenetic methods, In S. Heim and F. Mitelman (eds.) *Cancer cytogenetics*, 3rd edition. Hoboken, NJ: Wiley-Blackwell (2009), pp. 9–16.

Glenn, T.C., Field guide to next-generation DNA sequencers, *Mol Ecol Resour* **11**(5): 759–769 (2011).

Grossmann, V., A. Kohlmann, H.U. Klein, S. Schindela, S. Schnittger, F. Dicker, M. Dugas, W. Kern, T. Haferlach, and C. Haferlach, Targeted next-generation sequencing detects point mutations, insertions, deletions and balanced chromosomal rearrangements as well as identifies novel leukemia-specific fusion genes in a single procedure, *Leukemia* **25**(4): 671–680 (2011).

Ha, K.C., E. Lalonde, L. Li, L. Cavallone, R. Natrajan, M.B. Lambros, C. Mitsopoulos, J. Hakas, I. Kozarewa, K. Fenwick, and C.J. Lord, Identification of gene fusion transcripts by transcriptome sequencing in BRCA1-mutated breast cancers and cell lines, *BMC Med Genom* **4**(1): 1 (2011).

Hanahan, D. and R.A. Weinberg, The hallmarks of cancer, *Cell* **100**(1): 57–70 (2000).

Harbers M. and P. Carninci, Tag-based approaches for transcriptome research and genome annotation, *Nat Meth* **2**(7): 495–502 (2005).

Harsha, H.C. and A. Pandey, Phosphoproteomics in cancer, *Molecular Oncol* **4**(6): 482–495 (2010).

Heim, S., N. Mandahl, U. Kristoffersson, F. Mitelman, B. Rööser, A. Rydholm, and H. Willén, Reciprocal translocation t (3; 12)(q27; q13) in lipoma, *Canc Genet Cytogenet* **23**(4): 301–304 (1986).

Iyer, M.K., A.M. Chinnaiyan, and C.A. Maher, ChimeraScan: a tool for identifying chimeric transcription in sequencing data, *Bioinformatics* **27**(20): 2903–2904 (2011).

Kalyana-Sundaram, S., S. Shankar, S. DeRoo, M.K. Iyer, N. Palanisamy, A.M. Chinnaiyan, and C. Kumar-Sinha, Gene fusions associated with recurrent amplicons represent a class of passenger aberrations in breast cancer *Neoplasia* **14**(8): 702–IN13 (2012).

Kaye, F.J., Mutation-associated fusion cancer genes in solid tumors, *Mol Cancer Ther* **8**(6): 1399–1408 (2009).

Kim, D. and S.L. Salzberg, TopHat-Fusion: an algorithm for discovery of novel fusion transcripts, *Genome Biol* **12**(8): 1 (2011).

Kim, H., S.B. Yoo, J.Y. Choe, J.H. Paik, X. Xu, H. Nitta, W. Zhang, T.M. Grogan, C.T. Lee, S. Jheon, and J.H. Chung, Detection of ALK gene rearrangement in non-small cell lung cancer: a comparison of fluorescence *in situ* hybridization and chromogenic *in situ* hybridization with correlation of ALK protein expression, *J Thorac Oncol* **6**(8): 1359–1366 (2011).

Kim, J., S. Kim, S. Ko, Y.H. In, H.G. Moon, S.K. Ahn, M.K. Kim, M. Lee, J.H. Hwang, Y.S. Ju, and J.I. Kim, Recurrent fusion transcripts detected by whole-transcriptome sequencing of 120 primary breast cancer samples, *Gene Chromosome Canc* **54**(11): 681–691 (2015).

Langer-Safer, P.R., M. Levine, and D.C. Ward, Immunological method for mapping genes on Drosophila polytene chromosomes, *Proc Nat Acad Sci* **79**(14): 4381–4385 (1982).

Latysheva, N.S. and M.M. Babu, Discovering and understanding oncogenic gene fusions through data intensive computational approaches, *Nucleic Acids Res* 21: gkw282 (2016).

Leow, P.C., C.S. Ku, R. Soo, and R. Soong, Technological advances in the detection of novel fusion genes. eLS (2012).

Li, Y., J. Chien, D.I. Smith, and J. Ma, FusionHunter: identifying fusion transcripts in cancer using paired-end RNA-seq, *Bioinformatics* **27**(12): 1708–1710 (2011).

Liu, J., L. Weng, Y. Ming, B. Yin, S. Liu, N. Wu, and Z. Wu, Fusion genes and their detection through next generation sequencing in malignant hematological disease and solid tumors, *Diagnostic Pathology: Open Access* (2016).

Løvf, M., G.O. Thomassen, A.C. Bakken, R. Celestino, T. Fioretos, G.E. Lind, R.A. Lothe, and R.I. Skotheim, Fusion gene microarray reveals cancer type-specificity among fusion genes, *Gene Chromosome Canc* **50**(5): 348–357 (2011).

Madrid, M.A. and R.W. Lo, Chromogenic *in situ* hybridization (CISH): a novel alternative in screening archival breast cancer tissue samples for HER-2/neu status, *Breast Canc Res* **6**(5): 1 (2004).

Maher, C.A., C. Kumar-Sinha, X. Cao, S. Kalyana-Sundaram, B. Han, X. Jing, L. Sam, T. Barrette, N. Palanisamy, and A.M. Chinnaiyan, Transcriptome sequencing to detect gene fusions in cancer, *Nature* **458**(7234): 97–101 (2009a).

Maher, C.A., N. Palanisamy, J.C. Brenner, X. Cao, S. Kalyana-Sundaram, S. Luo, I. Khrebtukova, T.R. Barrette, C. Grasso, J. Yu, and R.J. Lonigro, Chimeric transcript discovery by paired-end transcriptome sequencing, *Proc Nat Acad Sci* **106**(30): 12353–12358 (2009b).

Mark, J., R. Dahlenfors, C. Ekedahl, and G. Stenman, The mixed salivary gland tumor — a normally benign human neoplasm frequently showing specific chromosomal abnormalities, *Canc Genet Cytogenet* **2**(3): 231–241 (1980).

McPherson, A., F. Hormozdiari, A. Zayed, R. Giuliany, G. Ha, M.G. Sun, M. Griffith, A.H. Moussavi, J. Senz, N. Melnyk, and M. Pacheco, deFuse: an algorithm for gene fusion discovery in tumor RNA-Seq data, *PLoS Comput Biol* **7**(5): e1001138 (2011).

Mertens, F., B. Johansson, T. Fioretos, and F. Mitelman, The emerging complexity of gene fusions in cancer, *Nat Rev Canc* **15**(6): 371–381 (2015).

Mertens, F and J. Tayebwa, Evolving techniques for gene fusion detection in soft tissue tumours, *Histopathology* **64**(1): 151–162 (2014).

Mitelman, F., B. Johansson, and F. Mertens, The impact of translocations and gene fusions on cancer causation, *Nat Rev Canc* **7**(4): 233–245 (2007).

Nitta, H., W. Zhang, B.D. Kelly, M. Miller, L. Pestic-Dragovich, C. Bieniarz, T.J. Vasicek, T. Marafioti, L. Rimsza, and T.M. Grogan, Automated bright-field break-apart *in situ* hybridization (ba-ISH) application: ALK and MALT1 genes as models, *Methods* **52**(4): 352–358 (2010).

Ohno, S., M. Babonits, F. Wiener, J. Spira, G. Klein, and M. Potter, Nonrandom chromosome changes involving the Ig gene-carrying chromosomes 12 and 6 in pristane-induced mouse plasmacytomas, *Cell* **18**(4): 1001–1007 (1979).

Ozsolak, F. and P.M. Milos, RNA sequencing: advances, challenges and opportunities, *Nat Rev Genet* **12**(2): 87–98 (2011).

Panagopoulos, I., S. Torkildsen, L. Gorunova, A. Tierens, G.E. Tjønnfjord, and S. Heim, Comparison between Karyotyping-FISH-reverse transcription PCR and RNA-sequencing-fusion gene identification programs in the detection of *KAT6A-CREBBP* in acute myeloid leukemia, F. Bertolini, ed., *PLoS ONE* **9**(5): e96570 (2014).

Penault-Llorca, F., M. Bilous, M. Dowsett, W. Hanna, R.Y. Osamura, J. Rüschoff, and M. van de Vijver, Emerging technologies for assessing HER2 amplification, *Am J Clin Pathol* **132**(4): 539–548 (2009).

Peter, M., E. Gilbert, and O. Delattre, A multiplex real-time PCR assay for the detection of gene fusions observed in solid tumors, *Lab Investig* **81**(6): 905–912 (2001).

Pinkel, D. and D.G. Albertson, Array comparative genomic hybridization and its applications in cancer, *Nat Genet* **37**: S11–S17 (2005).

Rikova, K., A. Guo, Q. Zeng, A. Possemato, J. Yu, H. Haack, J. Nardone, K. Lee, C. Reeves, Y. Li, and Y. Hu, Global survey of phosphotyrosine signaling identifies oncogenic kinases in lung cancer, *Cell* **131**(6): 1190–1203 (2007).

Rizzo, J.M. and M.J. Buck, Key principles and clinical applications of "next-generation" DNA sequencing *Can Prev Res* **5**(7): 887–900 (2012).

Robesova, B., M. Bajerova, K. Liskova, J. Skrickova, M. Tomiskova, S. Pospisilova, J. Mayer, and D. Dvorakova, TaqMan based real time PCR assay targeting EML4-ALK fusion transcripts in NSCLC, *Lung Canc* **85** (1): 25–30 (2014).

Rowley, J.D., Identificaton of a translocation with quinacrine fluorescence in a patient with acute leukemia, *Ann Genet* **16**(2): 109–112 (1973a).

Rowley, J.D., Letter: A new consistent chromosomal abnormality in chronic myelogenous leukaemia identified by quinacrine fluorescence and Giemsa staining, *Nature* **243**(5405): 290–293 (1973b).

Schildhaus, H.U., K.F. Deml, K. Schmitz, M. Meiboom, E. Binot, S. Hauke, S. Merkelbach-Bruse, and R. Büttner, Chromogenic *in situ* hybridization is a reliable assay for detection of ALK rearrangements in adenocarcinomas of the lung. *Mod Pathol* **26**(11): 1468–1477 (2013).

Schrock, E.D., S. Du, Manoir, T. Veldman, and B. Schoell, Multicolor spectral karotyping of human chromosomes, *Science* **273**(5274): 494 (1996).

Seidal, T., J. Mark, B. Hagmar, and L. Angervall, Alveolar rhabdomyosarcoma: a cytogenetic and correlated cytological and histological study, *Acta Pathol Microbiol Immunol Scand A* **90**(5): 345–354 (1982).

Shyr, D. and Q. Liu, Next generation sequencing in cancer research and clinical application, *Biological Procedures Online* **15**(1): 1 (2013).

Sinclair, P.B., E.P. Nacheva, M. Leversha, N. Telford, J. Chang, A. Reid, A. Bench, K. Champion, B. Huntly, and A.R. Green, Large deletions at the t(9; 22) breakpoint are common and may identify a poor-prognosis subgroup of patients with chronic myeloid leukemia, *Blood* **95**(3): 738–743 (2000).

Soda, M., Y.L. Choi, M. Enomoto, S. Takada, Y. Yamashita, S. Ishikawa, S.I. Fujiwara, H. Watanabe, K. Kurashina, H. Hatanaka, and M. Bando, Identification of the transforming EML4–ALK fusion gene in non-small-cell lung cancer, *Nature* **448**(7153): 561–566 (2007).

Speicher, M.R., S.G. Ballard, and D.C. Ward, Karyotyping human chromosomes by combinatorial multi-fluor FISH, *Nat Genet* **12**(4): 368–375.

Stenman, G., J. Sandros, R. Dahlenfors, M. Juberg-Ode, and J. Mark, 6q-and loss of the Y chromosome — two common deviations in malignant human salivary gland tumors, *Can Genet Cytogenet* **22**(4): 283–293 (1986).

Stephens, P.J., D.J. McBride, M.L. Lin, I. Varela, E.D. Pleasance, J.T. Simpson, L.A. Stebbings, C. Leroy, S. Edkins, L.J. Mudie, and C.D. Greenman, Complex landscapes of somatic rearrangement in human breast cancer genomes, *Nature* **462**(7276): 1005–1010 (2009).

Supper, J., C. Gugenmus, J. Wollnik, T. Drueke, M. Scherf, A. Hahn, K. Grote, N. Bretschneider, B. Klocke, C. Zinser, K. Cartharius, and M. Seifert, Detecting and visualizing gene fusions, *Methods* **59**(1): S24–S28 (2013).

Tanke, H.J., J. Wiegant, Van R.P. Gijlswijk, V. Bezrookove, H. Pattenier, R.J. Heetebrij, E.G. Talman, A.K. Raap, and J. Vrolijk, New strategy for multi-colour fluorescence *in situ* hybridisation: COBRA: COmbined Binary RAtio labelling, *Eur J Hum Genet* **7**(1): 2–11 (1999).

Tomlins, S.A., S.M. Aubin, J. Siddiqui, R.J. Lonigro, Sefton-L. Miller, S. Miick, S. Williamsen, P. Hodge, J. Meinke, A. Blase, and Y. Penabella, Urine TMPRSS2: ERG fusion transcript stratifies prostate cancer risk in men with elevated serum PSA, *Sci Transl Med* **3**(94): 94ra72 (2011).

Tomlins, S.A., D.R. Rhodes, S. Perner, S.M. Dhanasekaran, R. Mehra, X.W. Sun, S. Varambally, X. Cao, J. Tchinda, R. Kuefer, and C. Lee, Recurrent fusion of TMPRSS2 and ETS transcription factor genes in prostate cancer, *Science* **310**(5748): 644–648 (2005).

Tsoka, S. and C.A. Ouzounis, Recent developments and future directions in computational genomics, *FEBS Lett* **480**(1): 42–48 (2000).

Turc-Carel, C., Dal P. Cin, U. Rao, C. Karakousis, and A.A. Sandberg, Cytogenetic studies of adipose tissue tumors. I. A benign lipoma with reciprocal translocation t(3; 12)(q28; q14), *Canc Genet Cytogenet* **23**(4): 283–289 (1986).

Turc-Carel, C, I. Philip, M.P. Berger, T. Philip and G.M. Lenoir, Chromosomal translocations in Ewing's sarcoma, *N Engl J Med* **309**: 497–498 (1983).

Urakami, K., Y. Shimoda, K. Ohshima, T. Nagashima, M. Serizawa, T. Tanabe, J. Saito, T. Usui, Y. Watanabe, A. Naruoka, and S. Ohnami, Next generation sequencing approach for detecting 491 fusion genes from human cancer, *Biomed Res* **37**(1): 51–62 (2016).

Van Dongen, J.J., E.A. Macintyre, J.A. Gabert, E. Delabesse, V. Rossi, G. Saglio, E. Gottardi, A. Rambaldi, G. Dotti, F. Griesinger, and A. Parreira, Standardized RT-PCR analysis of fusion gene transcripts from chromosome aberrations in acute leukemia for detection of minimal residual disease Report of the BIOMED-I Concerted Action: Investigation of minimal residual disease in acute leukemia, *Leukemia* **13**: 1901–1928 (1999).

Wachtel, M., M. Dettling, E. Koscielniak, S. Stegmaier, J. Treuner, K. Simon-Klingenstein, P. Bühlmann, F.K. Niggli, and B.W. Schäfer, Gene expression signatures identify rhabdomyosarcoma subtypes and detect a novel t (2; 2) (q35; p23) translocation fusing PAX3 to NCOA1, *Can Res* **64**(16): 5539–5545 (2004).

Walters, D.K., T. Mercher, T.L. Gu, O'T. Hare, J.W. Tyner, M. Loriaux, V.L. Goss, K.A. Lee, C.A. Eide, M.J. Wong, and E.P. Stoffregen, Activating alleles of JAK3 in acute megakaryoblastic leukemia, *Canc Cell* **10**(1): 65–75 (2006).

Wang, K., D. Singh, Z. Zeng, S.J. Coleman, Y. Huang, G.L. Savich, X. He, P. Mieczkowski, S.A. Grimm, C.M. Perou, and MacLeod J.N., MapSplice: accurate mapping of RNA-seq reads for splice junction discovery, *Nucleic Acids Res* **38**(18): e178 (2010).

Wang, R., Y. Pan, C. Li, H. Hu, Y. Zhang, H. Li, X. Luo, J. Zhang, Z. Fang, Y. Li, and L. Shen, The use of quantitative real-time reverse transcriptase PCR for 5′ and 3′ portions of ALK transcripts to detect ALK rearrangements in lung cancers, *Clin Canc Res* **18**(17): 4725–4732 (2012b).

Wang, L., T. Motoi, R. Khanin, A. Olshen, F. Mertens, J. Bridge, P.D. Cin, C.R. Antonescu, S. Singer, M. Hameed, and J.V. Bovee, Identification of a novel, recurrent HEY1-NCOA2 fusion in mesenchymal chondrosarcoma based on a genome-wide screen of exon-level expression data, *Gene Chromosome Canc* **51**(2): 127–139 (2012a).

Wang, Q., J. Xia, P. Jia, W. Pao, and Z. Zhao, Application of next generation sequencing to human gene fusion detection: computational tools, features and perspectives, *Briefings Bioinform* **14**(4): 506–519 (2013).

Wang, Y, N. Wu, J. Liu, Z. Wu, and D. Dong, FusionCancer: a database of cancer fusion genes derived from RNA-seq data, *Diagn Pathol* **10**(1): 1 (2015).

Wang, Z., M. Gerstein, and Snyder M., RNA-seq: a revolutionary tool for transcriptomics, *Nat Rev Genet* **10**(1): 57–63 (2009).

Watson, I.R., K. Takahashi, P.A. Futreal, and L. Chin, Emerging patterns of somatic mutations in cancer, *Nat Rev Genet* **14**(10): 703–718 (2013).

West, R.B., B.P. Rubin, M.A. Miller, S. Subramanian, G. Kaygusuz, K. Montgomery, S. Zhu, R.J. Marinelli, De A. Luca, Downs-E. Kelly, and J.R. Goldblum, A landscape effect in tenosynovial giant-cell tumor from activation of CSF1 expression by a translocation in a minority of tumor cells, *Proc Nat Acad Sci USA*, **103**(3): 690–695 (2006).

4

The Receptor Tyrosine Kinase ALK — Its Fusion Partners and Their Implication in Various Cancers

*Ganesan Padmavathi, Krishan Kumar Thakur, Anand Anip, Devivasha Bordoloi and Ajaikumar B. Kunnumakkara**

INTRODUCTION

Anaplastic lymphoma kinase (ALK), an important receptor tyrosine kinase (RTK) protein belonging to the insulin receptor superfamily, is known to be frequently modified through point mutations and chromosomal rearrangements and is involved in variety of cancers including both solid and hematologic malignancies (Crescenzo *et al.*, 2015; Mossé, 2016; Mano, 2012). In general, a strong expression of ALK was observed in neuronal

*Author for correspondence: Cancer Biology Laboratory, Department of Biosciences and Bioengineering, Indian Institute of Technology Guwahati, Assam 781039, India. kunnumakkara@iitg.ernet.in

tissues signifying a possible role in the development of central and peripheral nervous tissues during the foetal development and no expression was found in other normal tissues (Mossé, 2016; Crescenzo *et al.*, 2015; Mariño-Enríquez *et al.*, 2013). Despite the fact that the exact role of ALK is ambiguous, identification of t(2;5) involving ALK gene in ALCL was a paradigm for further discoveries in the role of ALK rearrangements in cancer development and management (Mossé, 2016; Crescenzo *et al.*, 2015; Mano, 2012). Since the discovery of nucleophosmin (NPM)-ALK, more than 20 ALK fusion partners have been identified in various cancers and numerous preclinical and clinical studies have been carried out to identify potent ALK inhibitors for the treatment of such cancers (Crescenzo *et al.*, 2015). The partner genes of ALK fusions detected in various cancers (such as acute myelomonocytic leukemia (AML), ALCL, colorectal carcinomas (CRC), IMTs of different origin, large B-cell lymphomas, lung cancers, renal cell carcinoma and thyroid carcinomas) include ATIC, C2orf44, CAD, CARS, CLTC, DCTN1, EML4, FN1, HIP1, KIF5B, KLC1, MSN, MYH9, NPM, PPFIBP1, RANB2, SEC31A, SQSTM1, STRN, TFG, TPM3/4, TRAF1, TRP, VCL, etc. (Figure 4.1). All the translocations were found to be resulting in the constitutive activation of kinase domain of ALK thus mediating tumorigenesis. Moreover, it has been proved that ALK fusion kinases exert oncogenic property mainly through the deregulation of

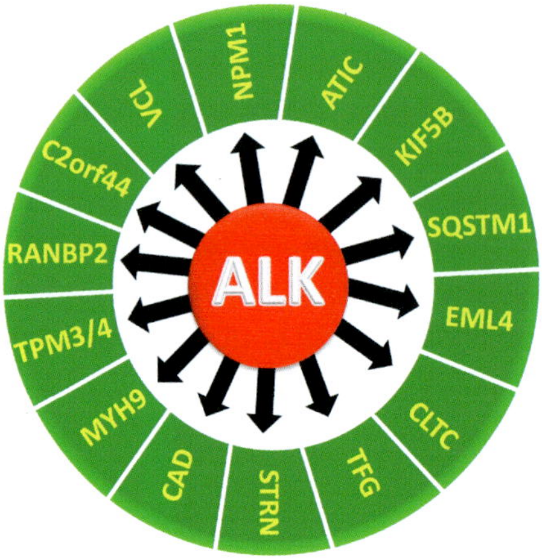

Figure 4.1: Different fusion partners of ALK.

PI3K-Akt, STAT3 and JNK-cJun, MEK-ERK signaling pathways and tyrosine kinase inhibitors were found as potent antagonists of these chimeric proteins (Mariño-Enríquez *et al.*, 2013; Leventaki *et al.*, 2007; Wasik *et al.*, 2009). Therefore, this chapter deals with the rearrangements of ALK gene and its downstream targets in the initiation and progression of tumors.

NPM1-ALK

Rearrangement of chromosomes 5 and 2 t(2;5)(p23;q35) results in the formation of NPM-ALK fusion gene involving amino-terminal (117 amino acid residues) of NPM and cytoplasmic portion of ALK was the first identified translocation of ALK gene (Figure 4.2) (Morris *et al.*, 1994; Takahashi *et al.*, 2008; Bischof *et al.*, 1997). Also, it is regarded as a signature translocation of CD30+ ALCL and is present in 44% of T cell ALCL, 45% of null cell ALCL, 8% of B cell ALCL and produces a hyperphosphorylated, constitutively active, 80 kD chimeric RTK (Shiota *et al.*, 1995; Drexler *et al.*, 2000; Van Roosbroeck *et al.*, 2010; Feldman *et al.*, 2013; Damm-Welk *et al.*, 2009). However, it was not the primary molecular event in the development of extranodal ALCL and Hodgkin's disease and moreover, NPM-ALK fusion transcripts had been detected in peripheral blood cells of healthy individuals supporting the hypothesis that chromosomal rearrangements as a single molecular alteration may not be adequate for the development of malignant diseases (Ott *et al.*, 1998; Weiss *et al.*, 1995; Weber-Matthiesen *et al.*, 1996; Trümper *et al.*, 1998). Subsequently, it has been found that NPM segment-mediated oligomerization induced tyrosine kinase activity and interaction of NPM-ALK with growth factor receptor bound protein 2 (GRB2) which regulated the NPM-ALK-mediated phosphorylation of Src homology-2 domain-containing phosphatase 2 (SHP-2) were associated with the malignant transformation (Figure 4.3) (Fujimoto *et al.*, 1996; Bischof *et al.*, 1997; Riera *et al.*, 2010).

In addition, it has been proved that ectopic expression of NPM-ALK in rat 1a fibroblasts promoted anchorage-independent growth in soft agar; induced cell proliferation through increased G0/G1 to S-phase transition; and elevated the expression of various genes involved in cell proliferation

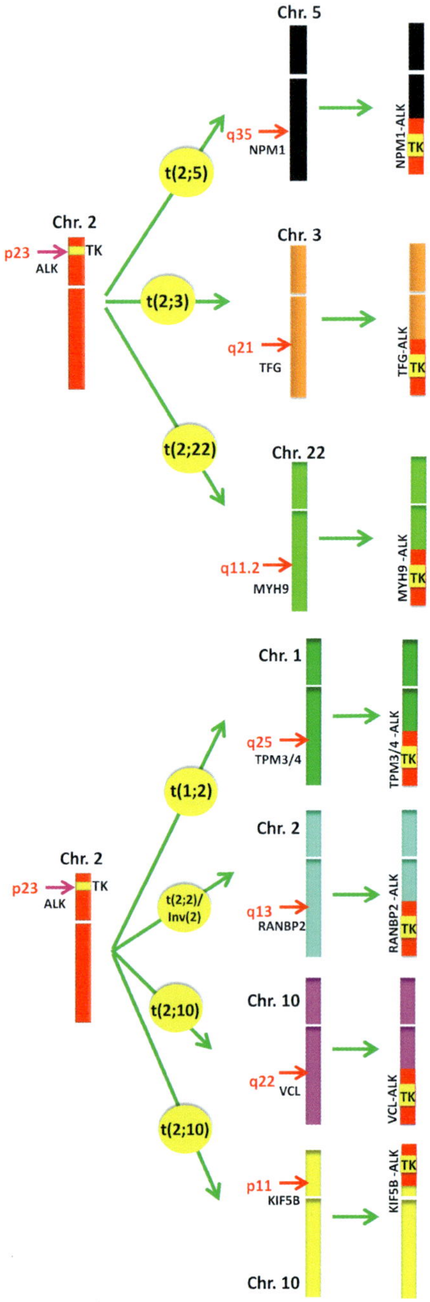

Figure 4.2: Schematic representation of ALK gene rearrangement with partner genes.

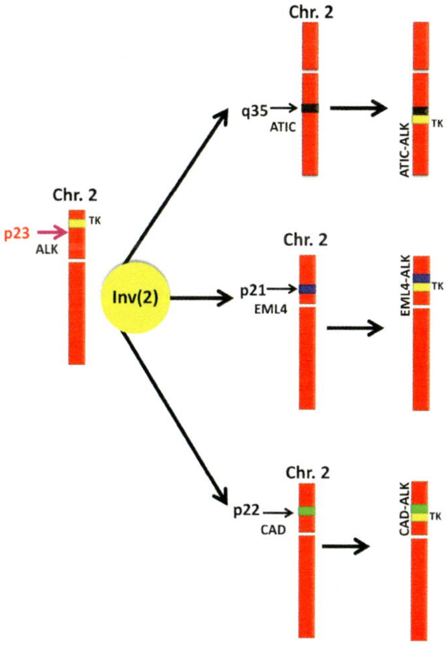

Figure 4.2: *(Continued)*

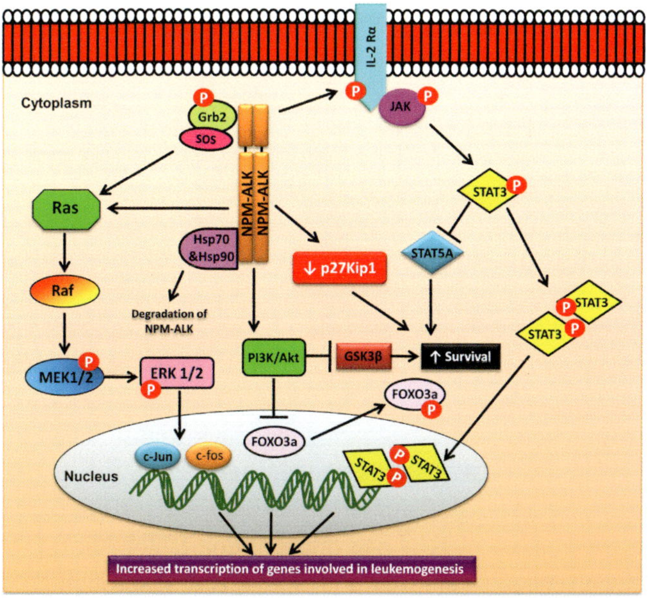

Figure 4.3: NPM-ALK fusion induced leukemogenesis and associated molecular targets.

like cyclin A, cyclin D1, fos, jun, and c-myc (Wellmann *et al.*, 1997). Apart from this, another cell cycle regulator protein CDC25A was also observed to be deregulated by this oncoprotein thereby mediating cell proliferation (Fernandez-Vidal *et al.*, 2009). In addition, it also increased the DNA binding activity of AP-1 thus inducing AP-1-dependent transcriptional activation (Wellmann *et al.*, 1997). Further, NPM-ALK was shown to up-regulate PI3K-Akt signaling cascade and down-regulate p27Kip1 eventually leading to malignant transformation (Figure 4.3) (Slupianek *et al.*, 2001; Slupianek and Skorski, 2004). This fusion-mediated deregulation of PI3K-Akt pathway resulted in the deactivation of forkhead box O3a (FOXO3a), a member of the forkhead family of transcription factors, through phosphorylation helping in hematopoietic transformation (Figure 4.3) (Gu *et al.*, 2004). Furthermore, very recently deregulation of SUMOylation pathway was found to play a major role in NPM-ALK+ lymphomagenesis through the prevention of ubiquitin-mediated degradation of the chimeric oncoprotein. This can be reverted with the help of SUMO1/Sentrin specific peptidase 1 (SENP1) protease. Therefore, it is apparent that targeting SUMOylation would give better treatment options to NPM-ALK+ lymphomas (Figure 4.4) (Vishwamitra *et al.*, 2015). Adding to this, DNA mismatch repair (MMR) pathway was also found to be abrogated by NPM-ALK induced phosphorylation of MSH2 protein (Bone *et al.*, 2015). It also increased the levels of immunophilin co-chaperone Cyclophilin 40 (Cyp40); elevated the expression of growth-promoting receptor ICOS and deregulated the activity of glycogen synthase kinase 3 beta (GSK3β) through PI3K-Akt-mediated phosphorylation which in turn promoted the survival of ALCL cells (Figure 4.3) (Pearson *et al.*, 2012; McDonnell *et al.*, 2012; Zhang *et al.*, 2011a). Likewise, interaction of this fusion protein with phosphoinositide kinase PIKfyve was shown to increase the invasiveness of the disease (Dupuis-Coronas *et al.*, 2011). Moreover, deregulation of c-Jun N-terminal kinase (JNK-cJun) and MEK-ERK signaling cascades were found to be associated with fusion positive ALCL and the reciprocal fusion protein was shown to increase the expression of platelet-derived growth factor receptor beta (PDGFRB) through JUN and transcription factor Jun B (JUNB) and to determine the shape and migration of ALCL cells through phosphorylation activation of VAV1 which in turn activated Cdc42 (Figure 4.4)

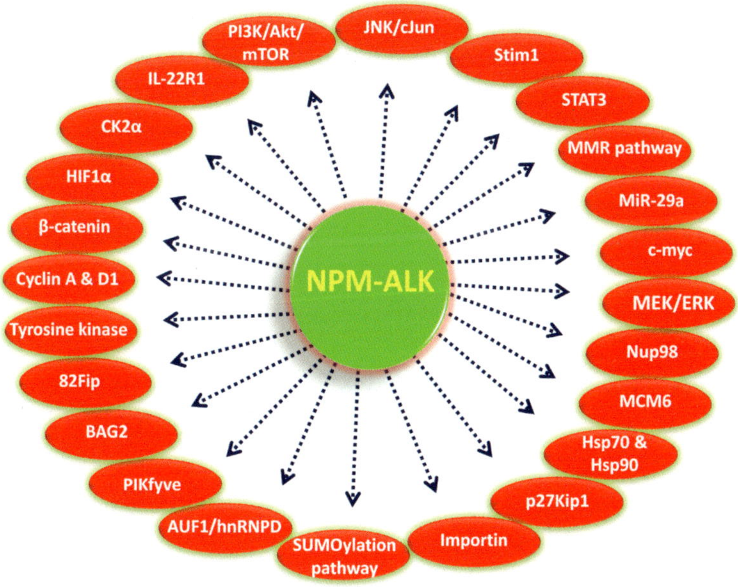

Figure 4.4: Molecular targets of NPM-ALK fusion gene.

(Leventaki *et al.*, 2007; Wasik *et al.*, 2009; Berghoff *et al.*, 2014; Ambrogio *et al.*, 2008). Furthermore, proteome-wide analysis identified a wide range of proteins associated with NPM-ALK induced lymphomagenesis including MCM6 involved in DNA repair; Nup98 and importin involved in subcellular protein transport; Stim1 involved in calcium signaling; 82Fip involved in RNA regulation; AUF1-hnRNPD involved in AU-rich element (ARE)-mediated mRNA degradation and BAG2 involved in proteosome degradation (Figure 4.4) (Wu *et al.*, 2009; Fawal *et al.*, 2006).

Other than the above mentioned molecular targets, NPM-ALK fusion was also found to provoke epigenetic silencing of STAT5A via STAT3 and DNA methylation that supports the binding of MeCP2 protein and blocks STAT5A transcription activator SP1 binding thereby leading to lymphomagenesis (Figure 4.3). However, inhibition of DNA methylation by DNA methyltransferase inhibitor recovered the STAT5A expression and resulted in the suppression of NPM-ALK gene (Zhang *et al.*, 2007). Similarly, it was also proved to deregulate the expression of IL-2Rγ, reconstitution of which reciprocally inhibited the expression of

NPM-ALK (Zhang *et al.*, 2011b). Further, the NPM-ALK oncoprotein was found to induce STAT3 activity through the phosphorylation-mediated degradation of STAT1 (Wu *et al.*, 2015). Ectopic expression of NPM-ALK in CD4(+) T lymphocytes was determined to induce the expression of IL-10, PD-L1-CD274, CD30 and to activate STAT3 and mammalian target of rapamycin complex 1 (mTORC1) signaling cascades leading to malignant transformation (Zhang *et al.*, 2013). Also, the NPM-ALK expressing lymphoid cells were found resistive to GC or dexamethasone (Dex) treatment due to constitutively active mTOR signaling and p70S6K. Rapamycin, inhibitor of mTOR pathway restored the sensitivity to GC and Dex treatment through the downregulation of mTOR and p70S6K (Gu *et al.*, 2008). Moreover, the tumorigenicity of NPM-ALK was described to be associated with hypoxia-induced factor 1 alpha (HIF1α), casein kinase 2α (CK2α) and β-catenin expressions and IL-22R1 was found to be yet another downstream effector of NPM-ALK which in turn activates STAT3 (Figure 4.4) (Marzec *et al.*, 2011; Armanious *et al.*, 2013; Bard *et al.*, 2008). In addition, Desjobert *et al.* (2011) showed that NPM-ALK expressing cells escaped apoptosis through the downregulation of miR-29a. Therefore, synthetic miR-29a may have a crucial role in the treatment of NPM-ALK expressing ALCL (Desjobert *et al.*, 2011). Several studies have attempted to identify modulators and inhibitors for this chimeric protein. For instance, Bonvini *et al.* (2002) showed the level of NPM-ALK chimera in ALCL to be controlled by its interaction with Hsp90 and Hsp70 suggesting them as a potential target for the treatment of ALCL; Kiss *et al.* (2015) proved lobatin B, an active phytochemical isolated from the medicinal plant *Neurolaena lobate*, to downregulate the expression of this fusion oncoprotein and to reduce the proliferation of ALCL cells; Hamedani *et al.* (2014) showed crizotinib, a small molecule kinase inhibitor to reduce the pSTAT3 levels and to induce apoptosis in ALCL cells; and Turturro *et al.* (2002) demonstrated that prolonged treatment of SUDHL-1 cells with herbimycin A, another protein kinase inhibitor, induced apoptosis by reducing the levels of NPM-ALK, Akt and p-Akt (Bonvini *et al.*, 2002; Kiss *et al.*, 2015; Hamedani *et al.*, 2014; Turturro *et al.*, 2002).

Above all, detailed studies on the advanced stage ALCL revealed that not only NPM-ALK but additional chromosomal abnormalities of ALK gene are also involved in the pathogenesis of ALCL (Lones *et al.*, 2006). Supporting this, in addition to NPM, few other fusion partners of ALK namely ATIC, CLTC, MSN, MYH9, SEC31A, TFG, TPM3/4 and TRAF1 were also identified to be associated with ALCL (Drexler *et al.*, 2000; Van Roosbroeck *et al.*, 2010; Feldman *et al.*, 2013, Damm-Welk *et al.*, 2009; Touriol *et al.*, 2000; Tort *et al.*, 2004). Unlike NPM-ALK, the other ALK fusions were less frequent (Drexler *et al.*, 2000).

ATIC-ALK and CLTC-ALK

ATIC-ALK is a product of chromosomal inversion inv(2)(p23q35) which was also associated with ALCL. 5-aminoimidazole-4-carboxamide ribonucleotide formyltransferase/IMP cyclohydrolase (ATIC) was found to be involved in purine biosynthesis and contains dimerization domain which has shown to be involved in the activation of kinase domain of ALK (Figure 4.2) (Colleoni *et al.*, 2000; Ma *et al.*, 2000). ATIC-ALK positive lymphoma cells were more sensitive to methotrexate, an anti-folate drug, due to the decreased ATIC enzymatic activity (Ma *et al.*, 2000).

Another type of ALK translocation t(2;17)(p23;q23) was detected in a distinct case of ALCL, plasma cell neoplasms and in rare IMTs where clathrin chain polypeptide-like (CLTCL) gene was fused to ALK which produces a 250 kD protein (Armstrong *et al.*, 2004; Touriol *et al.*, 2000; Patel *et al.*, 2007; Wang *et al.*, 2011). This chimeric protein was identified to be bound with clathrin-coated vesicles in the cytoplasm of CLTC-ALK positive cells. Like any other ALK fusion variants, this protein kinase is also constitutively active and contributed to the malignant transformation (Touriol *et al.*, 2000).

TFG-ALK

In rare cases of ALCL, t(2;3)(p23;q21) translocation involving ALK and TRK-fused gene (TFG) was detected (Figure 4.2). Three variants of the rearrangement TFG-ALK(S), TFG-ALK(L) and TFG-ALK(XL), with molecular weights of 85 kD, 97 kD and 113 kD, respectively, were identified in lymphoma. Like NPM, TFG also promoted the tyrosine kinase activity of ALK and formed complexes with various proteins like GRB2,

Shc, and PLC-gamma involved in the pathogenesis of ALCL (Hernández *et al.*, 1999, 2002).

MYH9-ALK

t(2;22)(p23;q11.2) translocation resulted in the MYH9-ALK chimera (Figure 4.2). Interestingly, unlike the other ALK chimeras, MYH9-ALK lacks the oligomerization domain thereby tyrosine kinase activity *in vitro*. However, it has been found to be phosphorylated *in vivo* at tyrosine residue through a possibly different mechanism from the other ALK-hybrids (Lamant *et al.*, 2003).

SQSTM1-ALK, another ALK fusion, was found to be associated with large B-cell lymphoma and STAT3 activation (d'Amore *et al.*, 2013; Takeuchi *et al.*, 2011).

TPM3/4-ALK

TPM3-ALK fusion is rarely reported in ALCL patients resulting from the translocation of ALK and non-muscular tropomyosin 3 (TPM3) gene on chromosome 1 and 2 t(1;2)(q25;p23) (Figure 4.2). Both TPM3-ALK and TPM4-ALK were also observed in IMTs (Lamant *et al.*, 1999; Lawrence *et al.*, 2000). Alike PLZF-RARA fusion gene, TPM3-ALK can also form homo or heterodimers via TPM coiled-coil domains which induce constitutive activation of kinases and other proteins like ALK, ERK1/2, and STAT3 (Lamant *et al.*, 1999; Shin *et al.*, 2012; Kinoshita *et al.*, 2007; Amano *et al.*, 2015). Further, this chimeric protein was believed to modify the cytoskeletal organization of tumor cells consequently increasing tumor invasion and metastasis (Armstrong *et al.*, 2007). Several tyrosine kinase inhibitors including herbimycin A were reported to suppress the tumor growth in TPM3-ALK transplant model (Giuriato *et al.*, 2007).

RANBP2-ALK

Mesenchymal proliferation of transformed myofibroblasts is defined as IMT with very low incidence rate. A novel chromosomal rearrangement t(2;2)(p23;q13) or inv(2)(p23q13) involving the ALK and Ran-binding protein 2 (RANBP2) genes has been reported to be involved in the pathogenesis of IMT (Figure 4.2) (Ma *et al.*, 2003; Patel *et al.*, 2007; Röttgers *et al.*, 2010; Li *et al.*, 2013). Interestingly, the RANBP2-ALK fusion bearing IMT cells were found to have a unique round cell transformation and an unusual nuclear membrane expression of ALK which was believed to be responsible for the poor prognosis of RANBP2-ALK positive IMTs (Chen *et al.*, 2008; Ma *et al.*, 2003). Other than IMTs, t(2;2)(p23;q13) was detected in AML as well, however, associated with a secondary alteration monosomy 7 (Lim *et al.*, 2014; Maesako *et al.*, 2014). Epithelioid inflammatory myofibroblastic sarcoma, a type of IMT expressing RANB2-ALK, was found to be highly aggressive and resistive to conventional therapies including surgery and doxorubicin treatment yet responded well to crizotinib, an ALK inhibitor therapy thus proving the therapeutic potential of ALK inhibitors in the management of otherwise aggressive IMTs (Kimbara *et al.*, 2014). However, in contrast to IMT, the inv(2) and monosomy 7 harboring AML developed resistance to crizotinib treatment by generating a G1269A point mutation in the kinase domain of ALK partner (Takeoka *et al.*, 2015). Additionally, more ALK translocations with different partner genes such as cysteinyl-tRNA synthetase (CARS), fibronectin 1 (FN1), protein-tyrosine phosphatase receptor-type F polypeptide-interacting protein-binding protein 1 (PPFIBP1) were also detected in IMT (Debelenko *et al.*, 2003; Ouchi *et al.*, 2015; Yoshida *et al.*, 2013).

STRN-ALK

This fusion involving striatin gene has been reported to occur in thyroid carcinomas, CRC and renal cell carcinoma with constitutive activation of ALK kinase domain which was driven by coiled-coil domain of STRN-mediated dimerization (Pérot *et al.*, 2014; Kelly *et al.*, 2014; Kusano *et al.*, 2016; Yakirevich *et al.*, 2016). The fusion kinase induced thyroid-stimulating hormone (TSH)-independent cell growth and transformation of thyroid cells. Moreover, it was also proved to be sufficient enough to initiate tumor growth *in vivo* (Kelly *et al.*, 2014).

EML4-ALK

Inv(2)(p21p23), suggested to form by either paracentric inversion or chromothripsis process, resulted in the fusion of echinoderm microtubule-associated protein-like 4 (EML4) gene and the ALK gene and recurrently detected in approximately 3–7% of non-small cell lung cancers (NSCLC) and rarely in CRC and large B-cell lymphomas (Figure 4.2) (Kodama *et al.*, 2014; Soda *et al.*, 2007; Sozzi *et al.*, 2009; Ma *et al.*, 2016; Houang *et al.*, 2015; Sakamoto *et al.*, 2016). Unlike other fusion genes associated with only hematological malignancies, EML4-ALK has been largely reported in pulmonary malignancies (Shinmura *et al.*, 2008). It was also detected in a patient presented with congenital pulmonary airway malformation (CPAM), an airway developmental disorder, with lung adenocarcinoma suggesting that testing for the EML4-ALK fusion in patients with CPAM would give a beneficial treatment option of using ALK inhibitors which would prevent neoplastic transformation (Tetsumoto *et al.*, 2013). Interestingly, initially thought to be restricted to carcinomas, eventually EML4-ALK has been discovered to be involved in the development of sarcomas as well (Sokai *et al.*, 2014).

More than 15 variants of this fusion have been identified based on the breakpoint regions and their protein length (Bayliss *et al.*, 2016). Among them, variant 1 (fusion of intron 13 of EML4 to intron 19 of ALK), variant 2 (fusion of intron 20 of EML4 gene to intron 19 of ALK) and variant 3 (fusion of intron 6 of EML4 to intron 19 of ALK) were the most common variants: v2 being the largest isoform with two thirds of EML4 gene and v3 being the smallest isoform with two subtypes 3a and 3b (Choi *et al.*, 2008; Bayliss *et al.*, 2016). Richards *et al.* (2014) identified a stabilizing domain, namely, tandem atypical propeller in EMLs (TAPE) in EML family of proteins and showed that translocation induced truncation of this TAPE domain as in some variants of EML4-ALK fusions would result in less stable isoforms and make them liable for Hsp90 inhibitors-mediated degradation. Therefore, knowing the type of EML4-ALK variant and the TAPE domain status will be useful in predicting the treatment outcome (Richards *et al.*, 2014). Similar to any other ALK fusion partners, EML4 also resulted in the constitutive activation of ALK tyrosine kinase activity through its trimerization domain (TD) and also proved to be associated with elevated levels of ALK in lung adenocarcinomas (Mano *et al.*, 2015; Katayama *et al.*, 2011; Zhang *et al.*, 2010; Bayliss *et al.*, 2016). Ectopic expression of this fusion gene increased the activation of ERK and STAT3 signaling pathways, however, failed to induce Akt-signaling in NIH 3T3 lung cancer cells (Takezawa *et al.*, 2011). Further through its kinase activity, EML4-ALK prompted the phosphorylation of Akt and ERK proteins *in vitro* which was significantly suppressed when treated with ALK inhibitors (Bayliss *et al.*, 2016). In addition, it was also shown to induce growth factor independence in Ba/F3 cells (Bayliss *et al.*, 2016). Among various inhibitors used to inhibit fusion induced ALK activity, the tyrosine kinase inhibitor (TKI) crizotinib was proved effective in both preclinical and clinical studies and was approved for NSCLC treatment (Bayliss *et al.*, 2016). However, prolonged use of crizotinib was shown to induce resistance through development of gatekeeper mutations in the tyrosine kinase domain of EML4-ALK; increased ALK expression; increased epithelial–mesenchymal transition (EMT) thus increasing the invasiveness of the disease; and enhanced levels of substitute receptor tyrosine kinases (RTKs) like EGFR, HER2, HER3, IGF-1R, KIT and SRC, etc. (Katayama *et al.*, 2011; Yamada *et al.*, 2012; Kim *et al.*, 2013; Guo *et al.*, 2015; Bayliss *et al.*, 2016; Tanizaki *et al.*, 2012). Therefore, treatment with second-generation ALK TKIs, Hsp90 inhibitors or combination of both were believed to give a better prognosis in EML4-ALK positive crizotinib-resistant lung cancer patients (Katayama *et al.*, 2011; Heuckmann *et al.*, 2012; Kim *et al.*, 2013). In certain EML4-ALK positive lung cancers, neither amplification nor gatekeeper mutations had been found. However, other mechanisms like EGFR activation and paracrine survival signals from the tumor microenvironment elicited resistance to standard ALK-TKI therapy indicating the requirement of ALK plus EGFR TKIs for the better clinical outcome in such cases (Yamada *et al.*, 2012; Yamaguchi *et al.*, 2014). Likewise, as EML4-ALK fusion highly activated the RAS-MAPK pathway, inhibition of both the kinases ALK and MEK will restore the sensitivity of tumor cells to treatment (Hrustanovic *et al.*, 2015). Further, EML4-ALK was shown to increase the expression of programmed death-ligand 1 (PD-L1) through the activation of PI3K-Akt and MEK-ERK pathways thus escaping the immune check point by inducing apoptosis of T cells in tumor cells and DC-CIK cells co-culture system insisting the need of anti-PD-1-PD-L1 immune therapy in addition to regular TKIs for both TKI- sensitive and resistant NSCLC patients (Hong *et al.*, 2015; Ota *et al.*, 2015). Strikingly, it was confirmed that EML4-ALK positive NSCLC patients exhibited higher rate of glucose metabolism than that of EML4-ALK negative patients. Further investigation on the connection between ALK translocation and glucose metabolism revealed that EML4-ALK oncoprotein increases hexokinase II (HK2) expression by activating the transcription factor HIF1α in normoxia conditions thus proving increased glucose metabolism to be one of the driving factors of fusion-mediated cancer progression (Ma *et al.*, 2016).

In a couple of studies involving 280 female and 95 male NSCLC patients with no history of smoking, the EML4-ALK fusion was found to be correlated with early disease onset and undifferentiated carcinomas (Ren *et al.*, 2015; Guo *et al.*, 2014). In addition, EML4-ALK + NSCLC patients were also found to be associated with reduced levels of thymidylate synthase (TYMS), a rate-limiting enzyme in *de novo* DNA synthesis which is known to induce increased disease progression, therefore responded to first-line pemetrexed chemotherapy (Xu *et al.*, 2015).

DCTN1, TRP, KLC1 and HIP1 are the other genes identified to participate in ALK translocation and were associated with the development of lung cancer (Hong *et al.*, 2014; Iyevleva *et al.*, 2015; Togashi *et al.*, 2012; Choi *et al.*, 2014).

KIF5B-ALK

Ligation of kinesin family member 5B (KIF5B) to the kinase protein ALK, engineered by the t(2;10)(p23;p11) translocation was first identified in lung adenocarcinoma (Figure 4.2). This chimeric KIF5B-ALK was found to increase the proliferation, migration and invasion of non-small cell lung cancer cells through the aberrant activation of STAT3 and protein kinase B (Takeuchi *et al.*, 2009; Wong *et al.*, 2011). Small molecule TKIs such as PF-1066, X-376 and X-396 were found effective against this fusion protein (Lovly *et al.*, 2011).

CAD-ALK and C2orf44-ALK

A subset of CRCs was found to exhibit an inversional abnormality within the chromosome 2 denoted as inv(2)(p22-21p23) which produces CAD-ALK fusion oncogene (Figure 4.2) (Amatu *et al.*, 2015; Lee *et al.*, 2015). carbamoyl-phosphate synthetase 2, aspartate transcarbamylase, and dihydroorotase (CAD) is involved in the pyrimidine pathway through its gluymine amidotransferase [GATase], carbamoyl-phosphate synthase [CPSase], dihydroorotase [DHOase] and aspartate transcarbamylase [ATCase] activities and loses its ATCase domain when fused with kinase domain of ALK (Lee *et al.*, 2015). Other than CAD-ALK, another chromosomal translocation involving C2orf44 (chromosome 2, open reading frame 44) also known as WD repeat and coiled coil containing protein (WDCP) was identified in CRC which also induced the constitutive activation of ALK through oligomerization (Yokoyama and Miller, 2015).

VCL-ALK

Rearrangement of 3′ kinase domain of ALK with 5′ vinculin (VCL) gene was identified to be resulted from t(2;10)(p23;q22) translocation (Figure 4.2). Expression of the resultant oncoprotein was localized to cytoplasmic and subplasmalemmal regions and was associated with renal medullary carcinoma and renal cell carcinoma with sickle cell trait suggesting kidney to be a new organ site for ALK fusion-mediated neoplasms (Debelenko *et al.*, 2011; Mariño-Enríquez *et al.*, 2011; Smith *et al.*, 2014). Moreover, unlike the other ALK fusions, VCL-ALK lacks the self-association domain instead contains talin binding domains of VCL and the fusion tyrosine kinase was found to cross-phosphorylate talins of neighboring VCL-ALK proteins on a talin scaffold which gives it oncogenic properties (Mariño-Enríquez *et al.*, 2011). Other than renal cancers, this fusion gene was also detected in epithelioid fibrous histiocytoma (Jedrych *et al.*, 2015).

CONCLUSION

In summary, ample amount of evidences suggested the importance of ALK fusion genes in the development and progression of various cancers and their effective management with small molecule tyrosine kinase inhibitors targeted to fusion kinase proteins. However, attaining complete regression of cancer remains questionable as the prolonged use of such inhibitors induced chemoresistance which was mediated through mutations in the tyrosine kinase domain and activation of alternate survival pathways. Therefore, combination of TKIs targeting both chimeric tyrosine kinases and other survival pathways is believed to give better prognosis. Moreover, further studies are required to elucidate the inducers of chromosomal translocations and their downstream targets for the prevention, early diagnosis and treatment of ALK fusion governed neoplasms.

CONFLICT OF INTEREST

The authors express no conflict of interest.

REFERENCES

Amano, Y., R. Ishikawa, T. Sakatani, J. Ichinose, M. Sunohara, K. Watanabe, H. Kage, J. Nakajima, T. Nagase, N. Ohishi, and D. Takai, Oncogenic TPM3-ALK activation requires dimerization through the coiled-coil structure of TPM3, *Biochem Biophys Res Commun* **457**(3): 457–460 (2015).

Amatu, A., A. Somaschini, G. Cerea, R. Bosotti, E. Valtorta, P. Buonandi, G. Marrapese, S. Veronese, D. Luo, Z. Hornby, P. Multani, D. Murphy, R. Shoemaker, C. Lauricella, L. Giannetta, M. Maiolani, A. Vanzulli, E. Ardini, A. Galvani, A. Isacchi, A. Sartore-Bianchi, and S. Siena, Novel CAD-ALK gene rearrangement is drugable by entrectinib in colorectal cancer, *Br J Canc* **113**(12): 1730–1734 (2015).

Ambrogio, C., C. Voena, A.D. Manazza C. Martinengo, C. Costa, T. Kirchhausen, E. Hirsch, G. Inghirami, and R. Chiarle, The anaplastic lymphoma kinase controls cell shape and growth of anaplastic large cell lymphoma through Cdc42 activation, *Canc Res* **68**(21): 8899–8907 (2008).

Armanious, H., P. Gelebart, M. Anand, and R. Lai, Identification of a novel cross-talk between casein kinase 2α and NPM-ALK in ALK-positive anaplastic large cell lymphoma, *Cell Signal* **25**(2): 381–388 (2013).

Armstrong, F., M.M. Duplantier, P. Trempat, C. Hieblot, L. Lamant, E. Espinos, C. Racaud-Sultan, M. Allouche, E. Campo, G. Delsol, and C. Touriol, Differential effects of X-ALK fusion proteins on proliferation, transformation, and invasion properties of NIH3T3 cells, *Oncogene* **23**(36): 6071–6082 (2004).

Armstrong, F., L. Lamant, C. Hieblot, G. Delsol, and C. Touriol, TPM3-ALK expression induces changes in cytoskeleton organization and confers higher metastatic capacities than other ALK fusion proteins, *J Canc* **43**(4): 640–646 (2007).

Bard, J.D., P. Gelebart, M. Anand, H.M. Amin, and R. Lai, Aberrant expression of IL-22 receptor 1 and autocrine IL-22 stimulation contribute to tumorigenicity in ALK+ anaplastic large cell lymphoma, *Leukemia* **22**(8): 1595–1603 (2008).

Bayliss, R., J. Choi, D.A. Fennell, A.M. Fry, and M.W. Richards, Molecular mechanisms that underpin EML4-ALK driven cancers and their response to targeted drugs, *Cell Mol Life Sci* **73**(6): 1209–1224 (2016).

Berghoff, A.S., P. Birner, B. Streubel, L. Kenner, and M. Preusser, ALK gene aberrations and the JUN/JUNB/PDGFR axis in metastatic NSCLC, *APMIS* **122**(9): 867–872 (2014).

Bischof, D., K. Pulford, D.Y. Mason, and S.W. Morris, Role of the nucleophosmin (NPM) portion of the non-Hodgkin's lymphoma-associated NPM-anaplastic lymphoma kinase fusion protein in oncogenesis, *Mol Cell Biol* **17**(4): 2312–2325 (1997).

Bone, K.M., P. Wang, F. Wu, C. Wu, L. Li, J.T. Bacani, S.E. Andrew, and R. Lai, NPM-ALK mediates phosphorylation of MSH2 at tyrosine 238, creating a functional deficiency in MSH2 and the loss of mismatch repair, *Blood Canc J* 5:e311 (2015).

Bonvini, P., T. Gastaldi, B. Falini, and A. Rosolen, Nucleophosmin-anaplastic lymphoma kinase (NPM-ALK), a novel Hsp90-client tyrosine kinase: down-regulation of NPM-ALK expression and tyrosine phosphorylation in ALK(+) CD30(+) lymphoma cells by the Hsp90 antagonist 17-allylamino, 17-demethoxygeldanamycin, *Canc Res* **62**(5): 1559–1566 (2002).

Chen, S.T. and J.C. Lee, An inflammatory myofibroblastic tumor in liver with ALK and RANBP2 gene rearrangement: combination of distinct morphologic, immunohistochemical, and genetic features, *Hum Pathol* **39**(12): 1854–1858 (2008).

Choi, Y.L., M.E. Lira, M. Hong, R.N. Kim, S.J. Choi, J.Y. Song, K. Pandy, D.L. Mann, J.A. Stahl, H.E. Peckham, Z. Zheng, J. Han, M. Mao, and J. Kim, A novel fusion of TPR and ALK in lung adenocarcinoma, *J Thorac Oncol* **9**(4): 563–566 (2014).

Choi, Y.L., K. Takeuchi, M. Soda, K. Inamura, Y. Togashi, S. Hatano, M. Enomoto, T. Hamada, H. Haruta, H. Watanabe, K. Kurashina, H. Hatanaka, T. Ueno, S. Takada, Y. Yamashita, Y. Sugiyama, Y. Ishikawa, and H. Mano, Identification of novel isoforms of the EML4-ALK transforming gene in non-small cell lung cancer, *Canc Res* **68**(13): 4971–4976 (2008).

Colleoni, G.W., J.A. Bridge, B. Garicochea, J. Liu, D.A. Filippa, and M. Ladanyi, ATIC–ALK: A novel variant ALK gene fusion in anaplastic large cell lymphoma resulting from the recurrent cryptic chromosomal inversion, inv(2)(p23q35), *Am J Pathol* **156**(3): 781–789 (2000).

Crescenzo, R. and G. Inghirami, Anaplastic lymphoma kinase inhibitors, *Curr Opin Pharmacol* **23**: 39–44 (2015).

Damm-Welk, C., W. Klapper, I. Oschlies, S. Gesk, S. Röttgers, J. Bradtke, R. Siebert, A. Reiter, and W. Woessmann, Distribution of NPM1-ALK and X-ALK fusion transcripts in paediatric anaplastic large cell lymphoma: a molecular-histological correlation, *Br J Haematol* **146**(3): 306–309 (2009).

d'Amore, E.S., C. Visco, A. Menin, B. Famengo, P. Bonvini, and Lazzari E. STAT3 pathway is activated in ALK-positive large B-cell lymphoma carrying SQSTM1-ALK rearrangement and provides a possible therapeutic target, *Am J Surg Pathol* **37**(5): 780–786 (2013).

Debelenko, L.V., D.C. Arthur, S.D. Pack, L.J. Helman, D.S. Schrump, and M. Tsokos, Identification of CARS-ALK fusion in primary and metastatic lesions of an inflammatory myofibroblastic tumor, *Lab Invest* **83**(9): 1255–1265 (2003).

Debelenko, L.V., S.C. Raimondi, N. Daw, B.R. Shivakumar, D. Huang, M. Nelson, and J.A. Bridge, Renal cell carcinoma with novel VCL-ALK fusion: new representative of ALK-associated tumor spectrum, *Mod Pathol* **24**(3): 430–442 (2014).

Desjobert, C., M.H. Renalier, J. Bergalet, E. Dejean, N. Joseph, A. Kruczynski, J. Soulier, E. Espinos, F. Meggetto, J. Cavaillé, G. Delsol, and L. Lamant, MiR-29a down-regulation in ALK-positive anaplastic large cell lymphomas contributes to apoptosis blockade through MCL-1 overexpression, *Blood* **117**(24): 6627–6637 (2011).

Drexler, H.G., S.M. Gignac, R. von Wasielewski, M. Werner, and W.G. Dirks, Pathobiology of NPM–ALK and variant fusion genes in anaplastic large cell lymphoma and other lymphomas, *Leukemia* **14**(9): 1533–1559 (2000).

Dupuis-Coronas, S., F. Lagarrigue, D. Ramel, G. Chicanne, E. Saland, F. Gaits-Iacovoni, B. Payrastre, H. Tronchère, The nucleophosmin-anaplastic lymphoma kinase oncogene interacts, activates, and uses the kinase PIKfyve to increase invasiveness, *J Biol Chem* **286**(37): 32105–32114 (2011).

Fawal, M., F. Armstrong, S. Ollier, H. Dupont, C. Touriol, B. Monsarrat, G. Delsol, B. Payrastre, and D. Morello, A "liaison dangereuse" between AUF1/hnRNPD and the oncogenic tyrosine kinase NPM–ALK, *Blood* **108**(8): 2780–2788 (2006).

Feldman, A.L., G. Vasmatzis, Y.W. Asmann, J. Davila, S. Middha, B.W. Eckloff, S.H. Johnson, J.C. Porcher, S.M. Ansell, and A. Caride, Novel TRAF1-ALK fusion identified by deep RNA sequencing of anaplastic large cell lymphoma, *Genes Chromosomes Canc* **52**(11): 1097–1102 (2013).

Fernandez-Vidal, A., A. Mazars, E.F. Gautier G. Prévost, B. Payrastre, and S. Manenti, Upregulation of the CDC25A phosphatase down-stream of the NPM/ALK oncogene participates to anaplastic large cell lymphoma enhanced proliferation, *Cell Cycle* **8**(9): 1373–1379 (2009).

Fujimoto, J., M. Shiota, T. Iwahara, N. Seki, H. Satoh, S. Mori, and T. Yamamoto, Characterization of the transforming activity of p80, a hyperphosphorylated protein in a Ki-1 lymphoma cell line with chromosomal translocation t(2;5), *Proc Natl Acad Sci USA* **93**(9): 4181–4186 (1996).

Giuriato, S., N. Faumont, E. Bousquet, M. Foisseau, A. Bibonne, M. Moreau, T. Al Saati, D.W. Felsher, G. Delsol, and F. Meggetto, Development of a conditional bioluminescent transplant model for TPM3-ALK-induced tumorigenesis as a tool to validate ALK-dependent cancer targeted therapy, *Canc Biol Ther* **6**(8): 1318–1323 (2007).

Gu, L., J. Gao, Q. Li, Y.P. Zhu, C.S. Jia, R.Y. Fu, Y. Chen, Q.K. Liao, and Z. Ma, Rapamycin reverses NPM–ALK-induced glucocorticoid resistance in lymphoid tumor cells by inhibiting mTOR signaling pathway, enhancing G1 cell cycle arrest and apoptosis, *Leukemia* **22**(11): 2091–2096 (2008).

Gu, T.L., Z. Tothova, B. Scheijen, J.D. Griffin, D.G. Gilliland, and D.W. Sternberg, NPM-ALK fusion kinase of anaplastic large-cell lymphoma regulates survival and proliferative signaling through modulation of FOXO3a, *Blood* **103**(12): 4622–4629 (2004).

Guo, F., X. Liu, Q. Qing, Y. Sang, C. Feng, X. Li, L. Jiang, P. Su, and Y. Wang, EML4-ALK induces epithelial-mesenchymal transition consistent with cancer stem cell properties in H1299 non-small cell lung cancer cells, *Biochem Biophys Res Commun* **459**(3): 398–404 (2015).

Guo, Y., J. Ma, X. Lyu, H. Liu, B. Wei, J. Zhao, S. Fu, L. Ding, and J. Zhang, Non-small cell lung cancer with EML4-ALK translocation in Chinese male never-smokers is characterized with early-onset, *BMC Canc* **14**: 834 (2014).

Hamedani, F.S., M. Cinar, Z. Mo, M.A. Cervania, H.M. Amin, and S. Alkan, Crizotinib (PF-2341066) induces apoptosis due to downregulation of pSTAT3 and BCL-2 family proteins in NPM–ALK(+) anaplastic large cell lymphoma, *Leuk Res* **38**(4): 503–508 (2014).

Hernández, L., S. Beà, B. Bellosillo, M. Pinyol, B. Falini, A. Carbone, G. Ott, A. Rosenwald, A. Fernández, K. Pulford, D. Mason, S.W. Morris, E. Santos, and E. Campo, Diversity of genomic breakpoints in TFG-ALK translocations in anaplastic large cell lymphomas: identification of a new TFG-ALK(XL) chimeric gene with transforming activity, *Am J Pathol* **160**(4): 1487–1494 (2002).

Hernández, L., M. Pinyol, S. Hernández, S. Beà, K. Pulford, A. Rosenwald, L. Lamant, B. Falini, G. Ott, D.Y. Mason, G. Delsol, and E. Campo, TRK-fused gene (TFG) is a new partner of ALK in anaplastic large cell lymphoma producing two structurally different TFG-ALK translocations, *Blood* **94**(9): 3265–3268 (1999).

Heuckmann, J.M., H. Balke-Want, F. Malchers, M. Peifer, M.L. Sos, M. Koker, L. Meder, C.M. Lovly, L.C. Heukamp, W. Pao, R. Küppers, and R.K. Thomas, Differential protein stability and ALK inhibitor sensitivity of EML4-ALK fusion variants, *Clin Canc Res* **18**(17): 4682–4690 (2012).

Hong, M., R.N. Kim, J.Y. Song, S.J. Choi, E. Oh, M.E. Lira, M. Mao, K. Takeuchi, J. Han, J. Kim, and Y.L. Choi, HIP1-ALK, a novel fusion protein identified in lung adenocarcinoma, *J Thorac Oncol* **9**(3): 419–422 (2014).

Hong, S., N. Chen, W. Fang, J. Zhan, Q. Liu, S. Kang, X. He, L. Liu, T. Zhou, J. Huang, Y. Chen, T. Qin, Y. Zhang, Y. Ma, Y. Yang, Y. Zhao, Y. Huang, and L. Zhang, Upregulation of PD-L1 by EML4–ALK fusion protein mediates the immune escape in ALK positive NSCLC: Implication for optional anti-PD-1/PD-L1 immune therapy for ALK–TKIs sensitive and resistant NSCLC patients, *Oncoimmunology* **5**(3): e1094598 (2015).

Houang, M., C.W. Toon, A. Clarkson, L. Sioson, K. de Silva, N. Watson, N.R. Singh, A. Chou, and A.J. Gill, ALK and ROS1 overexpression is very rare in colorectal adenocarcinoma, *Appl Immunohistochem Mol Morphol* **23**(2): 134–138 (2015).

Hrustanovic, G., V. Olivas, E. Pazarentzos, A. Tulpule, S. Asthana, C.M. Blakely, R.A. Okimoto, L. Lin, D.S. Neel, A. Sabnis, J. Flanagan, E. Chan, M. Varella-Garcia, D.L. Aisner, A. Vaishnavi, S.H. Ou, E.A. Collisson, E. Ichihara, P.C. Mack, C.M. Lovly, N. Karachaliou, R. Rosell, J.W. Riess, R.C. Doebele, and T.G. Bivona, RAS–MAPK dependence underlies a rational polytherapy strategy in EML4-ALK-positive lung cancer, *Nat Med* **21**(9): 1038–1047 (2015).

Iyevleva, A.G., G.A. Raskin, V.I. Tiurin, A.P. Sokolenko, N.V. Mitiushkina, S.N. Aleksakhina, A.R. Garifullina, T.N. Strelkova, V.O. Merkulov, A.O. Ivantsov, K.M. Kuligina, ESh, Pozharisski, A.V. Togo, and

E.N. Imyanitov, Novel ALK fusion partners in lung cancer, *Canc Lett* **362**(1): 116–121 (2015).

Jedrych, J., M. Nikiforova, T.F. Kennedy, and J. Ho, Epithelioid cell histiocytoma of the skin with clonal ALK gene rearrangement resulting in VCL-ALK and SQSTM1-ALK gene fusions, *Br J Dermatol* **172**(5): 1427–1429 (2015).

Katayama, R., T.M. Khan, C. Benes, E. Lifshits, H. Ebi, V.M. Rivera, W.C. Shakespeare, A.J. Iafrate, J.A. Engelman, and A.T. Shaw, Therapeutic strategies to overcome crizotinib resistance in non-small cell lung cancers harboring the fusion oncogene EML4-ALK, *Proc Natl Acad Sci USA* **108**(18): 7535–7540 (2011).

Kelly, L.M., G. Barila, P. Liu, V.N. Evdokimova, S. Trivedi, F. Panebianco, M. Gandhi, S.E. Carty, S.P. Hodak, J. Luo, S. Dacic, Y.P. Yu, M.N. Nikiforova, R.L. Ferris, D.L. Altschuler, and Y.E. Nikiforov, Identification of the transforming STRN-ALK fusion as a potential therapeutic target in the aggressive forms of thyroid cancer, *Proc Natl Acad Sci USA* **111**(11): 4233–4238 (2014).

Kim, H.R., W.S. Kim, Y.J. Choi C.M. Choi, J.K. Rho, and J.C. Lee, Epithelial-mesenchymal transition leads to crizotinib resistance in H2228 lung cancer cells with EML4–ALK translocation, *Mol Oncol* 7(6): 1093–1102 (2013).

Kimbara, S., K. Takeda, H. Fukushima, T. Inoue, H. Okada, Y. Shibata, U. Katsushima, A. Tsuya, S. Tokunaga, H. Daga, T. Okuno, and T. Inoue, A case report of epithelioid inflammatory myofibroblastic sarcoma with RANBP2-ALK fusion gene treated with the ALK inhibitor, crizotinib, *Jpn J Clin Oncol* **44**(9): 868–871 (2014).

Kinoshita, Y., T. Tajiri, S. Ieiri, K. Nagata, T. Taguchi, S. Suita, K. Yamazaki, I. Yoshino, Y. Maehara, K. Kohashi, H. Yamamoto, Y. Oda, and M. Tsuneyoshi, A case of an inflammatory myofibroblastic tumor in the lung which expressed TPM3-ALK gene fusion, *Pediatr Surg Int* **23**(6): 595–599 (2007).

Kiss, I., C. Unger, C.N. Huu, A.G. Atanasov, N. Kramer, W. Chatruphonprasert, S. Brenner, R. McKinnon, A. Peschel, A. Vasas, I. Lajter, R. Kain, P. Saiko, T. Szekeres, L. Kenner, M.R. Hassler, R. Diaz, R. Frisch, V.M. Dirsch, W. Jäger, R. de Martin, V.N. Bochkov, C.M. Passreiter, B. Peter-Vörösmarty, R.M. Mader, M. Grusch, H. Dolznig, B. Kopp, I. Zupko, J. Hohmann, and G. Krupitza, Lobatin B inhibits NPM/ALK and NF-κB attenuating anaplastic-large-cell-lymphomagenesis and lymphendothelial tumor intravasation, *Canc Lett* **356**(2 Pt B): 994–1006 (2015).

Kodama, T., N. Motoi, H. Ninomiya, H. Sakamoto, K. Kitada, T. Tsukaguchi, Y. Satoh, K. Nomura, H. Nagano, N. Ishii, Y. Terui, K. Hatake, and Y. Ishikawa, A novel mechanism of EML4-ALK rearrangement mediated by chromothripsis in a patient-derived cell line, *J Thorac Oncol* **9**(11): 1638–1646 (2014).

Kusano, H., Y. Togashi, J. Akiba, F. Moriya, K. Baba, N. Matsuzaki, Y. Yuba, Y. Shiraishi, H. Kanamaru, N. Kuroda, S. Sakata, K. Takeuchi, and H. Yano, Two cases of renal cell carcinoma harboring a novel STRN-ALK fusion Gene, *Am J Surg Pathol* **40**(6): 761–769 (2016).

Lamant, L., N. Dastugue, K. Pulford, G. Delsol, and B. Mariamé, A new fusion gene TPM3-ALK in anaplastic large cell lymphoma created by a (1;2)(q25;p23) translocation, *Blood* **93**(9): 3088–3095 (1999).

Lamant, L., R.D. Gascoyne, M.M. Duplantier, F. Armstrong, A. Raghab, M. Chhanabhai, E. Rajcan-Separovic, J. Raghab, G. Delsol, and E. Espinos, Non-muscle myosin heavy chain (MYH9): a new partner fused to ALK in anaplastic large cell lymphoma, *Genes Chromosomes Canc* **37**(4): 427–432 (2003).

Lawrence, B., A. Perez-Atayde, M.K. Hibbard, B.P. Rubin, P. Dal Cin, J.L. Pinkus, G.S. Pinkus, S. Xiao, E.S. Yi, C.D. Fletcher, and J.A. Fletcher, TPM3-ALK and TPM4-ALK oncogenes in inflammatory myofibroblastic tumors, *Am J Pathol* **157**(2): 377–384 (2000).

Lee, J., H.C. Kim, J.Y. Hong, K. Wang, S.Y. Kim, J. Jang, S.T. Kim, J.O. Park, H.Y. Lim, W.K. Kang, Y.S. Park, J. Lee, W.Y. Lee, Y.A. Park, J.W. Huh, S.H. Yun, I.G. Do, S.H. Kim, S. Balasubramanian, P.J. Stephens, J.S. Ross, G.G. Li, Z. Hornby, S.M. Ali, V.A. Miller, K.M. Kim, and S.H. Ou, Detection of novel and potentially actionable anaplastic lymphoma kinase (ALK) rearrangement in colorectal adenocarcinoma by immunohistochemistry screening, **6**(27): 24320–24332 (2015).

Leventaki, V., E. Drakos, L.J. Medeiros, M.S. Lim, K.S. Elenitoba-Johnson, F.X. Claret, and G.Z. Rassidakis, NPM-ALK oncogenic kinase promotes cell-cycle progression through activation of JNK/cJun signaling in anaplastic large-cell lymphoma, *Blood* **110**(5): 1621–1630 (2007).

Li, J., W.H. Yin, K. Takeuchi, H. Guan, Y.H. Huang, and J.K. Chan, Inflammatory myofibroblastic tumor with RANBP2 and ALK gene rearrangement: a report of two cases and literature review, *Diagn Pathol* **8**:147 (2013).

Lim, J.H., S. Jang, C.J. Park, Y.U. Cho, J.H. Lee, K.H. Lee, J.O. Lee, J.Y. Shin, J.I. Kim, J. Huh, and E.J. Seo, RANBP2-ALK fusion combined with monosomy 7 in acute myelomonocytic leukemia, *Canc Genet* **207**(1–2): 40–45 (2014).

Lones, M.A., N.A. Heerema, M.M. Le Beau, S.L. Perkins, M.E. Kadin, C.R. Kjeldsberg, R. Sposto, A. Meadows, S. Siegel, J. Buckley, J. Finlay, M. Abromowitch, M.S. Cairo, and W.G. Sanger, Complex secondary chromosome abnormalities in advanced stage anaplastic large cell lymphoma of children and adolescents: a report from CCG-E08, *Canc Genet Cytogenet* **171**(2): 89–96 (2006).

Lovly, C.M., J.M. Heuckmann, E. de Stanchina, H. Chen, R.K. Thomas, C. Liang, and W. Pao, Insights into ALK-driven cancers revealed through development of novel ALK tyrosine kinase inhibitors, *Canc Res* **71**(14): 4920–4931 (2011).

Ma, Y., C. Yu, E.M. Mohamed, H. Shao, L. Wang, G. Sundaresan, J. Zweit, M. Idowu, and X. Fang, A causal link from ALK to hexokinase II overexpression and hyperactive glycolysis in EML4–ALK -positive lung cancer, *Oncogene* (2016).

Ma, Z., J. Cools, P. Marynen, X. Cui, R. Siebert, S. Gesk, B. Schlegelberger, B. Peeters, C. De Wolf-Peeters, I. Wlodarska, and S.W. Morris, Inv(2)(p23q35) in anaplastic large-cell lymphoma induces constitutive anaplastic lymphoma kinase (ALK) tyrosine kinase activation by fusion to ATIC, an enzyme involved in purine nucleotide biosynthesis, *Blood* **95**(6): 2144–2149 (2000).

Ma, Z., D.A. Hill, M.H. Collins, S.W. Morris, J. Sumegi, M. Zhou, C. Zuppan, and J.A. Bridge, Fusion of ALK to the Ran-binding protein 2 (RANBP2) gene in inflammatory myofibroblastic tumor, *Genes Chromosomes Canc* **37**(1): 98–105 (2003).

Maesako, Y., K. Izumi, S. Okamori, K. Takeoka, C. Kishimori, A. Okumura, G. Honjo, T. Akasaka, and H. Ohno, inv(2)(p23q13)/RAN-binding protein 2 (RANBP2)-ALK fusion gene in myeloid leukemia that developed in an elderly woman, *Int J Hematol* **99**(2): 202–207 (2014).

Mano, H., ALKoma: a cancer subtype with a shared target, *Canc Discov* **2**(6): 495–502 (2012).

Mano, H., The EML4–ALK oncogene: targeting an essential growth driver in human cancer, *Proc Jpn Acad Ser B Phys Biol Sci* **91**(5): 193–201 (2015).

Mariño-Enríquez, A. and P. Dal, Cin ALK as a paradigm of oncogenic promiscuity: different mechanisms of activation and different fusion partners drive tumors of different lineages, *Canc Genet* **206**(11): 357–373 (2013).

Mariño-Enríquez, A., W.B. Ou, C.B. Weldon, J.A. Fletcher, and A.R. Pérez-Atayde, ALK rearrangement in sickle cell trait-associated renal medullary carcinoma, *Genes Chromosomes Canc* **50**(3): 146–153 (2011).

Marzec, M., X. Liu, W. Wong, Y. Yang, T. Pasha, K. Kantekure, P. Zhang, A. Woetmann, M. Cheng, N. Odum, and M.A. Wasik, Oncogenic kinase NPM/ALK induces expression of HIF1α mRNA, *Oncogene* **30**(11): 1372–1378 (2011).

McDonnell, S.R., S.R. Hwang, V. Basrur, K.P. Conlon, D. Fermin, E. Wey, C. Murga-Zamalloa, Z. Zeng, Y. Zu, K.S. Elenitoba-Johnson, and M.S. Lim, NPM–ALK signals through glycogen synthase kinase 3β to promote oncogenesis, *Oncogene* **31**(32): 3733–3740 (2012).

Morris, S.W., M.N. Kirstein, M.B. Valentine, K.G. Dittmer, D.N. Shapiro, D.L. Saltman, and A.T. Look, Fusion of a kinase gene, ALK, to a nucleolar protein gene, NPM, in non-Hodgkin's lymphoma, *Science* **263**(5151): 1281–1284 (1994).

Mossé, Y.P., Anaplastic lymphoma kinase as a cancer target in pediatric malignancies, *Clin Canc Res* **22**(3): 546–552 (2016).

Ota, K., K. Azuma, A. Kawahara, S. Hattori, E. Iwama, J. Tanizaki, T. Harada, K. Matsumoto, K. Takayama, S. Takamori, M. Kage, T. Hoshino, Y. Nakanishi, and I. Okamoto, Induction of PD-L1 expression by the EML4-ALK oncoprotein and downstream signaling pathways in non-small cell Lung cancer, *Clin Canc Res* **21**(17): 4014–4021 (2015).

Ott, G., T. Katzenberger, R. Siebert, J.F. DeCoteau, J.A. Fletcher, J.H. Knoll, J. Kalla, A. Rosenwald, M.M. Ott, K. Weber-Matthiesen, M.E. Kadin, and H.K. Müller-Hermelink, Chromosomal abnormalities in nodal and extranodal CD30+ anaplastic large cell lymphomas: infrequent detection of the t(2;5) in extranodal lymphomas, *Genes Chromosomes Canc* **22**(2): 114–121 (1998).

Ouchi, K., M. Miyachi, Y. Tsuma, K. Tsuchiya, T. Iehara, E. Konishi, A. Yanagisawa, and H. Hosoi, FN1: a novel fusion partner of ALK in an inflammatory myofibroblastic tumor, *Pediatr Blood Canc* **62**(5): 909–911 (2015).

Patel, A.S., K.M. Murphy, A.L. Hawkins, J.S. Cohen, P.P. Long, E.J. Perlman, and C.A. Griffin, RANBP2 and CLTC are involved in ALK rearrangements in inflammatory myofibroblastic tumors, *Canc Genet Cytogenet* **176**(2): 107–114 (2007).

Pearson, J.D., Z. Mohammed, J.T. Bacani, R. Lai, and R.J. Ingham, The heat shock protein-90 co-chaperone, Cyclophilin 40, promotes ALK-positive, anaplastic large cell lymphoma viability and its expression is regulated by the NPM-ALK oncoprotein, *BMC Canc* **12**: 229 (2012).

Pérot, G., I. Soubeyran, A. Ribeiro, B. Bonhomme, F. Savagner, N. Boutet-Bouzamondo, I. Hostein, F. Bonichon, Y. Godbert, and F. Chibon, Identification of a recurrent STRN/ALK fusion in thyroid carcinomas, *PLoS One* **9**(1): e87170 (2014).

Ren, W., B.O. Zhang, J. Ma, W. Li, J. Lan, H. Men, and Q. Zhang, EML4-ALK translocation is associated with early onset of disease and other clinicopathological features in Chinese female never-smokers with non-small-cell lung cancer, *Oncol Lett* **10**(6): 3385–3392 (2015).

Richards, M.W., E.W. Law, L.P. Rennalls, S. Busacca, L. O'Regan, A.M. Fry, D.A. Fennell, and R. Bayliss, Crystal structure of EML1 reveals the basis for Hsp90 dependence of oncogenic EML4-ALK by disruption of an atypical β-propeller domain, *Proc Natl Acad Sci USA* **111**(14): 5195–5200 (2014).

Riera, L., E. Lasorsa, C. Ambrogio, N. Surrenti, C. Voena, R. Chiarle, Involvement of Grb2 adaptor protein in nucleophosmin-anaplastic lymphoma kinase (NPM-ALK)-mediated signaling and anaplastic large cell lymphoma growth, *J Biol Chem* **285**(34): 26441–26450 (2010).

Röttgers, S., M. Gombert, A. Teigler-Schlegel, K. Busch, U. Gamerdinger, R. Slany, J. Harbott, and A. Borkhardt, ALK fusion genes in children with atypical myeloproliferative leukemia, *Leukemia* **24**(6): 1197–1200 (2010).

Sakamoto, K., H. Nakasone, Y. Togashi, S. Sakata, N. Tsuyama, S. Baba, A. Dobashi, R. Asaka, C.C. Tsai, S.S. Chuang, K. Izutsu, Y. Kanda, and K, Takeuchi, ALK-positive large B-cell lymphoma: identification of EML4-ALK and a review of the literature focusing on the ALK immunohistochemical staining pattern, *Int J Hematol* **103**(4): 399–408 (2016).

Shin, S., J. Kim, S.O. Yoon, Y.R. Kim, and K.A. Lee, ALK-positive anaplastic large cell lymphoma with TPM3-ALK translocation, *Leuk Res* **36**(7): e143–145 (2012).

Shinmura, K., S. Kageyama, H. Tao, T. Bunai, M. Suzuki, T. Kamo, K. Takamochi, K. Suzuki, M. Tanahashi, H. Niwa, H. Ogawa, and H. Sugimura EML4-ALK fusion transcripts, but no NPM-, TPM3-, CLTC-, ATIC-, or TFG-ALK fusion transcripts, in non-small cell lung carcinomas, *Lung Canc* **61**(2): 163–169 (2008).

Shiota, M., S. Nakamura, R. Ichinohasama, M. Abe, T. Akagi, M. Takeshita, N. Mori, J. Fujimoto, J. Miyauchi, A. Mikata, K. Nanba, T. Takami, H. Yamabe, Y. Takano, T. Izumo, T. Nagatani, N. Mohri, K. Nasu, H. Satoh, H. Katano, J. Fujimoto, T. Yamamoto, and S. Mori, Anaplastic large cell lymphomas expressing the novel chimeric protein p80NPM/ALK: a distinct clinicopathologic entity, *Blood* **86**(5): 1954–1960 (1995).

Slupianek, A., M. Nieborowska-Skorska, G. Hoser, A. Morrione, M. Majewski, L. Xue, S.W. Morris, M.A. Wasik, and T. Skorski, Role of phosphatidylinositol 3-kinase-Akt pathway in nucleophosmin/anaplastic lymphoma kinase-mediated lymphomagenesis, *Canc Res* **61**(5): 2194–2199 (2001).

Slupianek, A. and T. Skorski, NPM/ALK downregulates p27Kip1 in a PI-3K-dependent manner, *Exp Hematol* **32**(12): 1265–1271 (2004).

Smith, N.E., A.T. Deyrup, A. Mariño-Enriquez, J.A. Fletcher, J.A. Bridge, P.B. Illei, G.J. Netto, and P. Argani, VCL-ALK renal cell carcinoma in children with sickle-cell trait: the eighth sickle-cell nephropathy? *Am J Surg Pathol* **38**(6): 858–863 (2014).

Soda, M., Y.L. Choi, M. Enomoto, S. Takada, Y. Yamashita, S. Ishikawa, S. Fujiwara, H. Watanabe, K. Kurashina, H. Hatanaka, M. Bando, S. Ohno, Y. Ishikawa, H. Aburatani, T. Niki, Y. Sohara, Y. Sugiyama, and H. Mano, Identification of the transforming EML4-ALK fusion gene in non-small-cell lung cancer, *Nature* **448**(7153): 561–566 (2007).

Sokai, A., M. Enaka, R. Sokai, S. Mori, S. Mori, M. Gunji, M. Fujino, and M. Ito, Pulmonary inflammatory myofibroblastic tumor harboring EML4-ALK fusion gene, *Jpn J Clin Oncol* **44**(1): 93–96 (2014).

Sozzi, G., M.P. Martelli, D. Conte, P. Modena, V. Pettirossi, S.A. Pileri, and B. Falini, The EML4-ALK transcript but not the fusion protein can be expressed in reactive and neoplastic lymphoid tissues, *Haematologica* **94**(9): 1307–1311 (2009).

Takahashi, D., Y. Nagatoshi, J. Nagayama, J. Inagaki, N. Itonoaga, M. Takeshita, and J. Okamura, Anaplastic large cell lymphoma in leukemic presentation: a case report and a review of the literature, *J Pediatr Hematol Oncol* **30**(9): 696–700 (2008).

Takeoka, K., A. Okumura, Y. Maesako, T. Akasaka, and H. Ohno, Crizotinib resistance in acute myeloid leukemia with inv(2)(p23q13)/RAN binding protein 2 (RANBP2) anaplastic lymphoma kinase (ALK) fusion and monosomy 7, *Canc Genet* **208**(3): 85–90 (2015).

Takeuchi, K., Y.L. Choi, Y. Togashi, M. Soda, S. Hatano, K. Inamura, S. Takada, T. Ueno, Y. Yamashita, Y. Satoh, S. Okumura, K. Nakagawa, Y. Ishikawa, and H. Mano, KIF5B-ALK, a novel fusion oncokinase identified by an immunohistochemistry-based diagnostic system for ALK-positive lung cancer, *Clin Canc Res* **15**(9): 3143–3149 (2009).

Takeuchi, K., M. Soda, Y. Togashi, Y. Ota, Y. Sekiguchi, S. Hatano, R. Asaka, M. Noguchi, and H. Mano, Identification of a novel fusion, SQSTM1-ALK, in ALK-positive large B-cell lymphoma, *Haematologica* **96**(3): 464–467 (2011).

Takezawa, K., I. Okamoto, K. Nishio, P.A. Jänne, and K. Nakagawa, Role of ERK-BIM and STAT3-survivin signaling pathways in ALK inhibitor-induced apoptosis in EML4-ALK-positive lung cancer, *Clin Canc Res* **17**(8): 2140–2148 (2011).

Tanizaki, J., I. Okamoto, T. Okabe, K. Sakai, K. Tanaka, H. Hayashi, H. Kaneda, K. Takezawa, K. Kuwata, H. Yamaguchi, E. Hatashita, K. Nishio, and

K. Nakagawa, Activation of HER family signaling as a mechanism of acquired resistance to ALK inhibitors in EML4–ALK -positive non-small cell lung cancer, *Clin Canc Res* **18**(22): 6219–6226 (2012).

Tetsumoto, S., T. Kijima, E. Morii, S. Goya, T. Minami, H. Hirata, R. Takahashi, S. Kohmo, K. Inoue, I. Nagatomo, Y. Takeda, H. Kida, I. Tachibana, and A. Kumanogoh, Echinoderm microtubule-associated protein-like 4 (EML4)-anaplastic lymphoma kinase (ALK) rearrangement in congenital pulmonary airway malformation, *Clin Lung Cancer* **14**(4): 457–460 (2013).

Togashi, Y., M. Soda, S. Sakata, E. Sugawara, S. Hatano, R. Asaka, T. Nakajima, H. Mano, and K. Takeuchi, KLC1-ALK: a novel fusion in lung cancer identified using a formalin-fixed paraffin-embedded tissue only, *PLoS One* **7**(2): e31323 (2012).

Tort, F., E. Campo, B. Pohlman, and E. Hsi, Heterogeneity of genomic breakpoints in MSN-ALK translocations in anaplastic large cell lymphoma, *Hum Pathol* **35**(8): 1038–1041 (2004).

Touriol, C., C. Greenland, L. Lamant, K. Pulford, F. Bernard, T. Rousset, D.Y. Mason, and G. Delsol, Further demonstration of the diversity of chromosomal changes involving 2p23 in ALK-positive lymphoma: 2 cases expressing ALK kinase fused to CLTCL (clathrin chain polypeptide-like), *Blood* **95**(10): 3204–3207 (2000).

Trümper, L., M. Pfreundschuh, F.V. Bonin, and H. Daus, Detection of the t(2;5)-associated NPM/ALK fusion cDNA in peripheral blood cells of healthy individuals, *Br J Haematol* **103**(4): 1138–1144 (1998).

Turturro, F., M.D. Arnold, A.Y. Frist, and K. Pulford, Model of inhibition of the NPM-ALK kinase activity by herbimycin A, *Clin Cancer Res* **8**(1): 240–245 (2002).

Van Roosbroeck, K., J. Cools, D. Dierickx, J. Thomas, P. Vandenberghe, M. Stul, J. Delabie, C. De Wolf-Peeters, P. Marynen, and I. Wlodarska, ALK-positive large B-cell lymphomas with cryptic SEC31A-ALK and NPM1-ALK fusions, *Haematologica* **95**(3): 509–513 (2010).

Vishwamitra, D., C.V. Curry, P. Shi, S. Alkan, and H.M. Amin, SUMOylation confers posttranslational stability on NPM-ALK Oncogenic Protein, *Neoplasia* **17**(9): 742–754 (2015).

Wang, W.Y., L. Gu, W.P. Liu, G.D. Li, H.J. Liu, and Z.G. Ma, ALK-positive extramedullary plasmacytoma with expression of the CLTC-ALK fusion transcript, *Pathol Res Pract* **207**(9): 587–591 (2011).

Wasik, M.A., Q. Zhang, M. Marzec, M. Kasprzycka, H.Y. Wang, and X. Liu, Anaplastic lymphoma kinase (ALK)-induced malignancies: novel mechanisms of cell transformation and potential therapeutic approaches, *Semin Oncol* **36**(2 Suppl 1): S27–S35 (2009).

Weber-Matthiesen, K., J. Deerberg-Wittram, A. Rosenwald, M. Poetsch, W. Grote, and B. Schlegelberger, Translocation t(2;5) is not a primary event in Hodgkin's disease. Simultaneous immunophenotyping and interphase cytogenetics, *Am J Pathol* **149**(2): 463–468 (1996).

Weiss, L.M., J.R. Lopategui, L.H. Sun, O.W. Kamel, C.H. Koo, and C. Glackin, Absence of the t(2;5) in Hodgkin's disease, *Blood* **85**(10): 2845–2847 (1995).

Wellmann, A., V. Doseeva, W. Butscher, M. Raffeld, P. Fukushima, M. Stetler-Stevenson, and K. Gardner, The activated anaplastic lymphoma kinase increases cellular proliferation and oncogene up-regulation in rat 1a fibroblasts, *FASEB J* **11**(12): 965–972 (1997).

Wong, D.W., E.L. Leung, S.K. Wong, V.P. Tin, A.D. Sihoe, L.C. Cheng, J.S. Au, L.P. Chung, and M.P. Wong, A novel KIF5B-ALK variant in nonsmall cell lung cancer, *Cancer* **117**(12): 2709–2718 (2011).

Wu, C., O. Molavi, H. Zhang, N. Gupta, A. Alshareef, K.M. Bone, K. Gopal, F. Wu, J.T. Lewis, D.N. Douglas, and N.M. Kneteman, R. Lai, STAT1 is phosphorylated and downregulated by the oncogenic tyrosine kinase NPM-ALK in ALK-positive anaplastic large-cell lymphoma, *Blood* **126**(3): 336–345 (2015).

Wu, F., P. Wang, L.C. Young, R. Lai, and L. Li, Proteome-wide identification of novel binding partners to the oncogenic fusion gene protein, NPM-ALK, using tandem affinity purification and mass spectrometry, *Am J Pathol* **174**(2): 361–370 (2009).

Xu, C.W., G. Wang, W.L. Wang, W.B. Gao, C.J. Han, J.S. Gao, L.Y. Zhang, Y. Li, L. Wang, Y.P. Zhang, Y.W. Tian, and D.D. Qi, Association between EML4-ALK fusion gene and thymidylate synthase mRNA expression in non-small cell lung cancer tissues, *Exp Ther Med* **9**(6): 2151–2154 (2015).

Yakirevich, E., M.B. Resnick, S. Mangray, M. Wheeler, C.L. Jackson, K.A. Lombardo, J. Lee, K.M. Kim, A.J. Gill, K. Wang, K. Gowen, J. Sun, V.A. Miller, P.J. Stephens, S.M. Ali, J.S. Ross, and H. Safran, Oncogenic ALK fusion in rare and aggressive subtype of colorectal adenocarcinoma as a potential therapeutic target, *Clin Canc Res* **22**(15): 3831–3840 (2016).

Yamada, T., S. Takeuchi, J. Nakade, K. Kita, T. Nakagawa, S. Nanjo, T. Nakamura, K. Matsumoto, M. Soda, H. Mano, T. Uenaka, and S. Yano, Paracrine receptor activation by microenvironment triggers bypass survival signals and ALK inhibitor resistance in EML4-ALK lung cancer cells, *Clin Canc Res* **18**(13): 3592–3602 (2012).

Yamaguchi, N., A.R. Lucena-Araujo, S. Nakayama, L.L. de Figueiredo-Pontes, D.A. Gonzalez, H. Yasuda, S. Kobayashi, D.B. Costa, Dual ALK and EGFR inhibition targets a mechanism of acquired resistance to the tyrosine kinase inhibitor crizotinib in ALK rearranged lung cancer, *Lung Canc* **83**(1): 37–43 (2014).

Yokoyama, N., and W.T. Miller, Molecular characterization of WDCP, a novel fusion partner for the anaplastic lymphoma tyrosine kinase ALK, *Biomed Rep* **3**(1): 9–13 (2015).

Yoshida, A., T. Shibata, K. Tsuta, S. Watanabe, and H. Tsuda, Inflammatory myofibroblastic tumor of the lung with a novel PPFIBP1-ALK fusion variant, *Histopathology* **63**(6): 881–883 (2013).

Zhang, Q., H. Wang, K. Kantekure, J.C. Paterson, X. Liu, A. Schaffer, C. Paulos, M.C. Milone, N. Odum, S. Turner, T. Marafioti, and M.A. Wasik, Oncogenic tyrosine kinase NPM–ALK induces expression of the growth-promoting receptor ICOS, *Blood* **118**(11): 3062–3071 (2011a).

Zhang, Q., H.Y. Wang, X. Liu, G. Bhutani, K. Kantekure, and M. Wasik, IL-2R common gamma-chain is epigenetically silenced by nucleophosphin-anaplastic lymphoma kinase (NPM-ALK) and acts as a tumor suppressor by targeting NPM-ALK, *Proc Natl Acad Sci USA* **108**(29): 11977–11982 (2011b).

Zhang, Q., H.Y. Wang, X. Liu, and M.A. Wasik, STAT5A is epigenetically silenced by the tyrosine kinase NPM1-ALK and acts as a tumor suppressor by reciprocally inhibiting NPM1-ALK expression, *Nat Med* **13**(11): 1341–1348 (2007).

Zhang, Q., F. Wei, H.Y. Wang, X. Liu, D. Roy, Q.B. Xiong, S. Jiang, A. Medvec, G. Danet-Desnoyers, C. Watt, E. Tomczak, M. Kalos, J.L. Riley, and M.A. Wasik, The potent oncogene NPM–ALK mediates malignant transformation of normal human CD4(+) T lymphocytes, *Am J Pathol* **183**(6): 1971–1980 (2013).

Zhang, X., S. Zhang, X. Yang, J. Yang, Q. Zhou, L. Yin, S. An, J. Lin, S. Chen, Z. Xie, M. Zhu, X. Zhang, and Y.L. Wu, Fusion of EML4 and ALK is associated with development of lung adenocarcinomas lacking EGFR and KRAS mutations and is correlated with ALK expression, *Mol Canc* **9**: 188.

5

Role of BCR-ABL Fusion Kinase in the Development of Leukemia

*Ganesan Padmavathi, Kishore Banik, Nand K. Roy, Javadi Monisha and Ajaikumar B. Kunnumakkara**

INTRODUCTION

CML is a malignant disorder characterized by the clonal proliferation of blood cells specifically myeloid cells in bone marrow, and myeloid cells, erythroid cells and platelets in peripheral blood (Sawyers, 1999). Identification of the Philadelphia chromosome in 1960 was a milestone in the diagnosis and treatment of this disease. This shortened chromosome 22 was believed to be the key responsible factor for the development of CML until 1973 when the chromosomal translocation t(9;22)

*Author for correspondence: Ajaikumar B. Kunnumakkara, Cancer Biology Laboratory, Department of Biosciences and Bioengineering, Indian Institute of Technology Guwahati, Assam 781039, India. kunnumakkara@iitg.ernet.in

(q34;q11) involving the BCR and Abelson murine leukemia (ABL) genes were first discovered (Figure 5.1) (Sawyers, 1999). More than 95% of the CML patients are reported to be t(9;22) carriers and rest are either complex or variant translocation carriers. Ultimately, all these translocations are resulting in the fusion oncogene BCR-ABL which produces a constitutively active cytoplasmic tyrosine kinase and activates various signaling cascades involved in cell survival and proliferation (Sawyers, 1999; Granatowicz *et al.*, 2015). Also, expression of this fusion oncogene was proved to severely affect the normal process of embryogenesis as the BCR-ABL inserted fertilized one-cell embryos failed to develop transgenic progeny when re-implanted into foster mothers (Heisterkamp *et al.*, 1991).

Interestingly, the activity of this oncoprotein is not exactly same in all leukemic patients. For example, some had long latency period whereas some cases were found with very short period of latency before the development of disease (Voncken *et al.*, 1995; Lugo *et al.*, 1990). Reason for this difference in activity was found to be the variation in BCR of the BCR-ABL fusion gene. Mainly, three well defined breakpoint cluster

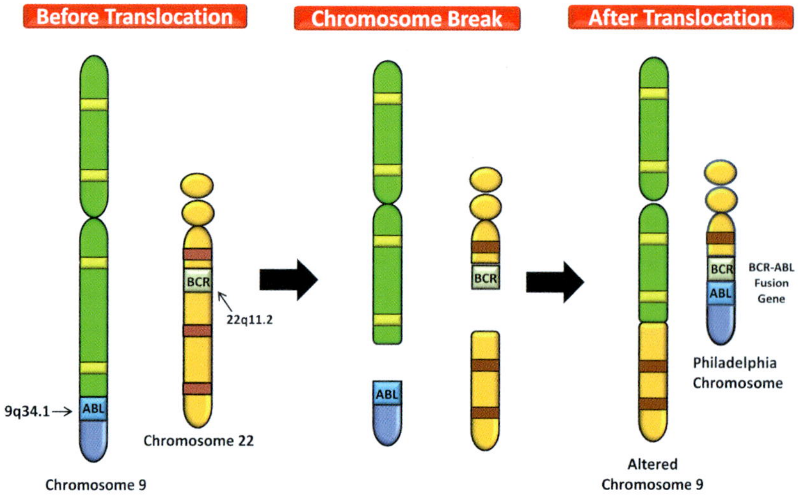

Figure 5.1: Translocation of BCR-ABL (t(9;22)(q34;q11)).

regions were reported to be involved in the gene fusion: a minor (m-BCR) in the first intron, a major BCR (M-BCR) between exons 12–16 and a μ-BCR in the 19th intron which resulted in three different oncoproteins with different molecular weight and different extent of kinase activity. Further, p190 (190 kDa), p210 (210 kDa) and p230 (230 kDa) were found to be the three chimeric proteins produced by ABL fusion with M-BCR, *m*-BCR and μ-BCR, respectively (Figure 5.2) (Ye *et al.*, 2014). The potency and kinase activity of p190 is much greater than p210 which correlated with the disease phenotypes. It was found that p190 is mainly associated with ALL and resulted in poor prognosis due to its higher tyrosine kinase activity whereas p210 was found to be associated more with CML (Voncken *et al.*, 1995; Lugo *et al.*, 1990; Ye *et al.*, 2014).

BCR-ABL fusion protein contains multiple domains with different functions. The ABL portion of the protein is same in all the three variants p190, p210 and p230 consisting of Src-homology (SH3 and SH2)

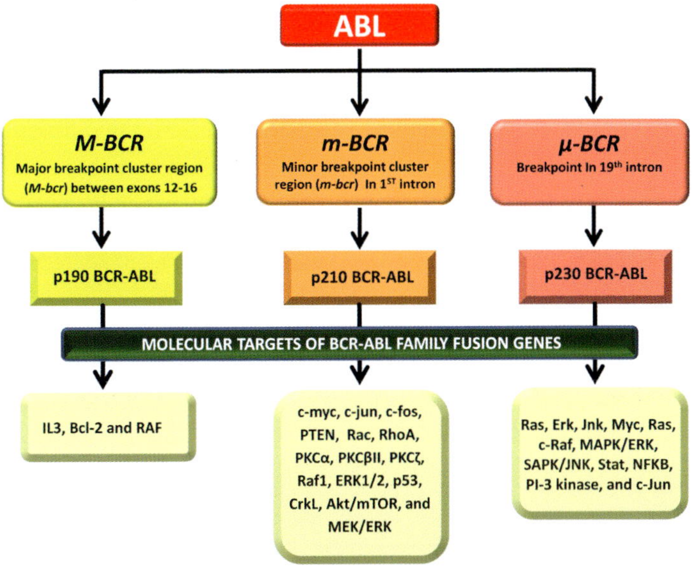

Figure 5.2: Different splice variants of BCR-ABL and their molecular targets.

domains, actin-binding domain, DNA-binding domain, tyrosine kinase domain, nuclear localization and export signals. SH2 domain helps in binding and phosphorylation of various signaling molecules like p62dok, c-Cbl and Rin1. Actin-binding domain facilitates the interaction with cytoskeleton and helps in the phosphorylation of cytoskeletal proteins (Advani and Pendergast, 2002). Unlike the ABL region, the extent of BCR regions varies significantly between p190, p210 and p230 due to the differential breakpoints. In general, the structural components of the BCR portion includes: a coiled-coil (CC) oligomerization domain and serine/threonine kinase domain which are common in all the three variants; pleckstrin homology (PH) domain and Dbl homology (DH) domain which are present only in p210 and p230; a calcium/phospholipid binding domain (CalB) and a Gap–Rac domain which are exclusive to p230 (Advani and Pendergast, 2002). The DH domain assists in guanine exchange between Rho family of small GTPases and the PH domain binds to various cellular proteins including PLCε, Zizimin1, tubulin and SMC1. Interaction of PH domain with phosphoinositides helps in the cellular localization of BCR-ABL (Miroshnychenko *et al.*, 2010).

Imatinib (INN), a small molecule tyrosine kinase inhibitor approved by Food & Drug Administration (FDA) in 2001 is used for the treatment of several cancers especially the Ph+ CML. Being a tyrosine kinase inhibitor (TKI), it has been found to effectively inhibit the chimeric tyrosine kinase activity of BCR-ABL which is exclusively present in cancer cells thus marking it to be a targeted therapy leaving the normal cells intact (Al-Hadiya *et al.*, 2014; Waller, 2014). Despite being effective in clinics, most often it is associated with adverse side effects like diarrhea, mild to moderate edema, myelosuppression, nausea and skin rashes. Moreover, chemoresistance developed against INN is yet another challenge requiring novel second- and third-generation TKIs for better management of such resistant disease (Waller, 2014).

p210 BCR-ABL

As mentioned earlier, p210 BCR-ABL is a subtype of BCR-ABL fusion gene produced by the fusion of ABL (a2) with the M-BCR (b2/b3) and found in 80–90% of CML patients (Tan *et al.*, 2012). The resulting fusion transcripts b2a2 and b3a2 generate 210 kDa protein isomers, which differ only in 25 amino acids coded by the b3 exon and a Glu903Asp substitution (Tan *et al.*, 2012; Hai *et al.*, 2014). Recent study showed that b3a2 rearrangement is more common in older patients and is associated with higher platelet count (Bennour *et al.*, 2013). However, the leukemogenic activities of these two isomers are found to be similar (Uchida *et al.*, 2009). The *in silico* modeling of these isomers revealed their variations in the secondary structural elements particularly in the SH3, SH2, SH1 and DNA-binding domains, which is expected to be the reason for the possible differences in their role during CML progression (Hai *et al.*, 2014). The 5′ non-coding sequence from BCR gene was found to regulate the transforming and tumorigenic activity of p210 BCR-ABL and p190 BCR-ABL (Gishizky *et al.*, 1991). The guanine nucleotide exchange factor (GEF) activity of p210 differentiates it from the p190 variant. Supporting this, the mutated p210 with no GEF activity has been shown to induce acute disease similar to that of p190 (Tala *et al.*, 2013). p210 has been shown to increase the tyrosine kinase activity which results in increased autophosphorylation and phosphorylation of various cellular proteins (Naldini *et al.*, 1986; Ben-Neriah *et al.*, 1986). Interestingly, expression of p210 transcript was detected in normal healthy individuals suggesting the fact that the expression of BCR-ABL alone is insufficient to induce the disease (Foley *et al.*, 2013; Ismail *et al.*, 2014). Further, the presence of p210 BCR-ABL with additional molecular alterations and chromosomal abnormalities is believed to drive the transition of CML from chronic phase to blast crisis (Gorska-Flipot *et al.*, 1990). However, further investigations are required to elucidate its exact association with the risk of developing leukemia (Ismail *et al.*, 2014).

p210 has been found to be complexed with a 53 kDa cellular protein in K562 cells and with p160, a BCR related gene product (Li *et al.*, 1988; Campbell *et al.*, 1990) and known to preferentially induce the proliferation of immature B-lineage cells even in myeloid lineage-enriched cultures (Young *et al.*, 1988). The autophosphorylation and the p160 BCR specific transphosphorylation activity of p210 fusion tyrosine kinase was found to be restricted to the tyrosine residues present in the first exon of BCR. This exon specific kinase activity of p210 was believed to modulate signal transduction activities of p160 BCR (Liu *et al.*, 1993). p210 BCR-ABL transfected Rat-1 cells, rodent fibroblast cells, attained major morphological transformation and exhibited tumorigenicity (Lugo and Witte, 1989). It also induced growth factor independent proliferation in lymphoid and myeloid cells through elevated expression of oncogenes like *c-myc*, *c-jun* and *c-fos* (Mandanas *et al.*, 1992). It has been proved that transforming activity of p210 tyrosine kinase requires autophosphorylation of Tyr1294 residue in the SH1 domain. However, it is not essential for the induction of growth factor-independence (Pendergast *et al.*, 1993a). p210 downregulated and delocalized the tumor suppressor phosphatase and tensin homolog (PTEN) which plays a crucial role in the development of CML (Panuzzo *et al.*, 2014; Morotti *et al.*, 2014) and the p210 induced transformation of hematopoietic cells was found to be mediated through the activation of small GTP-binding protein Rac (Skorski *et al.*, 1998). Besides inducing survival and proliferation of cells, p210 also increased the motility of cells which contributed to the invasiveness of the disease. Ectopic expression of p210 has been shown to induce amoeboid motility in Ba/F3 cells which was mediated through RhoA specific p210 BCR-ABL DH/PH domain, Rac1 activity and Vav1 in complex with BCR-ABL (Daubon *et al.*, 2012).

It has been shown that 12-O-tetradecanoylphorbol-13-acetate (TPA) treatment reduced the kinase activity of p210 in K562 cells which in turn reduced the cell proliferation and induced differentiation. It also inhibited the phosphorylation of p160 BCR in BCR-ABL/BCR complexes implicating that BCR-ABL induced phosphorylation of p160 BCR may play a major role in CML (Campbell *et al.*, 1993). The constitutive expression of p210 was found to be efficiently suppressed by oligonucleotides and/or transduced anti-sense sequences (Lewalle and Martiat, 1993). Moreover, sensitivity of p210 BCR-ABL to protein tyrosine phosphatase (PTPase) present in the granulocytes lysate was found to be equal to that of p190 BCR-ABL (Nishimura *et al.*, 1991). However, the cellular substrates varied significantly for these oncoproteins suggesting that the downstream pathways may also differ (Nishimura *et al.*, 1992). Treatment of KU812 and K562 cells with phenethyl isothiocyanate (PEITC), a natural isothiocyanate, was shown to increase the INN sensitivity through the downregulation of PKCα, PKCβII, PKCζ, Raf1 and ERK1/2 which ultimately inhibited the cross talk between p210 BCR-ABL and PKC signaling (Figure 5.2) (Roy *et al.*, 2015). Ectopic expression of KLWVIPQ, a heptapeptide which precisely recognized the IFN-α-sensitive CML cells has been shown to reduce the cell viability and induce apoptosis in IFN-α-sensitive KT-1/A3 cells through the downregulation of p210 and upregulation of p53 (Yang *et al.*, 2015). TKI treatment in p210 positive ALL patients was recently proved to induce E255V, D276G and F317L mutations in BCR-ABL1 kinase domain which may assist in the development of TKI resistance which leads to the poor prognosis (Molinos-Quintana *et al.*, 2015). As the oligomerization of p210 BCR-ABL at N-terminal CC domain was found to be essential for its tyrosine kinase activity, specific targeting of this CC domain by CC(mut3), a peptidomimetic delivered by leukemia-specific cell-penetrating peptide (CPP), inhibited BCR-ABL activity and induced apoptosis in CML cells (Bruno *et al.*, 2015). E35, a novel derivative of emodin, was shown to downregulate the levels of p210, phospho-p210 and its downstream targets including CrkL, Akt/mTOR and MEK-ERK signaling in imatinib mesylate (IM) resistant leukaemic cells (Li *et al.*, 2015a). Further, it has been proved that interaction of SH3 domain of p210 with the proline-rich region of apoptin, a chicken anemia viral protein that exhibits selective toxicity to cancer cells, can reduce its kinase activity. Additionally, a synthetic apoptin-derived decapeptide was also shown to effectively downregulate p210 and its downstream target c-Myc ultimately leading to inhibition of cell proliferation (Jangamreddy *et al.*, 2014).

p190 BCR-ABL

p190, also termed as p185 BCR-ABL, is the smallest of all the variants, detected in 60–75% of Ph+ ALL and in only 1% of CML (Yeung and Hughes, 2012; Melo *et al.*, 1994; Tan *et al.*, 2012). It has been proved to induce the expansion of lymphoid cells with a very high tumorigenic activity than the other fusion variants. It also induced growth factor independence *in vitro* (Advani and Pendergast, 2002). As already mentioned, it contains the coiled-coil dimerization domain, the GRJ32 binding site at Tyr177, and the phospho-serine/threonine rich SH2 binding domain which are crucial for the constitutive activation of ABL tyrosine kinase. The predominant expression of p190 BCR-ABL in ALL indicated that the small BCR structural components present in p190 may interact with various signaling cascades that are mainly involved in lymphoid and monocyte differentiation (Melo, 1996). p190 was also shown to inhibit interleukin-3 (IL3) deprivation induced apoptosis in 32Dcl3 cells through the upregulation anti-apoptotic protein Bcl-2 and RAF (Figure 5.2) (Salomoni *et al.*, 1998). Similar to p210, p190 also increased the motility of cells and augmented the invasiveness of the disease. Expression of p190 was shown to induce rolling movements through the formation of invadopodia which is attributed to complex formation of Vav1 and BCR-ABL, and Rac1 activity (Daubon *et al.*, 2012).

Co-expression of p190 and p210 was also found in CML, however, the frequency was very low (Tabassum *et al.*, 2014). It has also been found to be co-expressed with another fusion gene- ETV6-RUNX1 in a 3-year-old boy with B-cell ALL (B-ALL). In this patient, bone marrow was hypercellular and completely accumulated with agranular lymphoid blast cells. This patient showed a better prognosis after standard chemotherapy (Balatzenko *et al.*, 2013).

CML patients with p190 showed poor response to TKI therapy developing resistance to first generation TKIs (Verma *et al.*, 2009). However, treatment with second generation TKIs is believed to give better outcome (Molica *et al.*, 2015). Unfortunately, this TKI treatment alone was not sufficient due to chemoresistance and disease relapse (Lee *et al.*, 2011). p190 BCR-ABL fusion protein contains a unique amino acid sequence that do not belong to either of the fusion partners, thus specific to only BCR-ABL. Peptide vaccines derived from this unique region were shown to induce immune reaction mediated by CD4+ T cells against Ph+ ALL which can synergize TKI treatment and give better treatment outcome (Ippoliti *et al.*, 2012; Riva *et al.*, 2010).

p230 BCR-ABL

μ-BCR-ABL or p230 BCR-ABL chimera is a fusion of e19 BCR with a2 ABL. e19a2 is found in chronic neutrophilic leukaemia (CNL) and rarely in CML patients and mostly associated with benign clinical course unless there are additional genetic abnormalities (Oshikawa *et al.*, 2010; Advani and Pendergast, 2002). It fuses almost entire BCR with ABL thus contains a CalB domain and a GTPase activating p21rac (GAP) domain which are lacking in p190 and p210 variants (Advani and Pendergast, 2002; Pane *et al.*, 1996). p230 exhibits less tyrosine kinase activity than the other variants (Haskovec *et al.*, 1998) and the low levels of p230 in neutrophilic-chronic myeloid leukemia (CML-N) were found to be associated with indolent disease course and better prognosis (Verstovsek *et al.*, 2002). INN therapy suppressed the myeloproliferative disease in p230 overexpressing transgenic mice by reducing its expression (Inami *et al.*, 2006). However, the acquired E255K and G250E mutations in ABL kinase domain during INN therapy were found responsible for the treatment failure in p230 positive CML patients (Li *et al.*, 2015b).

Like the other two variants, p230 also induced growth factor independence in 32D cells, a lineage-restricted hematopoietic cell line. It also activated Ras, ERK and JNK signaling cascades in these cells indicating the similar survival, proliferative, and tumorigenic effects of three BCR-ABL variants. However, the tumorigenicity of p230 was limited in comparison with other variants in case of lineage-unrestricted primary mouse bone marrow cells (Quackenbush *et al.*, 2000). It has been found to be complexed with GRB2, indicating the probable association with Ras activation pathway (Wada *et al.*, 1995). All the three chimeras were proved to induce leukemogenesis through the phosphorylation and downstream activation of several proliferative signaling pathways like c-Jun, c-Raf, MAPK-ERK, Myc, NF-κB, PI3K, Ras, SAPK-JNK and STAT (Figure 5.3) (Cortez *et al.*, 1995, 1997; Pendergast *et al.*, 1993b; Salomoni *et al.*, 1998; Okuda *et al.*, 1994; Burgess *et al.*, 1998; Sawyers *et al.*, 1992; Shuai *et al.*, 1996; Ilaria and Van Etten, 1996; Skorski *et al.*, 1997; Reuther *et al.*, 1998). It also increased angiogenesis both *in vitro* and *in vivo* through the increased secretion of various angiogenic factors like VEGF, FGF-2, HGF, IL-8 and matrix metalloproteinases (MMPs) (Figure 5.2) (Janowska-Wieczorek *et al.*, 2002). The transforming activity of BCR-ABL was found to be mediated through the activation of PI3K-Akt signaling (Griffin, 2001).

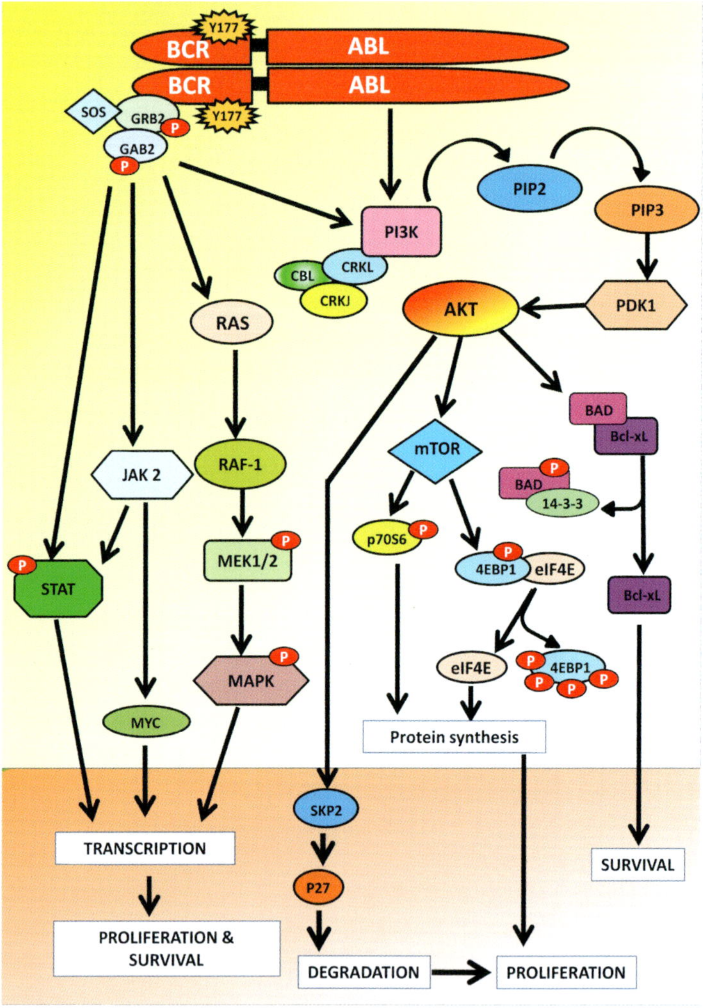

Figure 5.3: Molecular targets involved in BCR-ABL mediated leukemogenesis.

CONCLUSION

Taken together, increased frequency of BCR-ABL rearrangements resulted in poor survival. Various TKIs dramatically increased the treatment options which attributed to better prognosis of Ph+ leukemic patients. INN, dasatinib, nilotinib, hydroxyurea (HU), interferon alpha (IFN-α) with

HU and bone marrow transplantation are the treatment options available for this disease. However, most of these therapies are not effective due to the development of resistance and adverse side effects implicating the requirement of additional therapeutic options. Even though, combination of TKI with allogeneic hematopoietic stem cell transplantation (allo-HSCT) is believed to give better prognosis, the cost of the therapy is extremely high. Therefore, more extensive research is required to identify and explore novel, safe, potent and cost-effective therapy for this disease.

CONFLICT OF INTEREST

The authors express no conflict of interest.

REFERENCES

Advani, A.S. and A.M. Pendergast, Bcr-Abl variants: biological and clinical aspects, *Leuk Res* **26**: 713–720 (2002).

Al-Hadiya, B.M., A.H. Bakheit, and A.A. Abd-Elgalil, Imatinib mesylate, *Profiles Drug Subst Excip Relat Methodol* **39**: 265–297 (2014).

Balatzenko, G., M. Guenova, I. Kalinova, M. Belcheva, H. Hristozova, and V. Kaleva, Simultaneous occurrence of ETV6-RUNX1 and BCR-ABL1 (e1a2) transcripts in a child with B-cell acute lymphoblastic leukemia, *Canc Genet* **206**: 97–101 (2013).

Ben-Neriah, Y., G.Q. Daley, A.M. Mes-Masson, O.N. Witte, and D. Baltimore, The chronic myelogenous leukemia-specific P210 protein is the product of the bcr/abl hybrid gene, *Science* **233**: 212–214 (1986).

Bennour, A., I. Ouahchi, B. Achour, M. Zaier, Y.B. Youssef, A. Khelif, A. Saad, and H. Sennana, Analysis of the clinico-hematological relevance of the breakpoint location within M-BCR in chronic myeloid leukemia, *Med Oncol* **30**: 348 (2013).

Bruno, B.J. and C.S. Lim, Inhibition of bcr-abl in human leukemic cells with a coiled-coil protein delivered by a leukemia-specific cell-penetrating Peptide, *Mol Pharm* **12**: 1412–1421 (2015).

Burgess, G.S., E.A. Williamson, L.D. Cripe, S. Litz-Jackson, J.A. Bhatt, K. Stanley, M.J. Stewart, A.S. Kraft, H. Nakshatri, and H.S. Boswell, Regulation of the c-jun gene in p210 BCR-ABL transformed cells corresponds with activity of JNK, the c-jun N-terminal kinase, *Blood* **92**: 2450–2460 (1998).

Campbell, M.L., W. Li, and R.B. Arlinghaus, P210 BCR-ABL is complexed to P160 BCR and ph-P53 proteins in K562 cells, *Oncogene* **5**: 773–776 (1990).

Campbell, M.L., D. Lu, J.Q. Guo, and R.B. Arlinghaus, Inhibition of phosphorylation of p160 BCR within p210 BCR-ABL complexes during early stages of phorbol ester-induced differentiation of K562 cells, *Cell Growth Differ* **4**: 581–588 (1993).

Cortez, D., L. Kadlec, and A.M. Pendergast, Structural and signaling requirements for BCR-ABL-mediated transformation and inhibition of apoptosis, *Mol Cell Biol* **15**: 5531–5541 (1995).

Cortez, D., G. Reuther, and A.M. Pendergast, The Bcr-Abl tyrosine kinase activates mitogenic signaling pathways and stimulates G1-to-S phase transition in hematopoietic cells, *Oncogene* **15**: 2333–2342 (1997).

Daubon, T., T. Rochelle, N. Bourmeyster, and E. Génot, Invadopodia and rolling-type motility are specific features of highly invasive p190(bcr-abl) leukemic cells, *Eur J Cell Biol* **91**: 978–987 (2012).

Foley, S.B., Z.L. Hildenbrand, A.A. Soyombo, J.A. Magee, Y. Wu, K.I. Oravecz-Wilson, and T.S. Ross, Expression of BCR/ABL p210 from a knockin allele enhances bone marrow engraftment without inducing neoplasia, *Cell Rep* **5**: 51–60 (2013).

Gishizky, M.L., J. McLaughlin, A.M. Pendergast, and O.N. Witte, The 5′ non-coding region of the BCR/ABL oncogene augments its ability to stimulate the growth of immature lymphoid cells, *Oncogene* **6**: 1299–1306 (1991).

Gorska-Flipot, I., C. Norman, L. Addy, and M. Minden, Molecular pathology of chronic myelogenous leukemia, *Tumor Biol* **11** (Suppl): 25–43 (1990).

Granatowicz, A., C.I. Piatek, E. Moschiano, I. El-Hemaidi, J.D. Armitage, and M. Akhtari, An overview and update of chronic myeloid leukemia for primary care physicians, *Korean J Fam Med* **36**: 197–202 (2015).

Griffin, J.D., Phosphatidyl inositol signaling by BCR/ABL: opportunities for drug development, *Canc Chemother Pharmacol* **48**(Suppl 1): S11–S16 (2001).

Hai, A., N.A. Kizilbash, S.H. Zaidi, J. Alruwaili, and K. Shahzad, Differences in structural elements of Bcr-Abl oncoprotein isoforms in chronic myelogenous leukemia, *Bioinformation* **10**: 108–114 (2014).

Haskovec, C., C. Ponzetto, J. Polák, D. Maritano, Z. Zemanová, A. Serra, K. Michalová, H. Klamová, J. Cermák, and G. Saglio, P230 BCR/ABL protein may be associated with an acute leukaemia phenotype, *Br J Haematol* **103**: 1104–1108 (1998).

Heisterkamp, N., G. Jenster, D. Kioussis, P.K. Pattengale, and J. Groffen, Human bcr-abl gene has a lethal effect on embryogenesis, *Transgenic Res* **1**: 45–53 (1991).

Ilaria, R.L. Jr. and R.A. Van Etten, P210 and P190(BCR/ABL) induce the tyrosine phosphorylation and DNA binding activity of multiple specific STAT family members, *J Biol Chem* **271**: 31704–31710 (1996).

Inami, M., K. Inokuchi, H. Yamaguchi, K. Nakayama, A. Watanabe, N. Uchida, S. Tanosaki, and K. Dan, Oral administration of imatinib to P230 BCR/ABL-expressing transgenic mice changes clones with high BCR/ABL complementary DNA expression into those with low expression, *Int J Hematol* **84**: 346–353 (2006).

Ippoliti, M., M. Defina, A. Gozzini, C. Baratè, L. Aprile, A. Pietrini, A. Gozzetti, D. Raspadori, F. Lauria, and M. Bocchia, Identification of a novel p190-derived breakpoint Peptide suitable for Peptide vaccine therapeutic approach in ph+ acute lymphoblastic leukemia patients, *Leuk Res Treatment* **2012**: 150651 (2012).

Ismail, S.I., R.G. Naffa, A.M. Yousef, and M.T. Ghanim, Incidence of bcr-abl fusion transcripts in healthy individuals, *Mol Med Rep* **9**: 1271–1276 (2014).

Jangamreddy, J.R., S. Panigrahi, K. Lotfi, M. Yadav, S. Maddika, A.K. Tripathi, S. Sanyal, and M.J. Łos, Mapping of apoptin-interaction with BCR-ABL1, and development of apoptin-based targeted therapy, *Oncotarget* **5**: 7198–7211 (2014).

Janowska-Wieczorek, A., M. Majka, L. Marquez-Curtis, J.A. Wertheim, A.R. Turner, and M.Z. Ratajczak, Bcr-abl-positive cells secrete angiogenic factors including matrix metalloproteinases and stimulate angiogenesis *in vivo* in Matrigel implants, *Leukemia* **16**: 1160–1166 (2002).

Lee, H.J., J.E. Thompson, E.S. Wang, and M. Wetzler, Philadelphia chromosome-positive acute lymphoblastic leukemia: current treatment and future perspectives, *Cancer* **117**: 1583–1594 (2011).

Lewalle, P. and P. Martiat, Inhibition of P210 expression in chronic myeloid leukaemia: oligonucleotides and/or transduced antisense sequences, *Leuk Lymphoma* **11**(Suppl 1): 139–143 (1993).

Li, C., Y. Wang, D. Xu, P. Zhang, X. Ding, N. Zhang, M. Xiao, L. Huang, and L. Meng, E255K and G250E mutation appearing in a patient with e19a2 chronic myeloid leukemia resistant to imatinib, *Clin Lab* **61**: 183–186 (2015b).

Li, J., Y. Chen, B. Chen, C. Chen, B. Qiu, Z. Zheng, J. Zheng, T. Liu, W Wang, and J. Hu, Inhibition of 32Dp210 cells harboring T315I mutation by a novel derivative of emodin correlates with down-regulation of BCR-ABL and its downstream signaling pathways, *J Canc Res Clin Oncol* **141**: 283–293 (2015a).

Li, W.J., W.S. Kloetzer, and R.B. Arlinghaus, A novel 53 kDa protein complexed with P210bcr-abl in human chronic myelogenous leukemia cells, *Oncogene* **2**: 559–566 (1988).

Liu, J., M. Campbell, J.Q. Guo, D. Lu, Y.M. Xian, B.S. Andersson, and R.B. Arlinghaus, BCR-ABL tyrosine kinase is autophosphorylated or transphosphorylates P160 BCR on tyrosine predominantly within the first BCR exon, *Oncogene* **8**: 101–109 (1993).

Lugo, T.G., A.M. Pendergast, A.J. Muller, and O.N. Witte, Tyrosine kinase activity and transformation potency of bcr-abl oncogene products, *Science* **247**: 1079–1082 (1990).

Lugo, T.G. and O.N. Witte, The BCR-ABL oncogene transforms Rat-1 cells and cooperates with v-myc, *Mol Cell Biol* **9**: 1263–1270 (1989).

Mandanas, R.A., H.S. Boswell, L. Lu, and D. Leibowitz, BCR/ABL confers growth factor independence upon a murine myeloid cell line, *Leukemia* **6**: 796–800 (1992).

Melo, J.V., H. Myint, D.A. Galton, and J.M. Goldman, P190BCR-ABL chronic myeloid leukaemia: the missing link with chronic myelomonocytic leukaemia? *Leukemia* **8**: 208–211 (1994).

Melo, J.V., The diversity of BCR-ABL fusion proteins and their relationship to leukemia phenotype, *Blood* **88**: 2375–2384 (1996).

Miroshnychenko, D., A. Dubrovska, S. Maliuta, G. Telegeev, and P. Aspenström, Novel role of pleckstrin homology domain of the Bcr-Abl protein: analysis of protein-protein and protein-lipid interactions, *Exp Cell Res* **316**: 530–542 (2010).

Molica, M., I. Zacheo, D. Diverio, G. Alimena, and M. Breccia, Long-term outcome of chronic myeloid leukaemia patients with p210 and p190 co-expression at baseline, *Br J Haematol* **169**: 148–150 (2015).

Molinos-Quintana, A., V. Aquino, I. Montero, C. Pérez-de Soto, R. García-Lozano, J.A. Pérez-Simón, and J.M. Pérez-Hurtado, Emerging BCR/ABL1 mutations under treatment with tyrosine kinase inhibitors in paediatric acute lymphoblastic leukaemia, *Acta Haematol* **134**: 71–75 (2015).

Morotti, A., C. Panuzzo, S. Crivellaro, B. Pergolizzi, U. Familiari, A.H. Berger, G. Saglio, and P.P. Pandolfi, BCR-ABL disrupts PTEN nuclear-cytoplasmic shuttling through phosphorylation-dependent activation of HAUSP, *Leukemia* **28**: 1326–1333 (2014).

Naldini, L., A. Stacchini, D.M. Cirillo, M. Aglietta, F. Gavosto, and P.M. Comoglio, Phosphotyrosine antibodies identify the p210c-abl tyrosine kinase and proteins phosphorylated on tyrosine in human chronic myelogenous leukemia cells, *Mol Cell Biol* **6**: 1803–8011 (1986).

Nishimura, J., J. Okamura, K. Shibata, H. Takahira, Y. Yufu, S. Kato, J. Hirata, T. Umemura, and H. Nawata, Two bcr/abl fusion gene products, P210bcr/abl and P190bcr/abl, are equally sensitive to the protein tyrosine phosphatase of mature granulocytes, *Int J Hematol* **54**: 471–478 (1991).

Nishimura, J., K. Shibata, S. Sadamura, H. Takahira, J. Hirata, T. Umemura, H. Nawata, and J. Okamura, Differences in tyrosine phosphorylated proteins between cells expressing P210bcr/abl and P190bcr/abl, *Int J Hematol* **55**: 227–233 (1992).

Okuda, K., U. Matulonis, R. Salgia, Y. Kanakura, B. Druker, and J.D. Griffin, Factor independence of human myeloid leukemia cell lines is associated with increased phosphorylation of the proto-oncogene Raf-1, *Exp Hematol* **22**: 1111–1117 (1994).

Oshikawa, G., T. Kurosu, A. Arai, N. Murakami, and O Miura, Clonal evolution with double Ph followed by tetraploidy in imatinib-treated chronic myeloid leukemia with e19a2 transcript in transformation, *Canc Genet Cytogenet* **199**: 56–61 (2010).

Pane, F., F. Frigeri, M. Sindona, L. Luciano, F. Ferrara, R. Cimino, G. Meloni, G. Saglio, F. Salvatore, and B. Rotoli, Neutrophilic-chronic myeloid leukemia: a distinct disease with a specific molecular marker (BCR/ABL with C3/A2 junction), *Blood* **88**: 2410–2414 (1996).

Panuzzo, C., S. Crivellaro, G. Carrà, A. Guerrasio, G. Saglio, and A Morotti, BCR-ABL promotes PTEN downregulation in chronic myeloid leukemia, *PLoS One* **9**: e110682 (2014).

Pendergast, A.M., M.L. Gishizky, M.H. Havlik, and O.N. Witte, SH1 domain autophosphorylation of P210 BCR/ABL is required for transformation but not growth factor independence, *Mol Cell Biol* **13**: 1728–1736 (1993a).

Pendergast, A.M., L.A. Quilliam, L.D. Cripe, C.H. Bassing, Z. Dai, N. Li, A. Batzer, K.M. Rabun, C.J. Der, J. Schlessinger *et al.*, BCR-ABL-induced oncogenesis is mediated by direct interaction with the SH2 domain of the GRB-2 adaptor protein, *Cell* **75**: 175–185 (1993b).

Quackenbush, R.C., G.W. Reuther, J.P. Miller, K.D. Courtney, W.S. Pear, and A.M. Pendergast, Analysis of the biologic properties of p230 Bcr-Abl reveals unique and overlapping properties with the oncogenic p185 and p210 Bcr-Abl tyrosine kinases, *Blood* **95**: 2913–2921 (2000).

Reuther, J.Y., G.W. Reuther, D. Cortez, A.M. Pendergast, and A.S. Baldwin Jr., A requirement for NF-kappaB activation in Bcr-Abl-mediated transformation, *Genes Dev* **12**: 968–981 (1998).

Riva, G., M. Luppi, P. Barozzi, C. Quadrelli, S. Basso, D. Vallerini, E. Zanetti, M. Morselli, F. Forghieri, M. Maccaferri, F. Volzone, C. Del Giovane, R. D'Amico, F. Locatelli, G. Torelli, P. Comoli, and L. Potenza, Emergence of BCR-ABL-specific cytotoxic T cells in the bone marrow of patients with Ph+ acute lymphoblastic leukemia during long-term imatinib mesylate treatment, *Blood* **115**: 1512–1518 (2010).

Roy, M., R. Sarkar, A. Mukherjee, and S. Mukherjee, Inhibition of crosstalk between Bcr-Abl and PKC signaling by PEITC, augments imatinib sensitivity in chronic myelogenous leukemia cells, *Chem Biol Interact* **242**: 195–201 (2015).

Salomoni, P., M.A. Wasik, R.F. Riedel, K. Reiss, J.K. Choi, T. Skorski, and B. Calabretta, Expression of constitutively active Raf-1 in the mitochondria restores anti-apoptotic and leukemogenic potential of a transformation-deficient BCR/ABL mutant, *J Exp Med* **187**: 1995–2007 (1998).

Sawyers, C.L., W. Callahan, and O.N. Witte, Dominant negative MYC blocks transformation by ABL oncogenes, *Cell* **70**: 901–910 (1992).

Sawyers, C.L., Chronic myeloid leukemia, *N Engl J Med* **340**(17): 1330–1340 (1999).

Shuai, K., J. Halpern, J. ten Hoeve, X. Rao, and C.L. Sawyers, Constitutive activation of STAT5 by the BCR-ABL oncogene in chronic myelogenous leukemia, *Oncogene* **13**: 247–254 (1996).

Skorski, T., A. Bellacosa, M. Nieborowska-Skorska, M. Majewski, R. Martinez, J.K. Choi, R. Trotta, P. Wlodarski, D. Perrotti, T.O. Chan, M.A. Wasik, P.N. Tsichlis, and B. Calabretta, Transformation of hematopoietic cells by BCR/ABL requires activation of a PI-3k/Akt-dependent pathway, *EMBO J* **16**: 6151–6161 (1997).

Skorski, T., P. Wlodarski, L. Daheron, P. Salomoni, M. Nieborowska-Skorska, M. Majewski, M. Wasik, and B. Calabretta, BCR/ABL-mediated leukemogenesis requires the activity of the small GTP-binding protein Rac, *Proc Natl Acad Sci USA* **95**: 11858–11862 (1998).

Tabassum, N., M. Saboor, R. Ghani, and M. Moinuddin, Heterogeneity of BCR-ABL rearrangement in patients with chronic myeloid leukemia in Pakistan, *Pak J Med Sci* **30**: 850–853 (2014).

Tala, I., R. Chen, T. Hu, E.R. Fitzpatrick, D.A. Williams, and I.P. Whitehead, Contributions of the RhoGEF activity of p210 BCR/ABL to disease progression, *Leukemia* **27**: 1080–1089 (2013).

Tan, Y., X. Chen, X. Qi, G. Li, J. Wang, S. Bian, Z. Xu, and H. Wang, Acute lymphoblastic leukemia expressing b3a2 (p210), e1a2 (p190), and variant e1a2 BCR-ABL transcripts: a case report and review of the literature, *Acta Haematol* **128**: 119–123 (2012).

Uchida, N., H. Hanawa, K. Dan, K. Inokuchi, and T. Shimada, Leukemogenesis of b2a2-type p210 BCR/ABL in a bone marrow transplantation mouse model using a lentiviral vector, *J Nippon Med Sch* **76**: 134–147 (2009).

Verma, D., H.M. Kantarjian, D. Jones, R. Luthra, G. Borthakur, S. Verstovsek, M.B. Rios, and J. Cortes, Chronic myeloid leukemia (CML) with P190 BCR-ABL: analysis of characteristics, outcomes, and prognostic significance, *Blood* **114**: 2232–2235 (2009).

Verstovsek, S., H. Lin, H. Kantarjian, G. Saglio, D. De Micheli, F. Pane, G. Garcia-Manero, M. Intrieri, B. Rotoli, F. Salvatore, J.Q. Guo, M. Talpaz, G. Specchia, G. Pizzolo, A.M. Liberati, J. Cortes, R.C. Quackenbush, and R.B. Arlinghaus, Neutrophilic-chronic myeloid leukemia: low levels of p230 BCR/ABL mRNA and undetectable BCR/ABL protein may predict an indolent course, *Cancer* **94**: 2416–2425 (2002).

Voncken, J.W., V. Kaartinen, P.K. Pattengale, W.T. Germeraad, J. Groffen, and N. Heisterkamp, BCR/ABL P210 and P190 cause distinct leukemia in transgenic mice, *Blood* **86**: 4603–4611 (1995).

Wada, H., S. Mizutani, J. Nishimura, Y. Usuki, M. Kohsaki, M. Komai, H. Kaneko, S. Sakamoto, D. Delia, A. Kanamaru, *et al.*, Establishment and molecular characterization of a novel leukemic cell line with Philadelphia chromosome expressing p230 BCR/ABL fusion protein, *Canc Res* **55**: 3192–3196 (1995).

Waller, C.F., Imatinib mesylate, *Recent Results Cancer Res* **201**: 1–25 (2014).

Yang, F.L., F.Z. Chen, X.X. Wan, X. Zhou, M.J. Zhou, H.C. Chen, J.J. Fu, and D.Z. Zhang, Effects of a particular heptapeptide on the IFN-α-sensitive CML cells, *Biomed Res Int* **2015**: 325026 (2015).

Ye, Y.X., J. Zhou, Y.H. Zhou, Y. Zhou, X.B. Song, J. Wang, L. Lin, B.W. Ying, and X.J. Lu, Clinical significance of BCR-ABL fusion gene subtypes in chronic myelogenous and acute lymphoblastic leukemias, *Asian Pac J Canc Prev* **15**: 9961–9966 (2014).

Yeung, D.T. and T.P. Hughes, Therapeutic targeting of BCR-ABL: prognostic markers of response and resistance mechanism in chronic myeloid leukaemia, *Crit Rev Oncog* **17**: 17–30 (2012).

Young, J.C. and O.N. Witte, Selective transformation of primitive lymphoid cells by the BCR/ABL oncogene expressed in long-term lymphoid or myeloid cultures, *Mol Cell Biol* **8**: 4079–4087 (1988).

6

BRD4-NUT Fusion Oncoprotein and Its Significance in the Initiation and Progression of NUT Midline Carcinoma

*Ganesan Padmavathi, Devivasha Bordoloi, Kishore Banik and Ajaikumar B. Kunnumakkara**

INTRODUCTION

Bromodomain (BRD) family of proteins contains evolutionarily conserved domain modules which can recognize acetyl-lysine residues through its central hydrophobic cavity. This acetyl-lysine binding activity of BRD was proved to regulate various protein–protein interactions and assist in chromatin structure modification and transcriptional activation by

*Author for correspondence: Ajaikumar B. Kunnumakkara, Cancer Biology Laboratory, Department of Biosciences and Bioengineering, Indian Institute of Technology Guwahati, Assam 781039, India. kunnumakkara@iitg.ernet.in

cooperating with acetylated histone protein (Zeng and Zhou, 2002). Till date, more than 50 unique human BRDs were identified in merely 40 proteins and were further divided into groups based on the sequence length and similarity they share (Sanchez and Zhou, 2009). Bromodomain and extra-terminal (BET) is one of the major BRDs containing protein families comprising BRD2, BRD3, BRD4 and BRDT proteins (Sanchez and Zhou, 2009). These proteins act as important elements of transcription factor complexes and have been implicated in the pathogenesis of different diseases including inflammations, viral infections and cancers (Filippakopoulos *et al.*, 2010; Sanchez and Zhou, 2009).

For instance, BRD3 and BRD4 proteins, members of BET family were involved in gene fusion with a novel nuclear protein in testis (NUT) gene and associated with NUT midline carcinoma (NMC) of different origins (French *et al.*, 2003, 2008). Normally, the BRD4 with its two bromodomains functions through selective interaction with acetylated histones H3 and H4 and is associated with mitotic chromosomes like any other member of BET family (Dey *et al.*, 2003). Moreover, it has been shown to induce cell growth through interaction with positive transcription elongation factor complex (P-TEFb) and increased mitotic progression (Filippakopoulos *et al.*, 2010). Interestingly, the BRD4-NUT fusion protein is the only known oncogenic form of BRD4 which reduces the chromatin acetylation, blocks differentiation and drives tumor progression (Stathis *et al.*, 2016; French, 2012).

BRD4-NUT

A recurrent translocation of chromosome 15 and 19 denoted as t(15;19)(q14;p13.1) is frequently observed in two thirds of NMC, an aggressive and poorly differentiated squamous cell carcinoma of different midline origins including head and neck, lung, etc., and is believed to be a promising diagnostic biomarker and therapeutic target for the treatment of NMC (Figure 6.1). It is also detected in few cases of pediatric head and neck tumors and lung cancers (Bhaijee *et al.*, 2011; Yan *et al.*, 2011; Haruki *et al.*, 2005; French *et al.*, 2003; French, 2010, 2012). This chromosomal rearrangement produced a fusion of almost entire sequence of NUT protein and N-terminal component of BRD4 resulting in BRD4-NUT

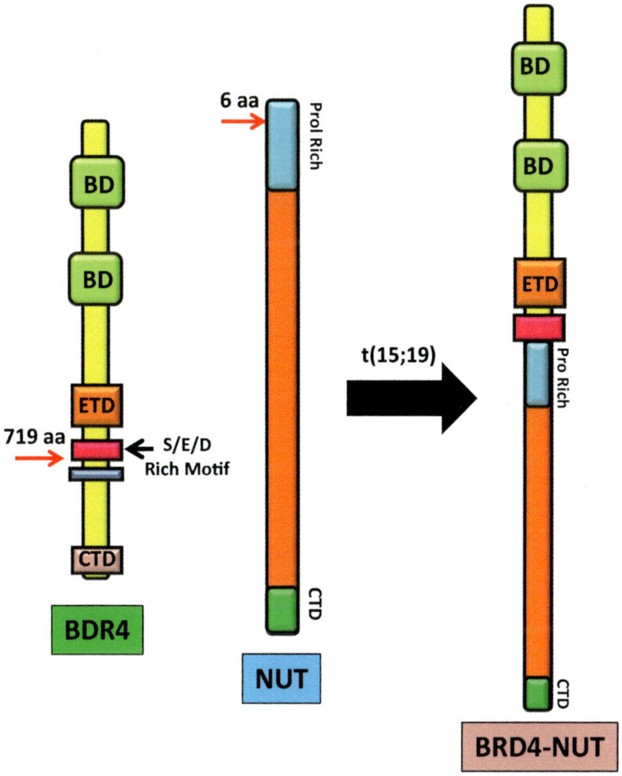

Figure 6.1: Formation of BRD4-NUT fusion protein. BD — bromodomain; ETD — extra terminal domain; CTD — C-terminal domain; S/E/D — Ser/Glu/Asp rich motif; Pro — proline; aa — amino acid.

chimera which blocked the differentiation through suppression of genes involved by hypomethylation and added growth advantage to the carcinoma cells (Parikh *et al.*, 2013; French *et al.*, 2003, 2008). In addition, it was found to correlate with highly aggressive, invariably lethal disease and to elevate the expression level of NUT which was the deciding factor of t(15;19) translocation-associated carcinoma (French *et al.*, 2003). Moreover, the disruption of normal BRD4 protein activity by BRD4-NUT oncoprotein hampered the cellular differentiation contributing to disease progression in NMC (Yan *et al.*, 2011). In addition, expression of this fusion oncogene was also correlated with the increased MYC expression thereby impeding the differentiation of NMC cells

(Grayson *et al.*, 2014). Adding to its oncogenic potential, Reynoird *et al.* (2010) reported that the interaction of NUT portion of BRD4-NUT with p300 triggers transcriptional inactivation of hyperacetylated chromatin domain thus inducing p300 sequestration-mediated inactivation of p53 and its target genes (Reynoird *et al.*, 2010; Wang and You, 2015). Moreover, fusion-mediated degradation of histone acetyltransferase could also be one of the possible mechanisms for the development of NMCs (French, 2012). Further, the fusion protein was shown to be associated with increased expression of sex determining region Y-box 2 (SOX2), a transcription factor, which was correlated with the BRD4-NUT-mediated oncogenic transformation in NMC (Wang *et al.*, 2014). From the available reports, it was apparent that bromodomains of BRD3/4 are responsible for the oncogenicity of BRD-NUT. Therefore, few studies reported the effectiveness of selective bromodomain inhibitors for the treatment of NMC. These inhibitors were shown to prevent BRD-NUT and chromatin binding thus triggering terminal differentiation of NMCs (French, 2012). OTX015 or MK-8628 is one such inhibitor which was proved effective both *in vitro* and *in vivo* against NMC and various other tumors by targeting BRD2/3/4/T. Results of preclinical studies were further confirmed in clinic where two out of four fusion positive advanced-stage NMC patients showed rapid tumor regression and one had stable disease upon treatment with 80 mg OTX015 or MK-8628 per day (Stathis *et al.*, 2016). Similarly, use of histone deacetylase inhibitors (HDACi) was also proved to induce differentiation and reduce cell growth through increased chromatin acetylation (Schwartz *et al.*, 2011). In addition, a 12-year-old NMC patient showed complete response to gemcitabine treatment following cisplatin and docetaxel suggesting combination therapy to be a better treatment option (Ueki *et al.*, 2014).

Recently, it was determined that different isoforms produced by the alternative splicing of the fusion gene play a crucial role in the pathogenesis by increasing disease complexity (Stirnweiss *et al.*, 2015; Thompson-Wicking *et al.*, 2013). In addition to BRDs, the NUT gene was also found to be involved in fusion with few other uncharacterized genes. For example, it has been found to rearrange with NSD3 gene in 1221 cells, a patient-derived NMC cell line. The NSD3-NUT fusion protein blocked differentiation and induced cell growth by binding with BRD4 which was reversed by bromodomain inhibitors. Moreover, it has been confirmed that NSD3 is also required for BRD4-NUT-mediated tumorigenesis in NMCs (French *et al.*, 2014). However, the exact molecular mechanism of these fusion proteins in the oncogenic progression of NMCs remains elusive suggesting the ultimate requirement of more extensive research on the downstream targets of BRD-NUT and NSD3-NUT.

CONFLICT OF INTEREST

The authors express no conflict of interest.

REFERENCES

Bhaijee, F., D.J. Pepper, K.T. Pitman, and D. Bell, New developments in the molecular pathogenesis of head and neck tumors: a review of tumor-specific fusion oncogenes in mucoepidermoid carcinoma, adenoid cystic carcinoma, and NUT midline carcinoma, *Ann Diagn Pathol* **15**(1): 69–77 (2011).

Dey, A., F. Chitsaz, A. Abbasi, T. Misteli, and K. Ozato, The double bromodomain protein Brd4 binds to acetylated chromatin during interphase and mitosis, *Proc Natl Acad Sci USA* **100**(15): 8758–8763 (2003).

Filippakopoulos, P., J. Qi, S. Picaud, Y. Shen, W.B. Smith, O. Fedorov, E.M. Morse, T. Keates, T.T. Hickman, I. Felletar, M. Philpott, S. Munro, M.R. McKeown, Y. Wang, A.L. Christie, N. West, M.J. Cameron, B. Schwartz, T.D. Heightman, N. La Thangue, C.A. French, O. Wiest, A.L. Kung, S. Knapp, and J.E. Bradner, Selective inhibition of BET bromodomains, *Nature* **468**(7327): 1067–1073 (2010).

French, C.A., I. Miyoshi, I. Kubonishi, H.E. Grier, A.R. Perez-Atayde, and J.A. Fletcher, BRD4-NUT fusion oncogene: a novel mechanism in aggressive carcinoma, *Canc Res* **63**(2): 304–307 (2003).

French, C.A., S. Rahman, E.M. Walsh, S. Kühnle, A.R. Grayson, M.E. Lemieux, N. Grunfeld, B.P. Rubin, C.R. Antonescu, S. Zhang, R. Venkatramani, P. Dal Cin, and P.M. Howley, NSD3-NUT fusion oncoprotein in NUT midline carcinoma: implications for a novel oncogenic mechanism, *Cancer Discov* **4**(8): 928–941 (2014).

French, C.A., C.L. Ramirez, J. Kolmakova, T.T. Hickman, M.J. Cameron, M.E. Thyne, J.L. Kutok, J.A. Toretsky, A.K. Tadavarthy, U.R. Kees, J.A. Fletcher, and J.C. Aster, BRD-NUT oncoproteins: a family of closely related nuclear proteins that block epithelial differentiation and maintain the growth of carcinoma cells, *Oncogene* **27**(15): 2237–2242 (2008).

French, C.A., NUT midline carcinoma, *Cancer Genet Cytogenet* **203**(1): 16–20 (2010).

French, C.A., Pathogenesis of NUT midline carcinoma, *Annu Rev Pathol* **7**: 247–265 (2012).

Grayson, A.R., E.M. Walsh, M.J. Cameron, J. Godec, T. Ashworth, J.M. Ambrose, A.B. Aserlind, H. Wang, G.I. Evan, M.J. Kluk, J.E. Bradner, J.C. Aster, and C.A. French, MYC, a downstream target of BRD-NUT, is necessary and sufficient for the blockade of differentiation in NUT midline carcinoma, *Oncogene* **33**(13): 1736–1742 (2014).

Haruki, N., K.S. Kawaguchi, S. Eichenberger, P.P. Massion, A. Gonzalez, A.F. Gazdar, J.D. Minna, D.P. Carbone, and T.P. Dang, Cloned fusion product from a rare t(15;19)(q13.2;p13.1) inhibit S phase *in vitro*, *J Med Genet* **42**(7): 558–564 (2005).

Parikh, S.A., C.A. French, B.A. Costello, R.S. Marks, R.S. Dronca, C.L. Nerby, A.C. Roden, V.G. Peddareddigari, J. Hilton, G.I. Shapiro, J.R. Molina, NUT midline carcinoma: an aggressive intrathoracic neoplasm, *J Thorac Oncol* **8**(10): 1335–1338 (2013).

Reynoird, N., B.E. Schwartz, M. Delvecchio, K. Sadoul, D. Meyers, C. Mukherjee, C. Caron, H. Kimura, S. Rousseaux, P.A. Cole, D. Panne, C.A. French, and S. Khochbin, Oncogenesis by sequestration of CBP/p300 in transcriptionally inactive hyperacetylated chromatin domains, *EMBO J* **29**(17): 2943–2952 (2010).

Sanchez, R. and M.M. Zhou, The role of human bromodomains in chromatin biology and gene transcription, *Curr Opin Drug Discov Devel* **12**(5): 659–665 (2009).

Schwartz, B.E., M.D. Hofer, M.E. Lemieux, D.E. Bauer, M.J. Cameron, N.H. West, E.S. Agoston, N. Reynoird, S. Khochbin, T.A. Ince, A. Christie, K.A. Janeway, S.O. Vargas, A.R. Perez-Atayde, J.C. Aster, S.E. Sallan, A.L. Kung, and J.E. Bradner, French CA, Differentiation of NUT midline carcinoma by epigenomic reprogramming, *Canc Res* **71**(7): 2686–2696 (2011).

Stathis, A., E. Zucca, M. Bekradda, C. Gomez-Roca, J.P. Delord, T. de La Motte Rouge, E. Uro-Coste, F. de Braud, G. Pelosi, and C.A. French, Clinical response of carcinomas harboring the BRD4-NUT oncoprotein to the targeted bromodomain inhibitor OTX015/MK-8628, *Canc Discov* **6**(5): 492–500 (2016).

Stirnweiss, A., K. McCarthy, J. Oommen, M.L. Crook, K. Hardy, U.R. Kees, S.D. Wilton, A. Anazodo, and A.H. Beesley, A novel BRD4-NUT fusion in an undifferentiated sinonasal tumor highlights alternative splicing as a contributing oncogenic factor in NUT midline carcinoma, *Oncogenesis* **4**: e174 (2015).

Thompson-Wicking, K., R.W. Francis, A. Stirnweiss, E. Ferrari, M.D. Welch, E. Baker, A.R. Murch, A.M. Gout, K.W. Carter, A.K. Charles, M.B. Phillips, U.R. Kees, and A.H. Beesley, Novel BRD4-NUT fusion isoforms increase the pathogenic complexity in NUT midline carcinoma, *Oncogene* **32**(39): 4664–4674 (2013).

Ueki, H., N. Maeda, M. Sekimizu, Y. Yamashita, S. Moritani, and K. Horibe, A case of NUT midline carcinoma with complete response to gemcitabine following cisplatin and docetaxel, *J Pediatr Hematol Oncol* **36**(8): e476–480 (2014).

Wang, R., W. Liu, C.M. Helfer, J.E. Bradner, J.L. Hornick, S.M. Janicki, C.A. French, and J. You, Activation of SOX2 expression by BRD4-NUT oncogenic fusion drives neoplastic transformation in NUT midline carcinoma, *Canc Res* **74**(12): 3332–3343 (2014).

Wang, R. and J. You, Mechanistic analysis of the role of bromodomain-containing protein 4 (BRD4) in BRD4-NUT oncoprotein-induced transcriptional activation, *J Biol Chem* **290**(5): 2744–2758 (2015).

Yan, J., J. Diaz, J. Jiao, R. Wang, and J. You, Perturbation of BRD4 protein function by BRD4-NUT protein abrogates cellular differentiation in NUT midline carcinoma, *J Biol Chem* **286**(31): 27663–27675 (2011).

Zeng, L. and M.M. Zhou, Bromodomain: an acetyl-lysine binding domain, *FEBS Lett* **513**(1): 124–128 (2002).

7

Importance of CBFB-MYH11 — A Chimeric Transcriptional Regulator in Leukemia

*Ganesan Padmavathi, Choudhary Harsha, Devivasha Bordoloi, Krishan Kumar Thakur and Ajaikumar B. Kunnumakkara**

INTRODUCTION

Approximately 5–8% of all cases of acute myeloid leukemia (AML) were found to be associated with a fusion gene known as CBFB-MYH11. This fusion gene is produced most commonly from the pericentric inversion inv(16)(p13; q22), and rarely from translocation t(16;16)(p13;q22) or from deletion del(16)(q22) (Akiyama *et al.*, 2015; Claxton *et al.*, 1996; Liu *et al.*, 1993; Usuki *et al.*, 1996). The associated AML was classified as acute myeloid leukemia subtype M4Eo (French–American–British

*Author for correspondence: Ajaikumar B. Kunnumakkara, Cancer Biology Laboratory, Department of Biosciences and Bioengineering, Indian Institute of Technology Guwahati, Assam 781039, India. kunnumakkara@iitg.ernet.in

classification subtype M4 with eosinophilia), which is characterized by the presence of myelomonocytic blasts and atypical eosinophils (Castilla *et al.*, 1996; Le Beau *et al.*, 1983; Hyde and Liu, 2010). The resulting fusion yielded CBFβ-SMMHC oncoprotein that comprised 165 amino acids of CBFB (core binding factor beta) and a C-terminal coiled-coil region of myosin heavy chain (MYH11) gene coding for smooth muscle myosin heavy chain (SMMHC) (Liu *et al.*, 1993; Durst *et al.*, 2003). It was known to block differentiation; maintain long-term hematopoietic stem cells (HSCs); and increased abnormal myeloid progenitors (AMPs) leading to the development of leukemia (Kuo *et al.*, 2006). Similar to several other fusion genes, CBFβ-SMMHC was also found to be associated with better clinical behavior exhibiting high rate of complete remission, longer 5-year relapse-free survival (RFS) and overall survival (OS). Loss of multidrug resistance protein (MRP) during inversion of chromosome 16 may be the responsible factor for the better prognosis associated with this fusion (Cao *et al.*, 2013; Dawson *et al.*, 2011; Kuss *et al.*, 1996). Till date, more than 10 transcript variants of CBFβ-SMMHC named types A–J have been identified to be associated with AML. Among them, type A was most commonly detected with the frequency of 85%. Unlike all other variants, the more frequent type A was found to coexist with RTK-KIT activating mutations which in turn were associated with poor prognosis (Albano *et al.*, 2014; Schwind *et al.*, 2013; Zhao *et al.*, 2012).The rare type D CBFB-MYH11 rearrangement was detected in few of the therapy related AML (t-AML) cases. In particular, it has been found to be associated with t-AML developed after the treatment with topoisomerase I and II inhibitors (Akiyama *et al.*, 2015; Dissing *et al.*, 1998).

One of the partner genes of inv(16), CBFB is a transcriptional regulator protein belongs to core binding factor (CBF) family. The CBF complex contains 3 alpha subunits, namely, RUNX1 (AML1, Cbfα2), RUNX2 (Cbfα1), and RUNX3 (Cbfα3) with DNA binding activity and only one beta subunit, namely, CBFβ with no DNA binding activity. Together these proteins are known to regulate transcription of various genes involved in cellular processes. For instance, the CBF transcription factor complex was proved to transcriptionally regulate the genes involved in hematopoiesis such as IL3, GM-CSF, CSF-1 receptor, myeloperoxidase and T cell receptors α and β (TCRα/β), etc. (Castilla *et al.*, 1996). Particularly, the wild-type β-subunit CBFβ was known to form heterodimer with DNA binding α-subunits and stabilized the CBFα-DNA interaction thus inducing the regulation of transcription of aforementioned genes (Tang *et al.*, 2000; Castilla *et al.*, 1996). Likewise, interaction of CBFβ with the other CBFα subunits RUNX2 and RUNX3 was also shown to regulate the expression of several genes involved in bone and gastrointestinal development respectively (Lopez-Camacho *et al.*, 2014). Besides stabilizing CBFα-DNA interaction, CBFβ was also shown to protect RUNX1 from ubiquitination-mediated degradation (Huang *et al.*, 2001). Moreover, through several *in vivo* studies, both RUNX1 and CBFβ have been confirmed to be essential for definitive hematopoiesis and embryonic blood circulation and were known to be frequently involved in chromosomal rearrangements thus inducing the development of AML (Castilla *et al.*, 1996; Hyde and Liu, 2010). Interestingly, Heilman *et al.* (2006) showed that intact CBFβ suppresses CBFβ-MYH11 induced AML in mice suggesting the need for therapies to specifically target the fusion protein and not the wild-type CBFβ (Heilman *et al.*, 2006). Further, this chapter deals with the role of inv(16) in the initiation and progression of AML.

ROLE OF CBFB-MYH11 IN LEUKEMOGENESIS

Ample amount of reports suggested CBFB-SMMHC as a dominant repressor of normal CBFβ-RUNX1 heterodimer activity thus blocking embryonic definitive hematopoiesis as well as adult hematopoietic stem cell differentiation to the myeloid and lymphoid lineages (Castilla *et al.*, 1996; Kundu *et al.*, 2002; Kundu and Liu, 2001; Hyde and Liu, 2010). Consecutively, it has been shown that CBFβ-SMMHC exhibits high affinity to RUNX1 through the high affinity binding domain (HABD) and hypothesized to impart oncogenic function which helps in the proliferation of immature myeloid progenitors (Figure 7.1). Supporting this, two hypotheses have been proposed for fusion-mediated repression of RUNX1 activity, first being sequestration of RUNX1 into the cytoskeletal filaments and second being the transcriptional repression mediated through recruitment of transcriptional corepressors by SMMHC portion of chimera (Adya *et al.*, 1998; Lukasik *et al.*, 2002; Shigesada *et al.*, 2004; Hyde and Liu, 2010; Huang *et al.*, 2004). Moreover, several other

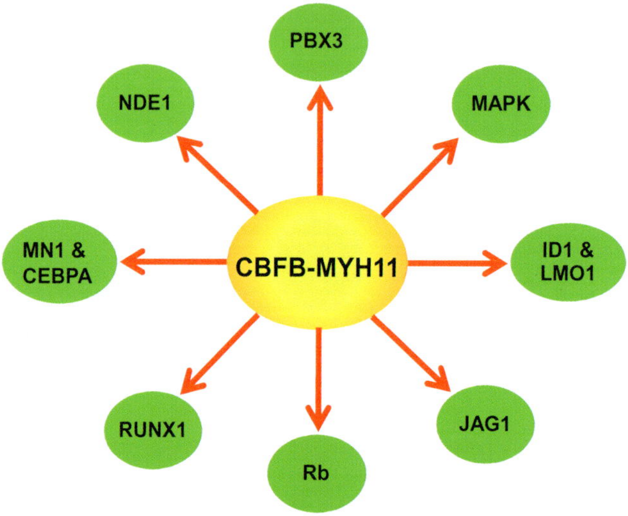

Figure 7.1: Molecular targets of CBFB-MYH11.

functions of this fusion gene have also been proposed over many years listing as localization of RUNX1 outside the nucleus, impaired transcription factor complex assembly and recruitment of histone deacetylases, all leading to the downregulation of RUNX1 and its target genes (Mandoli *et al.*, 2014). Further, CBFB-SMMHC was also proved to facilitate RUNX1-mediated transcriptional repression by forming a trimeric complex with RUNX1 and corepressor mSin3A (Lutterbach *et al.*, 1999). However, few *in vivo* studies proved that CBFβ-SMMHC-mediated dominant repression of RUNX1 is not the only key mechanism of leukemogenesis and suggested that besides RUNX1 repressing activity, CBFβ-SMMHC mutation must have some gain of function activities that contribute to this disease (Hyde and Liu, 2010; Hyde *et al.*, 2010). Contrastingly, the RUNX1 activity was shown to be crucial for CBFB-MYH11 induced leukemogenesis as the loss of RUNX1 in an *in vivo* mouse model repaired the CBFB-MYH11-mediated defects in differentiation and reduced the cell proliferation during both primitive and definitive hematopoiesis (Hyde *et al.*, 2015). Moreover, besides RUNX1, another CBFα subunit, RUNX2, was also shown to regulate inv(16) fusion-mediated leukemogenesis (Kuo *et al.*, 2009).

Even though the mechanism of CBFB-MYH11 fusion-induced leukemogenesis remains controversial, it is strongly believed that both CBF-mediated repression dependent and independent activities of this fusion gene play a critical role in the development leukemia (Hyde and Liu, 2010; Hyde *et al.*, 2010). In addition, it was evidenced that CBFB-MYH11 alone is not sufficient to initiate leukemia and requires multiple secondary mutations (Castilla *et al.*, 1999, 2004). In accordance with this, mice expressing both CBFβ-SMMHC and NRAS (G12D) mutations exhibited increased survival of preleukemic myeloid progenitors which was mediated by constitutive activation of MEK-ERK signaling cascade (Xue *et al.*, 2014). Furthermore, in addition to gene mutations, overexpression of PLAG1 and PLAGL2; trisomy 22 and 8 were also identified as secondary mutations in CBFB-MYH11 positive AML (Paschka *et al.*, 2013; Landrette *et al.*, 2005). Also, presence of breakpoint clusters in downstream MYH11 gene as observed in 90% of cases was resulted in the disruption of nuclear distribution gene E homolog 1 (NDE1) gene as well which is positioned in the opposing DNA strand. Therefore, it is believed that disruption of NDE1 may also cooperate with CBFB-MYH11 during pathogenesis (Van der Reijden *et al.*, 2010). Further, the CBFB-MYH11 was found to correlate with deregulation of RAS signaling pathway through coexisting mutations in KRAS, NRAS and in upstream regulators of RAS cascade such as FLT3, KIT, CBL and NF1 leading to the development of AML (Haferlach *et al.*, 2010). Moreover, it increased the calreticulin induced suppression of CEBPA, a granulocytic differentiation factor and blocked the differentiation process (Figure 7.1) (Helbling *et al.*, 2005).

Though initially thought to have only transcriptional repressor activity, recently this oncofusion was also proved to exhibit transcriptional activator effect and was found to upregulate the levels of various genes like ID1, LMO1 and JAG1 thus critically regulating the hematopoietic stem cell self-renewal process and stem cell phenotype maintenance (Figure 7.1) (Mandoli *et al.*, 2014). Interestingly, CBFβ-SMMHC fusion was shown to activate p38 MAPK pathway which leads to oncogene-induced senescence. However, secondary genetic mutations seem to inactivate the oncogene-mediated senescence process in leukemia (Wajapeyee *et al.*, 2010). Further, ectopic expression of this chimera was shown to induce cell cycle arrest at G1 to S transition through $p21^{CIP1/WAF1}$-mediated hypophosphorylation of Rb (Figure 7.1) (Cao *et al.*, 1997). In addition, it has been proved to alter the methylation profile and expression levels of certain genes crucial for leukemogenesis such as PBX3, MN1, etc. (Hájková *et al.*, 2014).

CONCLUSION

Taken together, all these reports proved CBFB-MYH11 to be an important driving factor for AML M4Eo and secondary mutations to be inducing factors for disease onset. Therefore, inhibitors that target specifically the fusion oncogene and secondary mutations may have a great potential in treating this disease. However, more extensive research is required to further elucidate the role of this fusion in the development of AML and the difference from other AML which would help in the better management of this disease.

CONFLICT OF INTEREST

The authors express no conflict of interest.

REFERENCES

Adya, N., T. Stacy, N.A. Speck, and P.P. Liu, The leukemic protein core binding factor beta (CBFbeta)-smooth-muscle myosin heavy chain sequesters CBFalpha2 into cytoskeletal filaments and aggregates, *Mol Cell Biol* **18**(12): 7432–7443 (1998).

Akiyama, H., M. Yamamoto, C. Sakashita, Y. Umezawa, T. Kurosu, N. Murakami, and O. Miura, Therapy-related leukemia with Inv(16)(p13.1q22) and type D CBFB/MYH11 developing after exposure to irinotecan-containing chemoradiotherapy, *Intern Med* **54**(6): 651–655 (2015).

Albano, F., L. Anelli, A. Zagaria, N. Coccaro, G. Tota, L. Impera, C.F. Minervini, A. Cellamare, M. Delia, A. Minervini, P. Casieri, and G. Specchia, Acute myeloid leukemia with t(16;16) (p13;q22) showing a new CBFB-MYH11 fusion transcript associated with an atypical leukemic blasts morphology, *Hum Pathol* **45**(3): 643–647 (2014).

Cao, T.T., M.H. Zhou, L. Yuan, Q. Wang, L.P. Dou, Y.Y. Xu, N. Wang, L.L. Wang, L. Yu, and Y. Jing, [Clinical analysis of acute myeloid leukemia with CBFB-MYH11-positive], *Zhongguo Shi Yan Xue Ye Xue Za Zhi* **21**(2): 305–310 (2013).

Cao, W., M. Britos-Bray, D.F. Claxton, C.A. Kelley, N.A. Speck, P.P. Liu, and A.D. Friedman, CBF beta-SMMHC, expressed in M4Eo AML, reduced CBF DNA-binding and inhibited the G1 to S cell cycle transition at the restriction point in myeloid and lymphoidcells, *Oncogene* **15**(11): 1315–1327 (1997).

Castilla, L.H., L. Garrett, N. Adya, D. Orlic, A. Dutra, S. Anderson, J. Owens, M. Eckhaus, D. Bodine, and P.P. Liu, The fusion gene Cbfb-MYH11 blocks myeloid differentiation and predisposes mice to acute myelomonocytic leukaemia, *Nat Genet* **23**(2): 144–146 (1999).

Castilla, L.H., P. Perrat, N.J. Martinez, S.F. Landrette, R. Keys, S. Oikemus, J. Flanegan, S. Heilman, L. Garrett, A. Dutra, S. Anderson, G.A. Pihan, L. Wolff, and P.P. Liu, Identification of genes that synergize with Cbfb-MYH11 in the pathogenesis of acute myeloid leukemia, *Proc Natl Acad Sci USA* **101**(14): 4924–4929 (2004).

Castilla, L.H., C. Wijmenga, Q. Wang, T. Stacy, N.A. Speck, M. Eckhaus, M. Marín-Padilla, F.S. Collins, A. Wynshaw-Boris, and P.P. Liu, Failure of embryonic hematopoiesis and lethal hemorrhages in mouse embryos heterozygous for a knocked-in leukemia gene CBFB-MYH11, *Cell* **87**(4): 687–696 (1996).

Claxton, D., Q.S. Xie, S. Patel, A.B. Deisseroth, and S. Kornblau, The gene product of CBFB-MYH11, *Leukemia* **10**(9): 1479–1485 (1996).

Dawson, A.J., S. Bal, B. McTavish, M. Tomiuk, I. Schroedter, A.N. Ahsanuddin, M.D. Seftel, R. Vallente, S. Mai, P.D. Cotter, K. Hovanes, M. Gorre, and S.R. Gunn, Inversion and deletion of 16q22 defined by array CGH, FISH, and RT-PCR in a patient with AML, *Canc Genet* **204**(6): 344–347 (2011).

Dissing, M., M.M. Le Beau, and J. Pedersen-Bjergaard, Inversion of chromosome 16 and uncommon rearrangements of the CBFB and MYH11 genes in therapy-related acute myeloid leukemia: rare events related to DNA-topoisomerase II inhibitors? *J Clin Oncol* **16**(5): 1890–1896 (1998).

Durst, K.L., B. Lutterbach, T. Kummalue, A.D. Friedman, and S.W. Hiebert, The inv(16) fusion protein associates with corepressors via a smooth muscle myosin heavy-chain domain, *Mol Cell Biol* **23**(2): 607–619 (2003).

Haferlach, C., F. Dicker, A. Kohlmann, S. Schindela, T. Weiss, W. Kern, S. Schnittger, and T. Haferlach, AML with CBFB-MYH11 rearrangement demonstrate RAS pathway alterations in 92% of all cases including a high frequency of NF1 deletions, *Leukemia* **24**(5): 1065–1069 (2010).

Hájková, H., M.H. Fritz, C. Haškovec, J. Schwarz, C. Šálek, J. Marková, Z. Krejčík, M. Dostálová Merkerová, A. Kostečka, M. Vostrý, O. Fuchs, K. Michalová, P. Cetkovský, and V. Beneš, CBFB-MYH11 hypomethylation signature and PBX3 differential methylation revealed by targeted bisulfite sequencing in patients with acute myeloid leukemia, *J Hematol Oncol* **7**: 66 (2014).

Heilman, S.A., Y.H. Kuo, C.S. Goudswaard, P.J. Valk, and L.H. Castilla, Cbfbeta reduces Cbfbeta-SMMHC-associated acute myeloid leukemia in mice, *Canc Res* **66**(23): 11214–11218 (2006).

Helbling, D., B.U. Mueller, N.A. Timchenko, J. Schardt, M. Eyer, D.R. Betts, M. Jotterand, S. Meyer-Monard, M.F. Fey, and T. Pabst, CBFB-SMMHC is correlated with increased calreticulin expression and suppresses the granulocytic differentiation factor CEBPA in AML with inv(16), *Blood* **106**(4): 1369–1375 (2005).

Huang, G., K. Shigesada, K. Ito, H.J. Wee, T. Yokomizo, and Y. Ito, Dimerization with PEBP2beta protects RUNX1/AML1 from ubiquitin-proteasome-mediated degradation, *EMBO J* **20**(4): 723–733 (2001).

Huang, G., K. Shigesada, H.J. Wee, P.P. Liu, M. Osato, and Y. Ito, Molecular basis for a dominant inactivation of RUNX1/AML1 by the leukemogenic inversion 16 chimera, *Blood* **103**(8): 3200–3207 (2004).

Hyde, R.K., Y. Kamikubo, S. Anderson, M. Kirby, L. Alemu, L. Zhao, and P.P. Liu, Cbfb/Runx1 repression-independent blockage of differentiation and accumulation of Csf2rb-expressing cells by Cbfb-MYH11, *Blood* **115**(7): 1433–1443 (2010).

Hyde, R.K., and P.P. Liu, RUNX1 repression-independent mechanisms of leukemogenesis by fusion genes CBFB-MYH11 and AML1-ETO (RUNX1-RUNX1T1), *J Cell Biochem* **110**(5): 1039–1045 (2010).

Hyde, R.K., L. Zhao, L. Alemu, and P.P. Liu, Runx1 is required for hematopoietic defects and leukemogenesis in Cbfb-MYH11 knock-in mice, *Leukemia* **29**(8): 1771–1778 (2015).

Kundu, M., A. Chen, S. Anderson, M. Kirby, L. Xu, L.H. Castilla, D. Bodine, and P.P. Liu, Role of Cbfb in hematopoiesis and perturbations resulting from expression of the leukemogenic fusion gene Cbfb-MYH11, *Blood* **100**(7): 2449–2456 (2002).

Kundu, M., and P.P. Liu, Function of the inv(16) fusion gene CBFB-MYH11, *Curr Opin Hematol* **8**(4): 201–205 (2001).

Kuo, Y.H., S.F. Landrette, S.A. Heilman, P.N. Perrat, L. Garrett, P.P. Liu, M.M. Le Beau, S.C. Kogan, and L.H. Castilla, Cbf beta-SMMHC induces distinct abnormal myeloid progenitors able to develop acute myeloid leukemia, *Cancer Cell* **9**(1): 57–68 (2006).

Kuo, Y.H., S.K. Zaidi, S. Gornostaeva, T. Komori, G.S. Stein, and L.H. Castilla, Runx2 induces acute myeloid leukemia in cooperation with Cbfbeta-SMMHC in mice, *Blood* **113**(14): 3323–3332 (2009).

Kuss, B.J., R.G. Deeley, S.P. Cole, C.L. Willman, K.J. Kopecky, S.R. Wolman, H.J. Eyre, and D.F. Callen, The biological significance of the multidrug resistance gene MRP in inversion 16 leukemias, *Leuk Lymphoma* **20**(5–6): 357–364 (1996).

Landrette, S.F., Y.H. Kuo, K. Hensen, B. Khosrovani, P.N. Perrat, W.J. Van de Ven, R. Delwel, and L.H. Castilla, Plag1 and Plagl2 are oncogenes that induce acute myeloid leukemia in cooperation with Cbfb-MYH11, *Blood* **105**(7): 2900–2907 (2005).

Le Beau, M.M., R.A. Larson, M.A. Bitter, J.W. Vardiman, H.M. Golomb, and J.D. Rowley, Association of an inversion of chromosome 16 with abnormal marrow eosinophils in acute myelomonocytic leukemia. A unique cytogenetic-clinicopathological association, *N Engl J Med* **309**(11): 630–636 (1983).

Liu, P., S.A. Tarlé, A. Hajra, D.F. Claxton, P. Marlton, M. Freedman, M.J. Siciliano, and F.S. Collins, Fusion between transcription factor CBF beta/PEBP2 beta and a myosin heavy chain in acute myeloid leukemia, *Science* **261**(5124): 1041–1044 (1993).

Lopez-Camacho, C., A.J. van Wijnen, J.B. Lian, J.L. Stein, and G.S. Stein, Core binding factor β (CBFβ) is retained in the midbody during cytokinesis, *J Cell Physiol* **229**(10): 1466–1474 (2014).

Lukasik, S.M., L. Zhang, T. Corpora, S. Tomanicek, Y. Li, M. Kundu, K. Hartman, P.P. Liu, T.M. Laue, R.L. Biltonen, N.A. Speck, and J.H. Bushweller, Altered affinity of CBF beta-SMMHC for Runx1 explains its role in leukemogenesis, *Nat Struct Biol* **9**(9): 674–679 (2002).

Lutterbach, B., Y. Hou, K.L. Durst, and S.W. Hiebert, The inv(16) encodes an acute myeloid leukemia 1 transcriptional corepressor, *Proc Natl Acad Sci USA* **96**(22): 12822–12827 (1999).

Mandoli, A., A.A. Singh, P.W. Jansen, A.T. Wierenga, H. Riahi, G. Franci, K. Prange, S. Saeed, E. Vellenga, M. Vermeulen, H.G. Stunnenberg, and J.H. Martens, CBFB-MYH11/RUNX1 together with a compendium of hematopoietic regulators, chromatin modifiers and basal transcription factors occupies self-renewal genes in inv(16) acute myeloid leukemia, *Leukemia* **28**(4): 770–778 (2014).

Paschka, P., J. Du, R.F. Schlenk, V.I. Gaidzik, L. Bullinger, A. Corbacioglu, D. Späth, S. Kayser, B. Schlegelberger, J. Krauter, A. Ganser, C.H. Köhne, G. Held, M. von Lilienfeld-Toal, H. Kirchen, M. Rummel, K. Götze, H.A. Horst, M. Ringhoffer, M. Lübbert, M. Wattad, H.R. Salih, A. Kündgen,

H. Döhner, and K. Döhner, Secondary genetic lesions in acute myeloid leukemia with inv(16) or t(16;16): a study of the German-Austrian AML Study Group (AMLSG), *Blood* **121**(1): 170–177 (2013).

Schwind, S., C.G. Edwards, D. Nicolet, K. Mrózek, K. Maharry, Y.Z. Wu, P. Paschka, A.K. Eisfeld, P. Hoellerbauer, H. Becker, K.H. Metzeler, J. Curfman, J. Kohlschmidt, T.W. Prior, J.E. Kolitz, W. Blum, M.J. Pettenati, P. Dal Cin, A.J. Carroll, M.A. Caligiuri, R.A. Larson, S. Volinia, G. Marcucci, and C.D. Bloomfield, Alliance for Clinical Trials in Oncology. inv(16)/t(16;16) acute myeloid leukemia with non-type A CBFB-MYH11 fusions associate with distinct clinical and genetic features and lack KIT mutations, *Blood* **121**(2): 385–391 (2013).

Shigesada, K., B. van de Sluis, and P.P. Liu, Mechanism of leukemogenesis by the inv(16) chimeric gene CBFB/PEBP2B-MHY11, *Oncogene* **23**(24): 4297–4307 (2004).

Tang, Y.Y., J. Shi, L. Zhang, A. Davis, J. Bravo, A.J. Warren, N.A. Speck, and J.H. Bushweller, Energetic and functional contribution of residues in the core binding factor beta (CBFbeta) subunit to heterodimerization with CBFalpha, *J Biol Chem* **275**(50): 39579–39588 (2000).

Usuki, K., M. Nakatsu, K. Kitazume, M. Endo, M. Osawa, S. Iki, M. Arai, and A. Urabe, CBFB/MYH11 fusion transcripts in a case of acute myelogenous leukemia (M1) with partial deletion of the long arm of chromosome 16, *Intern Med* **35**(4): 327–330 (1996).

Van der Reijden,, B.A., M. Massop, A. Simons, T. de Witte, M. Breuning, and J.H. Jansen. The NDE1 gene is disrupted by the inv(16) in 90% of cases with CBFB-MYH11-positive acute myeloid leukemia, *Leukemia* **24**(4): 857–859 (2010).

Wajapeyee, N., S.Z. Wang, R.W. Serra, P.D. Solomon, A. Nagarajan, X. Zhu, and M.R. Green, Senescence induction in human fibroblasts and hematopoietic progenitors by leukemogenic fusion proteins, *Blood* **115**(24): 5057–5060 (2010).

Xue, L., J.A. Pulikkan, P.J. Valk, and L.H. Castilla, NrasG12D oncoprotein inhibits apoptosis of preleukemic cells expressing Cbfβ-SMMHC via activation of MEK/ERK axis, *Blood* **124**(3): 426–436 (2014).

Zhao, L., J.J. Melenhorst, L. Alemu, M. Kirby, S. Anderson, M. Kench, S. Hoogstraten-Miller, L. Brinster, Y. Kamikubo, D.G. Gilliland, and P.P. Liu, KIT with D816 mutations cooperates with CBFB-MYH11 for leukemogenesis in mice, *Blood* **119**(6): 1511–1521 (2012).

8

Rearrangements Involving ETS Family of Genes and Their Role in Different Cancers

*Ganesan Padmavathi, Javadi Monisha, Kishore Banik, Choudhary Harsha, Devivasha Bordoloi and Ajaikumar B. Kunnumakkara**

INTRODUCTION

ETS, also known as E26 transformation-specific or E-twenty-six, is a transcription factor family comprising more than 28 genes grouped into subfamilies and is responsible for regulation of the expression of genes involved in different cellular processes including development, tissue remodeling, differentiation, proliferation and apoptosis (Feng *et al.*, 2014). With the highly conserved DNA-binding ETS domain, these transcription factors are well-known to recognize specific sequence motif

*Author for correspondence: Ajaikumar B. Kunnumakkara, Cancer Biology Laboratory, Department of Biosciences and Bioengineering, Indian Institute of Technology Guwahati, Assam 781039, India. kunnumakkara@iitg.ernet.in

5′-GGA(A/T)-3′, bind promoters of specific genes and assist in the assembly of transcription machinery thus regulating the expression of several important genes required in both normal and diseased conditions (Feng *et al.*, 2014; Hollenhorst *et al.*, 2011). For instance, these transcription factors were proved to maintain the expression levels of housekeeping genes; upregulate T-cell activation genes, Ewing's sarcoma genes and serum responsive genes; and downregulate prostate differentiation genes (Hollenhorst *et al.*, 2011). Moreover, among the 28 unique genes, few genes like ERG, friend leukemia virus integration 1 (FLI1) and ETS translocation variant 1 (ETV1) were commonly seen to be deregulated in various cancers like acute lymphoid leukemia (ALL), acute myeloid leukemia (AML), breast cancer, Ewing's sarcoma, melanoma and prostate cancer, etc. (Feng *et al.*, 2014; Tomlins *et al.*, 2005; Tognon *et al.*, 2002; Shurtleff *et al.*, 1995; Shimizu *et al.*, 1993; Jané-Valbuena *et al.*, 2010; de Alava *et al.*, 1998). Deregulation of ETS genes was generally found to appear as increased expression and amplification, translocations, cytoplasmic and stromal expression, post-translational modifications, etc. Such deregulations result in uncontrolled proliferation, angiogenesis, invasion and metastasis (Kar and Gutierrez-Hartmann, 2013). Additionally, ERG fusions were shown to positively regulate prostaglandin signaling which contributes towards cancer progression (Mohamed *et al.*, 2011). This chapter primarily focuses on the ETS gene fusions mediated oncogenesis.

ETS family of genes is found to be fused with a variety of genes including AML1, PDGFRβ, EWS and prostate specific TMPRSS2 gene, thus mediating the tumorigenesis of leukemia, prostate cancer, sarcomas, etc. (Figure 8.1) (Kar and Gutierrez-Hartmann, 2013).

TMPRSS2-ETS FUSIONS IN PROSTATE CANCER

Transmembrane protease serine 2 (TMPRSS2) is a prostate specific androgen responsive gene known to produce type II serine protease enzyme (Thangapazham *et al.*, 2014). Translocation of TMPRSS2 gene with ETS family members such as ETV1, ETV4, ETV5 and ERG has been implicated mainly in prostate cancer (Tomlins *et al.*, 2005; Helgeson *et al.*, 2008). Moreover, the resulting fusion genes were known to encode

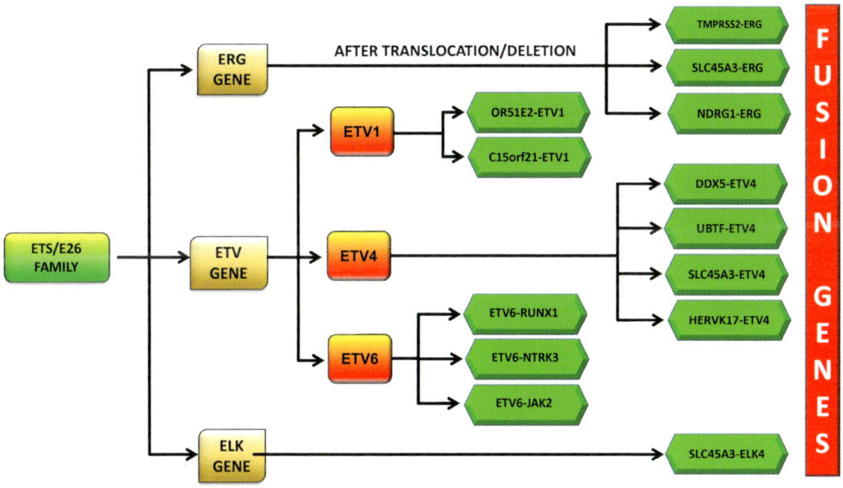

Figure 8.1: ETS/E26 family of genes involved in different gene fusions.

the complete ETS protein with hormonal control and elevate transcription factor activity thus inducing the expression of proliferative genes (Feng *et al.*, 2014; Thangapazham *et al.*, 2014). Among these, ERG is the most common fusion partner of TMPRSS2 found in almost 50% of prostate cancer patients (Kim *et al.*, 2014).

TMPRSS2-ERG

As mentioned earlier, the TMPRSS2-ERG fusion is produced due to interstitial deletion in chromosome 21 and is observed in approximately half of all prostate cancers as well as possesses strong correlation with higher pathological grades (Figure 8.1) (Kim *et al.*, 2014; Yi *et al.*, 2015; Gasi Tandefelt *et al.*, 2014). Aberrant expression of this fusion gene led to prostatic intraepithelial neoplasia (PIN) which can be further progressed to invasive carcinoma by accompanying molecular alterations like loss of PTEN (phosphatase and tensin homolog), increased levels of androgen receptors and constitutive activation of PI3K-Akt pathway, etc. implying the requirement of secondary mutations for the development of cancer (Fallahabadi *et al.*, 2016; Tomlins *et al.*, 2008; King *et al.*,

2009; Carver *et al.*, 2009; Zong *et al.*, 2009; Wang *et al.*, 2015). Supporting this, the loss of tumor suppressor NKX3.1 has also been found to cooperate with TMPRSS2-ERG fusion thus establishing itself as a potent secondary genetic modification in prostate tumorigenesis (Thangapazham *et al.*, 2014). Further, it was shown to activate *C-MYC*; suppress prostate epithelial differentiation by reduced proenzyme prostate-specific antigen (PSA), solute carrier family 45 member 3 (SLC45A3)/prostein expression and block the neuroendocrine and luminal cell differentiation leading to tumorigenesis (Figure 8.2) (Sun *et al.*, 2008; Mounir *et al.*, 2015). Recently, the regulation of micro RNAs was also determined to augment the process of tumorigenesis. For example, modulation of miR-200c expression by TMPRSS2-ERG was proved as a key factor in prostate tumorigenesis and miR-200b/a/429 to be the target genes of ERG fusion (Figure 8.2) (Culig, 2014; Kim *et al.*, 2014; Zhang *et al.*, 2016). In addition, the chimeric transcription factor was also proved to significantly upregulate the expression of matrix metallopeptidase 9 (MMP9) and plexin A2 (PLXNA2) leading to increased migration and invasion of PC3 cells and modulate EMT facilitators, namely, ZEB1 and ZEB2 leading to increased epithelial to mesenchymal transition (Figure 8.2) (Tian *et al.*, 2014; Leshem *et al.*, 2011).

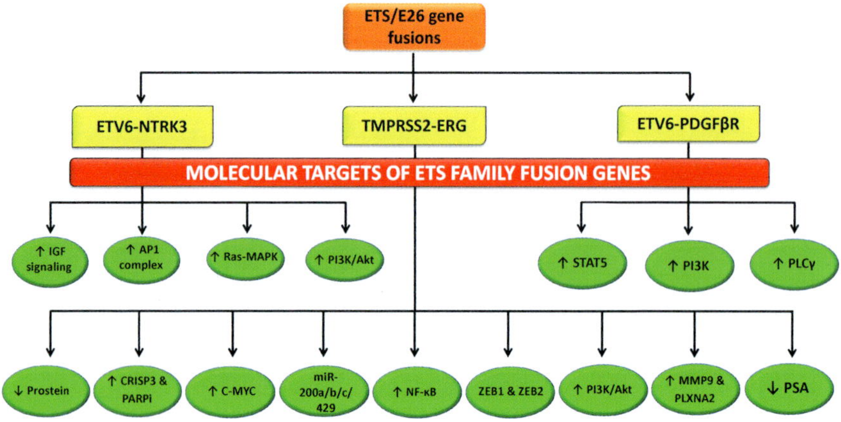

Figure 8.2: Molecular targets of ETS/E26 family fusion genes.

Further, it increased the expression of the important transcription factor nuclear factor-kappa B (NF-κB) which can be reverted by celastrol treatment (Shao *et al.*, 2013; Wang *et al.*, 2011). Likewise, a high level of cysteine-rich secretory protein-3 (CRISP3) was also found to correlate with TMPRSS2-ERG positive prostate carcinomas (Ribeiro *et al.*, 2011). Strikingly, the chimeric protein was shown to increase the poly ADP ribose polymerase inhibitors (PARPi) mediated radiosensitization in prostate cancer patients through inhibition of non-homologous end-joining (NHEJ) DNA repair mechanism (Chatterjee *et al.*, 2015). Also, it has been reported that the prostate cancer patients harboring TMPRSS2-ERG fusion show better response to androgen deprivation therapy (Graff *et al.*, 2015).

Fusion of TMPRSS2 gene with the other ETS family members ETV1 and ETV4 was also found to be implicated in prostate cancer. However, frequency of occurrence of such fusions was very less when compared to the TMPRSS2-ERG (Barros-Silva *et al.*, 2013; Wang *et al.*, 2012; Winnes *et al.*, 2007). The possible mechanism of these fusion genes in the development of prostate carcinoma could be the fusion-mediated deregulation of the ETS proteins (Tomlins *et al.*, 2006). However, detailed experimental studies are required to elucidate the exact molecular pathogenesis of TMPRSS2- ETS fusion-induced prostate cancer.

Other ETS Fusion Genes in Prostate Cancer

It was assumed that the TMPRSS2-ERG was the only ETS translocation associated with prostate cancers until other recurrent C15orf21-ETV1, DDX5-ETV4, EST14-ETV1, HERVK17-ETV4, NDRG1-ERG, OR51E2-ETV1, SLC45A3-ELK4, SLC45A3-ERG, SLC45A3-ETV1, SLC45A3-ETV4, SLC45A3-ETV5 and UBTF-ETV4 translocations have been identified (Figure 8.1) (Esgueva *et al.*, 2010; Pflueger *et al.*, 2009; Barros-Silva *et al.*, 2013; Rickman *et al.*, 2009; Han *et al.*, 2008; Attard *et al.*, 2008; Helgeson *et al.*, 2008). Following TMPRSS2, SLC45A3 is the second most common fusion partner of ERG which upon fusing with ERG reduced the expression of wild-type SLC45A3 significantly and led to poor clinical behavior (Perner *et al.*, 2013).

TEL-NTRK3 (ETV6-NTRK3)

The ETV6-NTRK3 fusion gene is formed as a result of t(12;15)(p13;q25) translocation and was first identified in congenital fibrosarcoma (Wai *et al.*, 2000; Knezevich *et al.*, 1998). Other than fibrosarcoma, this translocation was also commonly observed in congenital mesoblastic nephroma (CMN), secretory breast carcinoma (SBC), mammary analogue secretory carcinoma (MASC), acute myelogenous leukemia (AML) and thyroid cancer, etc. (Arce *et al.*, 2005; Chi *et al.*, 2012; Leeman-Neill *et al.*, 2014; Del Castillo *et al.*, 2015; Majewska *et al.*, 2015; Eguchi *et al.*, 1999). Further, it was found that the recurrent t(12;15) translocation linked the sterile alpha motif (SAM) oligomerization domain of the ETV6 (TEL) transcription factor to the protein tyrosine kinase domain of the neurotrophin-3 receptor NTRK3 resulting in a constitutively active chimeric tyrosine kinase (Chi *et al.*, 2012). The resulting fusion tyrosine kinase was found to possess high transforming activity which was mediated by SAM domain induced oligomerization and activation of insulin-like growth factor 1 (IGF) signaling (Figure 8.2) (Tognon *et al.*, 2004; Morrison *et al.*, 2002). In addition, the fusion protein resulted in the aberrant activation of MAPK pathway thus contributing to the radiation-induced thyroid carcinogenesis (Leeman-Neill *et al.*, 2014; Ricarte-Filho *et al.*, 2013). In breast cancers, ETV6-NTRK3 had been implicated in the transformation of mammary progenitors through activation of AP1 complex (Figure 8.2) (Li *et al.*, 2007). Moreover, tyrosine kinase effect of ETV6-NTRK was found to induce constitutive activation of Ras-MAPK and PI3K-Akt pathways, responsible for cell survival and transforming activity through the IRS-1 adapter protein (Figure 8.2) (Ricarte-Filho *et al.*, 2013; Lannon and Sorensen, 2005; Lannon *et al.*, 2004; Tognon *et al.*, 2001). It is also reported that ETV6-NTRK3 cooperates with c-Src. Therefore, treatment with a c-Src inhibitor would attenuate the constitutively active MAPK pathway (Jin *et al.*, 2007). Furthermore, the constitutive kinase activity of the chimera was shown to be deregulated by an ETV6-NTRK3 inhibitor-midostaurin (PKC412) thus inhibiting cell proliferation and inducing apoptosis (Chi *et al.*, 2012). This implicated that the tyrosine kinase inhibitors might have great potential in the management of ETV6-NTRK3 positive malignancies.

ETS FUSIONS IN LEUKEMIA

More than 40 chromosomal rearrangements involving ETS genes have been identified in hematological malignancies such as ALL, AML and CML. ETV6, also known as TEL, is one of the potent candidate genes frequently fused in leukemic diseases and the fusion partners include ABL, AML1, EVI1, JAK2, PDGFβR and TRKC, etc. All these translocations were known to retain ETS domain or PNT domain or both the domains of ETS proteins (Romana *et al.*, 1995a, 1995b; Peeters *et al.*, 1997; Golub *et al.*, 1994, 1996; Eguchi *et al.*, 1999; Papadopoulos *et al.*, 1995; Lacronique *et al.*, 1997; Kar and Gutierrez-Hartmann, 2013). Most of these fusions have produced constitutively active tyrosine kinase protein which was activated through the oligomerization governed by the PNT domain of TEL protein (Kar and Gutierrez-Hartmann, 2013). Similar to any other fusion tyrosine kinases, the downstream targets include STAT5, cyclins, anti-apoptotic proteins, etc. (Schwaller, 2000; Kar and Gutierrez-Hartmann, 2013).

TEL-AML1 (ETV6-RUNX1)

The most common TEL fusion observed in leukemia is TEL-AML1 fusion, also known as ETV6-RUNX1, is produced by the translocation of chromosomes 12 and 21 t(12;21)(p13;q22). The role of this fusion gene is discussed in detail in Chapter 19.

TEL-JAK2 (ETV6-JAK2)

Like PCM1-JAK2, this fusion is also reported in various haematological malignancies of both lymphoid and myeloid origins with t(9;12)(p24;p13) translocation which joins the tyrosine kinase domain of JAK2 to the helix-loop-helix (HLH) oligomerization domain or ETS DNA-binding domain of ETV6 resulting in constitutive tyrosine kinase activity (Peeters *et al.*, 1997; Onnebo *et al.*, 2012; Schwaller, 2012). STAT5 was found to be the mediator of TEL-JAK2 induced leukemogenesis (Schwaller *et al.*, 2000).

TEL-PDGFβR

As a result of recurrent t(5;12)(q33;p13) translocation, the oligomerization HLH domain of TEL is fused with the tyrosine kinase domain of the platelet-derived growth factor receptor-beta (PDGFβR) producing the chimeric TEL-PDGFβR transcript (Golub *et al.*, 1994; Tomasson *et al.*, 1999). Further, this fusion was found to be associated with the development of chronic myelomonocytic leukemia (CMML) suggesting it to be an early genetic event of AML progression (Golub *et al.*, 1994). Ectopic expression of this fusion gene was shown to develop myeloproliferative disease (MPD) in mice (Cain *et al.*, 2007). It was also found to induce growth factor independence and transformation in Ba/F3 cells via phosphorylation activation of STAT5, PI3K and PLCg (Figure 8.2) (Sternberg *et al.*, 2001; Carroll *et al.*, 1996; Cain *et al.*, 2007). Treatment with tyrosine kinase inhibitors was observed to increase the survival rate *in vivo* suggesting a promising treatment strategy (Tomasson *et al.*, 1999).

CONCLUSION

Altogether, the ETS family of transcription factors has been frequently observed to be involved in chromosomal translocations therefore mediating the initiation and progression of numerous neoplasms including both solid tumors and hematological malignancies. Most often, fusion of ETS genes resulted in the highly active transcription factors or tyrosine kinase proteins leading to the uncontrolled proliferation, angiogenesis, invasion and metastasis.

CONFLICT OF INTEREST

The authors express no conflict of interest.

REFERENCES

Arce, C., D. Cortes-Padilla, D.G. Huntsman, M.A. Miller, A. Dueñnas-Gonzalez, A. Alvarado, V. Pérez, D, Gallardo-Rincón, and F, Lara-Medina, Secretory carcinoma of the breast containing the ETV6-NTRK3 fusion gene in a male: case report and review of the literature, *World J Surg Oncol* **3**: 35 (2005).

Attard, G., J. Clark, L. Ambroisine, I.G. Mills, G. Fisher, P. Flohr, A. Reid, S. Edwards, G. Kovacs, D. Berney, C. Foster, C.E. Massie, A. Fletcher, J.S. De Bono, P. Scardino, J. Cuzick, and C.S. Cooper, Transatlantic Prostate Group. Heterogeneity and clinical significance of ETV1 translocations in human prostate cancer, *Br J Canc* **99**(2): 314–320 (2008).

Barros-Silva, J.D., P. Paulo, A.C. Bakken, N. Cerveira, M. Løvf, R. Henrique, C. Jerónimo, R.A. Lothe, R.I. Skotheim, and M.R. Teixeira, Novel 5′ fusion partners of ETV1 and ETV4 in prostate cancer, *Neoplasia* **15**(7): 720–726 (2013).

Cain, J.A., Z. Xiang, J. O'Neal, F. Kreisel, A. Colson, H. Luo, L. Hennighausen, and M.H. Tomasson, Myeloproliferative disease induced by TEL-PDGFRB displays dynamic range sensitivity to Stat5 gene dosage, *Blood* **109**(9): 3906–3914 (2007).

Carroll, M., M.H. Tomasson, G.F. Barker, T.R. Golub, and D.G. Gilliland, The TEL/platelet-derived growth factor beta receptor (PDGF beta R) fusion in chronic myelomonocytic leukemia is a transforming protein that self-associates and activates PDGF beta R kinase-dependent signaling pathways, *Proc Natl Acad Sci USA* **93**(25): 14845–14850 (1996).

Carver, B.S., J. Tran, A. Gopalan, Z. Chen, S. Shaikh, A. Carracedo, A. Alimonti, C. Nardella, S. Varmeh, P.T. Scardino, C. Cordon-Cardo, W. Gerald, and P.P. Pandolfi, Aberrant ERG expression cooperates with loss of PTEN to promote cancer progression in the prostate, *Nat Genet* **41**(5): 619–624 (2009).

Chatterjee, P., G.S. Choudhary, T. Alswillah, X. Xiong, W.D. Heston, C. Magi-Galluzzi, J. Zhang, E.A. Klein, and A. Almasan, The TMPRSS2-ERG gene fusion blocks XRCC4-mediated nonhomologous end-joining repair and radiosensitizes prostate cancer cells to PARP inhibition, *Mol Canc Ther* **14**(8): 1896–1906 (2015).

Chi, H.T., B.T. Ly, Y. Kano, A. Tojo, T. Watanabe, and Y. Sato, ETV6-NTRK3 as a therapeutic target of small molecule inhibitor PKC412, *Biochem Biophys Res Commun* **429**(1–2): 87–92 (2012).

Culig, Z., Words of wisdom: Re: TMPRSS2-ERG gene fusions induce prostate tumorigenesis by modulating microRNA miR-200c, *Eur Urol* **65**(5): 1011 (2014).

de Alava, E., A. Kawai, J.H. Healey, I. Fligman, P.A. Meyers, A.G. Huvos, W.L. Gerald, S.C. Jhanwar, P. Argani, C.R. Antonescu, F.J. Pardo-Mindan, J. Ginsberg, R. Womer, E.R. Lawlor, J. Wunder, I. Andrulis, P.H. Sorensen, F.G. Barr, and M. Ladanyi, EWS-FLI1 fusion transcript structure is an independent determinant of prognosis in Ewing's sarcoma, *J Clin Oncol* **16**(4): 1248–1255. Erratum in: *J Clin Oncol* **16**(8): 2895 (1998).

Del Castillo, M., F. Chibon, L. Arnould, S. Croce, A. Ribeiro, G. Perot, I. Hostein, S. Geha, C. Bozon, A. Garnier, M. Lae, A. Vincent-Salomon, and G. MacGrogan, Secretory breast carcinoma: A histopathologic and genomic spectrum characterized by a joint specific ETV6-NTRK3 gene fusion, *Am J Surg Pathol* **39**(11): 1458–1467 (2015).

Eguchi, M., M. Eguchi-Ishimae, A. Tojo, K. Morishita, K. Suzuki, Y. Sato, S. Kudoh, K. Tanaka, M. Setoyama, F. Nagamura, S. Asano, and N. Kamada, Fusion of ETV6 to neurotrophin-3 receptor TRKC in acute myeloid leukemia with t(12;15)(p13;q25), *Blood* **93**(4): 1355–1363 (1999).

Esgueva, R., S. Perner, C. J LaFargue, V. Scheble, C. Stephan, M. Lein, F.R. Fritzsche, M. Dietel, G. Kristiansen, and M.A. Rubin, Prevalence of TMPRSS2-ERG and SLC45A3-ERG gene fusions in a large prostatectomy cohort, *Mod Pathol* **23**(4): 539–546 (2010).

Fallahabadi, Z.R., M.R. Noori Daloii, R. Mahdian, F. Behjati, M.A. Shokrgozar, M. Abolhasani, M. Asgari, and H. Shahrokh, Frequency of PTEN alterations, TMPRSS2-ERG fusion and their association in prostate cancer, *Gene* **575**(2 Pt 3): 755–760 (2016).

Feng, F.Y., J.C. Brenner, M. Hussain, and A.M. Chinnaiyan, Molecular pathways: targeting ETS gene fusions in cancer, *Clin Canc Res* **20**(17): 4442–4448 (2014).

Gasi Tandefelt, D., J. Boormans, K. Hermans, and J. Trapman, ETS fusion genes in prostate cancer, *Endocr Relat Canc* **21**(3): R143–R152 (2014).

Golub, T.R., G.F. Barker, M. Lovett, and D.G. Gilliland, Fusion of PDGF receptor beta to a novel ets-like gene, tel, in chronic myelomonocytic leukemia with t(5;12) chromosomal translocation, *Cell* **77**(2): 307–316 (1994).

Golub, T.R., A. Goga, G.F. Barker, D.E. Afar, J. McLaughlin, S.K. Bohlander, J.D. Rowley, O.N. Witte, and D.G. Gilliland, Oligomerization of the ABL tyrosine kinase by the Ets protein TEL in human leukemia, *Mol Cell Biol* **16**(8): 4107–1416 (1996).

Graff, R.E., A. Pettersson, R.T. Lis, N. DuPre, K.M. Jordahl, E. Nuttall, J.R. Rider, M. Fiorentino, H.D. Sesso, S.A. Kenfield, M. Loda, E.L. Giovannucci, B. Rosner, P.L. Nguyen, C.J. Sweeney, and L.A. Mucci, Transdisciplinary prostate cancer partnership ToPCaP. The TMPRSS2:ERG fusion and response to androgen deprivation therapy for prostate cancer, *Prostate* **75**(9): 897–906 (2015).

Han, B., R. Mehra, S.M. Dhanasekaran, J. Yu, A. Menon, R.J. Lonigro, X. Wang, Y. Gong, L. Wang, S. Shankar, B. Laxman, R.B. Shah, S. Varambally, N. Palanisamy, S.A. Tomlins, C. Kumar-Sinha, and A.M. Chinnaiyan,

A fluorescence *in situ* hybridization screen for E26 transformation-specific aberrations: identification of DDX5-ETV4 fusion protein in prostate cancer, *Canc Res* **68**(18): 7629–7637 (2008).

Helgeson, B.E., S.A. Tomlins, N. Shah, B. Laxman, Q. Cao, J.R. Prensner, X. Cao, N. Singla, J.E. Montie, S. Varambally, R. Mehra, and A.M. Chinnaiyan, Characterization of TMPRSS2:ETV5 and SLC45A3:ETV5 gene fusions in prostate cancer, *Canc Res* **68**(1): 73–80 (2008).

Hollenhorst, P.C., L.P. McIntosh, and B.J. Graves, Genomic and biochemical insights into the specificity of ETS transcription factors, *Annu Rev Biochem* **80**: 437–471 (2011).

Jané-Valbuena, J., H.R. Widlund, S. Perner, L.A. Johnson, A.C. Dibner, W.M. Lin, A.C. Baker, R.M. Nazarian, K.G. Vijayendran, W.R. Sellers, W.C. Hahn, L.M. Duncan, M.A. Rubin, D.E. Fisher, and L.A. Garraway, An oncogenic role for ETV1 in melanoma, *Canc Res* **70**(5): 2075–2084 (2010).

Jin, W., C. Yun, A. Hobbie, M.J. Martin, P.H. Sorensen, and S.J. Kim, Cellular transformation and activation of the phosphoinositide-3-kinase-Akt cascade by the ETV6-NTRK3 chimeric tyrosine kinase requires c-Src, *Canc Res* **67**(7): 3192–3200 (2007).

Kar, A., A. Gutierrez-Hartmann, Molecular mechanisms of ETS transcription factor-mediated tumorigenesis, *Crit Rev Biochem Mol Biol* **48**(6): 522–543 (2013).

Kim, J., L. Wu, J.C. Zhao, H.J. Jin, and J. Yu, TMPRSS2-ERG gene fusions induce prostate tumorigenesis by modulating microRNA miR-200c, *Oncogene* **33**(44): 5183–5192 (2014).

King, J.C., J. Xu, J. Wongvipat, H. Hieronymus, B.S. Carver, D.H. Leung, B.S. Taylor, C. Sander, R.D. Cardiff, S.S. Couto, W.L. Gerald, and C.L. Sawyers, Cooperativity of TMPRSS2-ERG with PI3-kinase pathway activation in prostate oncogenesis, *Nat Genet* **41**(5): 524–526 (2009).

Knezevich, S.R., D.E. McFadden, W. Tao, J.F. Lim, and P.H. Sorensen, A novel ETV6-NTRK3 gene fusion in congenital fibrosarcoma, *Nat Genet* **18**(2): 184–187 (1998).

Lacronique, V., A. Boureux, V.D. Valle, H. Poirel, C.T. Quang, M. Mauchauffé, C. Berthou, M. Lessard, R. Berger, J. Ghysdael, and O.A. Bernard, A TEL-JAK2 fusion protein with constitutive kinase activity in human leukemia, *Science* **278**(5341): 1309–1312 (1997).

Lannon, C.L., M.J. Martin, C.E. Tognon, W. Jin, S.J. Kim, and P.H. Sorensen, A highly conserved NTRK3 C-terminal sequence in the ETV6-NTRK3 oncoprotein binds the phosphotyrosine binding domain of insulin receptor substrate-1: an essential interaction for transformation, *J Biol Chem* **279**(8): 6225–6234 (2004).

Lannon, C.L. and P.H. Sorensen, ETV6-NTRK3: a chimeric protein tyrosine kinase with transformation activity in multiple cell lineages, *Semin Canc Biol* **15**(3): 215–223 (2005).

Leeman-Neill, R.J., L.M. Kelly, P. Liu, A.V. Brenner, M.P. Little, T.I. Bogdanova, V.N. Evdokimova, M. Hatch, L.Y. Zurnadzy, M.N. Nikiforova, N.J. Yue, M. Zhang, K. Mabuchi, M.D. Tronko, and Y.E. Nikiforov, ETV6-NTRK3 is a common chromosomal rearrangement in radiation-associated thyroid cancer, *Canc* **120**(6): 799–807 (2014).

Leshem, O., S. Madar, I. Kogan-Sakin, I. Kamer, I. Goldstein, R. Brosh, Y. Cohen, J. Jacob-Hirsch, M. Ehrlich, S. Ben-Sasson, N. Goldfinger, R. Loewenthal, E. Gazit, V. Rotter, and R. Berger, TMPRSS2/ERG promotes epithelial to mesenchymal transition through the ZEB1/ZEB2 axis in a prostate cancer model, *PLoS One* **6**(7): e21650 (2011).

Li, Z., C.E. Tognon, F.J. Godinho, L. Yasaitis, H. Hock, J.I. Herschkowitz, C.L. Lannon, E. Cho, SJ. Kim, R.T. Bronson, C.M. Perou, P.H. Sorensen, and S.H. Orkin, ETV6-NTRK3 fusion oncogene initiates breast cancer from committed mammary progenitors via activation of AP1 complex, *Canc Cell* **12**(6): 542–558 (2007).

Majewska, H., A. Skálová, D. Stodulski, A. Klimková, P. Steiner, C. Stankiewicz, and W. Biernat, Mammary analogue secretory carcinoma of salivary glands: a new entity associated with ETV6 gene rearrangement, *Virchows Arch* **466**(3): 245–254 (2015).

Mohamed, A.A., S.H. Tan, C. Sun, S. Shaheduzzaman, Y. Hu, G. Petrovics, Y. Chen, I.A. Sesterhenn, H. Li, T. Sreenath, D.G. McLeod, A. Dobi, and S. Srivastava, ERG oncogene modulates prostaglandin signaling in prostate cancer cells, *Canc Biol Ther* **11**(4): 410–417 (2011).

Morrison, K.B., C.E. Tognon, M.J. Garnett, C. Deal, and P.H. Sorensen, ETV6-NTRK3 transformation requires insulin-like growth factor 1 receptor signaling and is associated with constitutive IRS-1 tyrosine phosphorylation, *Oncogene* **21**(37): 5684–5695 (2002).

Mounir, Z., F. Lin, V.G. Lin, J.M. Korn, Y. Yu, R. Valdez, O.H. Aina, G. Buchwalter, A.B. Jaffe, M. Korpal, P. Zhu, M. Brown, R.D. Cardiff, J.L. Rocnik, Y. Yang, and R. Pagliarini, TMPRSS2:ERG blocks neuroendocrine and luminal cell differentiation to maintain prostate cancer proliferation, *Oncogene* **34**(29): 3815–3825 (2015).

Onnebo, S.M., P. Rasighaemi, J. Kumar, C. Liongue, and A.C. Ward, Alternative TEL-JAK2 fusions associated with T-cell acute lymphoblastic leukemia and atypical chronic myelogenous leukemia dissected in zebrafish, *Haematologica* **97**(12): 1895–1903 (2012).

Papadopoulos, P., S.A. Ridge, C.A. Boucher, C. Stocking, and L.M. Wiedemann, The novel activation of ABL by fusion to an ets-related gene, TEL, *Canc Res* **55**(1): 34–38 (1995).

Peeters, P., S.D. Raynaud, J. Cools, I. Wlodarska, J. Grosgeorge, P. Philip, F. Monpoux, L. Van Rompaey, M. Baens, H. Van den Berghe, and P. Marynen, Fusion of TEL, the ETS-variant gene 6 (ETV6), to the receptor-associated kinase JAK2 as a result of t(9;12) in a lymphoid and t(9;15;12) in a myeloid leukemia, *Blood* **90**(7): 2535–2540 (1997).

Peeters, P., I. Wlodarska, M. Baens, A. Criel, D. Selleslag, A. Hagemeijer, H. Van den Berghe, and P. Marynen, Fusion of ETV6 to MDS1/EVI1 as a result of t(3;12)(q26;p13) in myeloproliferative disorders, *Canc Res* **57**(4): 564–569 (1997).

Perner, S., N.J. Rupp, M. Braun, M.A. Rubin, H. Moch, M. Dietel, N. Wernert, K. Jung, C. Stephan, and G. Kristiansen, Loss of SLC45A3 protein (prostein) expression in prostate cancer is associated with SLC45A3-ERG gene rearrangement and an unfavorable clinical course, *Int J Canc* **132**(4): 807–812 (2013).

Pflueger, D., D.S. Rickman, A. Sboner, S. Perner, C.J. LaFargue, M.A. Svensson, B.J. Moss, N. Kitabayashi, Y. Pan, A. de la Taille, R. Kuefer, A.K. Tewari, F. Demichelis, M.S. Chee, M.B. Gerstein, and M.A. Rubin, N-myc downstream regulated gene 1 (NDRG1) is fused to ERG in prostate cancer, *Neoplasia* **11**(8): 804–811 (2009).

Ribeiro, F.R., P. Paulo, V.L. Costa, J.D. Barros-Silva, J. Ramalho-Carvalho, C. Jerónimo, R. Henrique, G.E. Lind, R.I. Skotheim, R.A. Lothe, and M.R. Teixeira, Cysteine-rich secretory protein-3 (CRISP3) is strongly up-regulated in prostate carcinomas with the TMPRSS2-ERG fusion gene, *PLoS One* **6**(7): e22317 (2011).

Ricarte-Filho, J.C., S. Li, M.E. Garcia-Rendueles, C. Montero-Conde, F. Voza, J.A. Knauf, A. Heguy, A. Viale, T. Bogdanova, G.A. Thomas, C.E. Mason, and J.A. Fagin, Identification of kinase fusion oncogenes in post-Chernobyl radiation-induced thyroid cancers, *J Clin Invest* **123**(11): 4935–4944 (2013).

Rickman, D.S., D. Pflueger, B. Moss, V.E. VanDoren, C.X. Chen, A. de la Taille, R. Kuefer, A.K. Tewari, S.R. Setlur, F. Demichelis, and M.A. Rubin, SLC45A3-ELK4 is a novel and frequent erythroblast transformation-specific fusion transcript in prostate cancer, *Canc Res* **69**(7): 2734–2738 (2009).

Romana, S.P., H. Poirel, M. Leconiat, M.A. Flexor, M. Mauchauffé, P. Jonveaux, E.A. Macintyre, R. Berger, and O.A. Bernard, High frequency of t(12;21) in childhood B-lineage acute lymphoblastic leukemia, *Blood* **86**(11): 4263–4269 (1995a).

Romana, S.P., M. Mauchauffé, M. Le Coniat, I. Chumakov, D. Le Paslier, R. Berger, and O.A. Bernard, The t(12;21) of acute lymphoblastic leukemia results in a tel-AML1 gene fusion, *Blood* **85**(12): 3662–3670 (1995b).

Schwaller, J., E. Parganas, D. Wang, D. Cain, J.C. Aster, I.R. Williams, C.K. Lee, R. Gerthner, T. Kitamura, J. Frantsve, E. Anastasiadou, M.L. Loh, D.E. Levy, J.N. Ihle, and D.G. Gilliland, Stat5 is essential for the myelo- and lymphoproliferative disease induced by TEL/JAK2, *Mol Cell* **6**(3): 693–704 (2000).

Schwaller, J., Modeling ETV6-JAK2-induced leukemia: insights from the zebrafish, *Haematologica* **97**(12): 1783–1785 (2012).

Shao, L., Z. Zhou, Y. Cai, P. Castro, O. Dakhov, P. Shi, Y. Bai, H. Ji, W. Shen, and J. Wang, Celastrol suppresses tumor cell growth through targeting an AR-ERG-NF-κB pathway in TMPRSS2/ERG fusion gene expressing prostate cancer, *PLoS One* **8**(3): e58391 (2013).

Shimizu, K., H. Ichikawa, A. Tojo, Y. Kaneko, N. Maseki, Y. Hayashi, M. Ohira, S. Asano, and M. Ohki, An ets-related gene, ERG, is rearranged in human myeloid leukemia with t(16;21) chromosomal translocation, *Proc Natl Acad Sci USA* **90**(21): 10280–10284 (1993).

Shurtleff, S.A., A. Buijs, F.G. Behm, J.E. Rubnitz, S.C. Raimondi, M.L. Hancock, G.C. Chan, C.H. Pui, G. Grosveld, and J.R. Downing, TEL/AML1 fusion resulting from a cryptic t(12;21) is the most common genetic lesion in pediatric ALL and defines a subgroup of patients with an excellent prognosis, *Leukemia* **9**(12): 1985–1989 (1995).

Sternberg, D.W., M.H. Tomasson, M. Carroll, D.P. Curley, G. Barker, M. Caprio, A. Wilbanks, A. Kazlauskas, and D.G. Gilliland, The TEL/PDGFbetaR fusion in chronic myelomonocytic leukemia signals through STAT5-dependent and STAT5-independent pathways, *Blood* **98**(12): 3390–3397 (2001).

Sun, C., A. Dobi, A. Mohamed, H. Li, R.L. Thangapazham, B. Furusato, S. Shaheduzzaman, S.H. Tan, G. Vaidyanathan, E. Whitman, D.J. Hawksworth, Y. Chen, M. Nau, V. Patel, M. Vahey, J.S. Gutkind, T. Sreenath, G. Petrovics, I.A. Sesterhenn, D.G. McLeod, and S. Srivastava, TMPRSS2-ERG fusion, a common genomic alteration in prostate cancer activates C-MYC and abrogates prostate epithelial differentiation, *Oncogene* **27**(40): 5348–5353 (2008).

Thangapazham, R., F. Saenz, S. Katta, A.A. Mohamed, S.H. Tan, G. Petrovics, S. Srivastava, and A. Dobi, Loss of the NKX3.1 tumorsuppressor promotes the TMPRSS2-ERG fusion gene expression in prostate cancer, *BMC Canc* **14**: 16 (2014).

Tian, T.V., N. Tomavo, L. Huot, A. Flourens, E. Bonnelye, S. Flajollet, D. Hot, X. Leroy, Y. de Launoit, and M. Duterque-Coquillaud, Identification of novel TMPRSS2:ERG mechanisms in prostate cancer metastasis: involvement of MMP9 and PLXNA2, *Oncogene* **33**(17): 2204–2214 (2014).

Tognon, C., M. Garnett, E. Kenward, R. Kay, K. Morrison, and P H. Sorensen, The chimeric protein tyrosine kinase ETV6-NTRK3 requires both Ras-Erk1/2 and PI3-kinase-Akt signaling for fibroblast transformation, *Canc Res* **61**(24): 8909–8916 (2001).

Tognon, C., S.R. Knezevich, D. Huntsman, C.D. Roskelley, N. Melnyk, J.A. Mathers, L. Becker, F. Carneiro, N. MacPherson, D. Horsman, C. Poremba, and P.H. Sorensen, Expression of the ETV6-NTRK3 gene fusion as a primary event in human secretory breast carcinoma, *Cancer Cell* **2**(5): 367–376 (2002).

Tognon, C.E., C.D. Mackereth, A.M. Somasiri, L.P. McIntosh, and P.H. Sorensen, Mutations in the SAM domain of the ETV6-NTRK3 chimeric tyrosine kinase block polymerization and transformation activity, *Mol Cell Biol* **24**(11): 4636–4650 (2004).

Tomasson, M.H., I.R. Williams, R. Hasserjian, C. Udomsakdi, S.M. McGrath, J. Schwaller, B. Druker, and D.G. Gilliland, TEL/PDGFbetaR induces hematologic malignancies in mice that respond to a specific tyrosine kinase inhibitor, *Blood* **93**(5): 1707–1714 (1999).

Tomlins, S.A., B. Laxman, S. Varambally, X. Cao, J. Yu, B.E. Helgeson, Q. Cao, J.R. Prensner, M.A. Rubin, R.B. Shah, R. Mehra, and A.M. Chinnaiyan, Role of the TMPRSS2-ERG gene fusion in prostate cancer, *Neoplasia* **10**(2): 177–188 (2008).

Tomlins, S.A., R. Mehra, D.R. Rhodes, L.R. Smith, D. Roulston, B.E. Helgeson, X. Cao, J.T. Wei, M.A. Rubin, R.B. Shah, and A.M. Chinnaiyan TMPRSS2:ETV4 gene fusions define a third molecular subtype of prostate cancer, *Canc Res* **66**(7): 3396–3400 (2006).

Tomlins, S.A., D.R. Rhodes, S. Perner, S.M. Dhanasekaran, R. Mehra, X.W. Sun, S. Varambally, X. Cao, J. Tchinda, R. Kuefer, C. Lee, J.E. Montie, R.B. Shah, K.J. Pienta, M.A. Rubin, and A.M. Chinnaiyan, Recurrent fusion of TMPRSS2 and ETS transcription factor genes in prostate cancer, *Science* **310**(5748): 644–648 (2005).

Wai, D.H., S.R. Knezevich, T. Lucas, B. Jansen, R.J. Kay, and P.H. Sorensen, The ETV6-NTRK3 gene fusion encodes a chimeric protein tyrosine kinase that transforms NIH3T3 cells, *Oncogene* **19**(7): 906–915 (2000).

Wang, J., Y. Cai, L.J. Shao, J. Siddiqui, N. Palanisamy, R. Li, C. Ren, G. Ayala, and M. Ittmann, Activation of NF-{kappa}B by TMPRSS2/ERG Fusion

Isoforms through Toll-Like Receptor-4, *Cancer Res* **71**(4): 1325–1333 (2011).

Wang, J.J., Y.X. Liu, W. Wang, W. Yan, Y.P. Zheng, L.D. Qiao, D. Liu, and S. Chen, Fusion between TMPRSS2 and ETS family members (ERG, ETV1, ETV4) in prostate cancers from northern China, *Asian Pac J Cancer Prev* **13**(10): 4935–4938 (2012).

Wang, L., S.R. Williamson, S. Zhang, J. Huang, R. Montironi, D.D. Davison, M. Wang, J.L. Yao, A. Lopez-Beltran, A.O. Osunkoya, G.T. MacLennan, L.A. Baldridge, X. Du, and L. Cheng, Increased androgen receptor gene copy number is associated with TMPRSS2-ERG rearrangement in prostatic small cell carcinoma, *Mol Carcinog* **54**(9): 900–907 (2015).

Winnes, M., E. Lissbrant, J.E. Damber, and G. Stenman, Molecular genetic analyses of the TMPRSS2-ERG and TMPRSS2-ETV1 gene fusions in 50 cases of prostate cancer, *Oncol Rep* **17**(5): 1033–1036 (2007).

Yi, F.X., H. Li, Q. Wei, X. Li, and H. Zeng, [Relationship between TMPRSS2: ERG and the pathological grade of prostate cancer], *Zhonghua Nan Ke Xue* **21**(10): 887–891 (2015).

Zhang, Z., R.B. Lanz, L. Xiao, L. Wang, S.M. Hartig, M.M. Ittmann, Q. Feng, and B. He, The tumor suppressive miR-200b subfamily is an ERG target gene in human prostate tumors, *Oncotarget* **7**(25): 37993–38003 (2016).

Zong, Y., L. Xin, A.S. Goldstein, D.A. Lawson, M.A. Teitell, and O.N. Witte, ETS family transcription factors collaborate with alternative signaling pathways to induce carcinoma from adult murine prostate cells, *Proc Natl Acad Sci USA* **106**(30): 12465–12470 (2009).

9

Translocation of FET Family Members with Various Partner Genes and Their Role in Cancer Development

*Ganesan Padmavathi, Devivasha Bordoloi, Anand Anip, Krishan Kumar Thakur and Ajaikumar B. Kunnumakkara**

INTRODUCTION

DNA and RNA binding proteins fused in sarcoma (FUS), Ewing sarcoma (EWS) and TATA-box binding protein associated factor 15 (TAF15) compose the FET family and assist in mRNA biogenesis of thousands of transcripts (Schwartz *et al.*, 2015; Rossow and Janknecht, 2001). The FET

*Author for correspondence: Ajaikumar B. Kunnumakkara, Cancer Biology Laboratory, Department of Biosciences and Bioengineering, Indian Institute of Technology Guwahati, Assam 781039, India. kunnumakkara@iitg.ernet.in

family members were found to share highly conserved structural features with N-terminal LC domain, RGG domain, zinc finger (ZnF) domain, and RNA recognition motif (RRM) which were known to facilitate the self-assembly and nucleic acid interactions of FET proteins (Schwartz *et al.*, 2015). Besides DNA and RNA binding activities, FET proteins were also known to involve in oligomerization and protein–protein interactions (Schwartz *et al.*, 2013, 2015). Further, FET proteins have been confirmed to interact with RNA polymerase II and transcription factor II D (TFIID) complex thus regulating transcription and RNA splicing (Bertolotti *et al.*, 1996, 1998). In addition, these highly abundant nucleic acid binding proteins are commonly regarded as heterogeneous nuclear ribonucleoprotein particle (hnRNP) proteins and either occupied in nucleus or shuttle between nucleus and cytosol (Schwartz *et al.*, 2015; Rossow and Janknecht, 2001). Shuttling nature of these proteins was found to be supportive in RNA transport in complex from nucleus to other cellular compartments and making them as potential targets of tyrosine kinases and G-protein-coupled receptors (GPCRs) (Zinszner *et al.*, 1997; Felsch *et al.*, 1999; Kanai *et al.*, 2004). For instance, protein kinase C (PKC) was shown to negatively regulate the RNA binding property of FET proteins through phosphorylation of IQ domain (Deloulme *et al.*, 1997). Moreover, these proteins were also found to exert p300 acetyltransferase inhibitory effects and to mediate the DNA repair mechanisms thus maintaining genomic integrity (Wang *et al.*, 2008).

Translocations involving the LC domain of FET proteins were frequently detected in leukemia, carcinomas, sarcomas, etc. and were known to elevate the transcription of proliferative genes through the resulting chimeric transcriptional activators (Crozat *et al.*, 1993; Zinszner *et al.*, 1994; Ichikawa *et al.*, 1994; Schwartz *et al.*, 2015). Among the three proteins, FUS and EWS were most commonly found to participate in chromosomal rearrangements and the fusion partners include variety of transcription factors and other genes such as ATF1, CREB1, CREB3L1, CREB3L2, DDIT3, ERG, ETV1, ETV4, FEV, FLI1, NR4A3, PATZ1, PBX1, POU5F1, SP3, WT1 and ZNF384. The following section of this chapter deals with the various FET fusion genes and their implication in different cancers.

FUS-DDIT3 OR FUS-CHOP

FUS-DDIT3 also denoted as FUS-CHOP is a chimeric oncoprotein generated by t(12;16)(q13;p11) rearrangement and is the most common chromosomal translocation observed in liposarcomas, which are characterized by the accumulation of early adipocytic precursors (Figure 9.1) (Pérez-Mancera *et al.*, 2007, 2008; Rabbitts *et al.*, 1993; Turc-Carel *et al.*, 1986). t(12;16) rearrangement resulted in the fusion of entire coding sequence from DNA-binding CHOP gene to the 5′-terminal part of FUS thus producing FUS-CHOP chimera comprising DNA-binding and leucine zipper dimerization domains of CHOP and the transcriptional activation domain

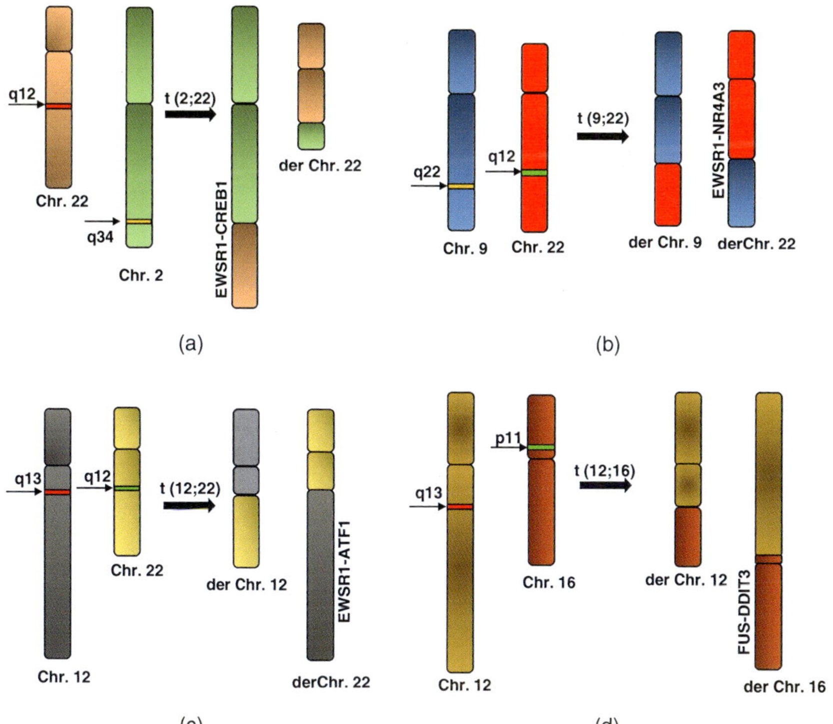

Figure 9.1: Chromosomal translocations involving FET family members: (A) EWSR1-CREB1; (B) EWSR1-NR4A3; (C) EWSR1-ATF1; (D) FUS-DDIT3.

of FUS but lacks RNA binding domain and the RGG triplet motif of FUS (Panagopoulos *et al.*, 2000; Crozat *et al.*, 1993). Moreover, it was confirmed that tight regulation of this fusion protein was correlated with the development of myxoid liposarcoma (MLS) (Åman *et al.*, 2016; Rodriguez *et al.*, 2013).

Proving its oncogenic potential, FUS-CHOP chimera was shown to block adipocyte differentiation process contributing to the accumulation of early adipocytic precursors by reducing the expression of peroxisome proliferator-activated receptors gamma (PPARγ) and C/EBPα, hampering C/EBPβ function and activating eukaryotic translation initiation factor 4E (eIF4E) (Pérez-Mancera *et al.*, 2007, 2008; Adelmant *et al.*, 1998). Further, it also enhanced the MLS tumor growth through reduced levels of MDA-7/IL-24 expression (Oikawa *et al.*, 2012). In addition, it was also proved to contribute to the metastatic potential of liposarcoma cells which was mediated by activated matrix-metalloproteinases (MMP) -2 and -9 and by increased levels of metastasis regulator, plasminogen activator inhibitor-1 (PAI-1) through the suppression of miR-486 (Patil *et al.*, 2014; Borjigin *et al.*, 2012). Moreover, indirect stimulation of fms related tyrosine kinase 1 (FLT1) by this fusion gene was detected in MLS suggesting a possible presence of intracrine signaling loop (Andersson *et al.*, 2010).

Through further analysis, the DDIT3-CHOP portion of the fusion gene was found to interact with cell cycle regulator protein cyclin-dependent kinase 2 (CDK2) thus implicating a crucial role of FUS-CHOP chimera in cancer cell growth (Bento *et al.*, 2009). Besides CDK2, various other cell cycle regulator genes including cyclins D1 and E and CDK4 were also found to be highly correlated with FUS-CHOP resulting in a complete deregulation of cell cycle (Olofsson *et al.*, 2004). Additionally, it also elevated the tumor associated IL6 which was found to be mediated by the increased expression of CEBPB (Göransson *et al.*, 2005). Further, the interaction of this fusion protein with the transcription factor NF-κB family member, NF-κB inhibitor zeta (NFKBIZ) resulted in the modulation of NF-κB-regulated genes like IL8 which may also contribute to fusion induced tumorigenesis (Göransson *et al.*, 2009).

FUS-ERG

FUS-ERG gene produced by the t(16;21)(p11;q22) was recurrently observed in several types of myeloid leukemia (Ichikawa *et al.*, 1994; Panagopoulos *et al.*, 1994; Kong *et al.*, 1997; Buchanan and Tirado, 2016). Kanazawa *et al.* (2005) identified a case of B cell leukemia (B-ALL) for the first time with TLS/FUS-ERG translocation thus proving FUS-ERG fusion is not only restricted to myeloid leukemia (Kanazawa *et al.*, 2005). Further, it was also detected in myeloid sarcoma and Ewing sarcoma-peripheral neuroectodermal tumor of the kidney (Berg *et al.*, 2009; Ueda *et al.*, 2016; Chen *et al.*, 2016). Despite being a transcriptional activator, ERG upon fusion with FUS-TLS exhibited only moderate transcriptional activation properties whereas TLS-FUS fusion domain (TFD) of the chimeric protein exhibited high transactivation properties and altered the DNA binding activities of the fusion protein thus mediating tumorigenesis (Prasad *et al.*, 1994). Moreover, FUS-ERG chimera was shown to have two N-terminal domains, namely, TR1 and TR2 both independently mediated the inhibition of differentiation and G-CSF-dependent proliferation of L-G cells; and the anchorage-independent growth of NIH 3T3 cells. In addition, these domains also independently regulated the expression of various genes representing the involvement of two independent and simultaneous oncogenic pathways in leukemogenesis (Ichikawa *et al.*, 1999). Similarly, fusion-mediated deregulation of CDK1 blocked the terminal differentiation of myeloid progenitor cells (MPCs) (Pan *et al.*, 2008). In addition, the fusion gene lacked the C-terminal RNA splicing activity of the wild-type TLS which can recruit serine-arginine (SR) family of splicing factors thus leading to splicing abnormality of important cellular regulators (Yang *et al.*, 2000b; Chansky *et al.*, 2001; Zou *et al.*, 2005). Interestingly, FUS-ERG also acts as a potent repressor of retinoic acid (RA) signaling pathway thus blocking the myeloid differentiation (Sotoca *et al.*, 2016). Above all, the fusion positive AML was found to exhibit strong resistance to standard chemotherapy as FUS-ERG transcripts were detected in short and long complete remission tumor samples as well as imposing the requirement of more advanced therapeutic options for the treatment of such diseases (Kong *et al.*, 1997).

FUS-CREB3L2 AND FUS-CREB3L1

Fusion of cAMP responsive element binding protein 3-like 2 (CREB3L2) gene of the CREB3 transcription factor family, FUS-CREB3L2, was frequently observed in malignant low-grade fibromyxoid sarcoma (LGFMS) with t(7;16)(q33;p11) rearrangement and was shown to correlate with increased expression of CD24 and forkhead box L1 (FOXL1) (Mertens *et al.*, 2005; Panagopoulos *et al.*, 2004, 2007; Möller *et al.*, 2011). However, in rare cases of LGFMS, a variant fusion FUS-CREB3L1 was also detected (Mertens *et al.*, 2005).

OTHER FUSION GENES INVOLVING FUS

t(2;16)(q35;p11) was identified in a 33-year-old Ewing sarcoma patient and was found to result in an in-frame fusion of FUS and FEV denoted as FUS-FEV (Ng *et al.*, 2007). Another translocation t(7;16)(q33;p11) producing FUS-BBF2H7 fusion was detected in low grade fibromyxoid sarcoma (Storlazzi *et al.*, 2003). Further, fusion of FUS with activating transcription factor 1 (ATF1) gene was found to be associated with fibrous histiocytoma (Raddaoui *et al.*, 2002).

EWSR1-FLI1

The EWS RNA-binding protein 1, abbreviated as EWSR1 gene, was known to govern the synthesis of EWS protein belonging to FET family, whose function is poorly understood. Like the other members of FET family, mutations involving EWSR1 gene also were shown to cause Ewing sarcoma (ES), a type of cancerous tumor, which develops in bones or soft tissues. The most common mutation that leads to 85% of Ewing sarcoma is the translocation of genetic material between chromosome 22 and chromosome 11, written as t(11;22)(q24;q12) resulting in EWSR1-FLI1 fusion gene. The protein produced from this fusion, called EWS-FLI exhibited the functions of both partner genes i.e. the DNA-binding function of the FLI protein as well as the transcription regulation function of the EWS protein. Abnormal expression of this fusion protein effects the regulation of variety of genes involved in the normal cellular processes and induces tumor angiogenesis, uncontrolled proliferation, abnormal maturation and survival of cells, supporting tumorigenesis (http://ghr.nlm.nih.gov/gene/EWSR1, Potikyan *et al.*, 2007). Further, the chimeric transcription factor EWSR1-FLI1 mediated the tumorigenesis process via aberrant transcriptional regulation of a wide range of genes such as Caveolin-1 (CAV1), DAX1, EWS susceptibility gene, EGR2, FOXO1, GLI1, GSTM4, IGF-1R, IGFBP, MK-STYX-STYXL1, NKX2-2, NR0B1, p21WAF1-CIP1, p53, PPP1R1A, PTPL1 and SOX2, etc. via both transcriptional and post-transcriptional mechanisms (Figure 9.2) (Baer *et al.*, 2004; Prieur

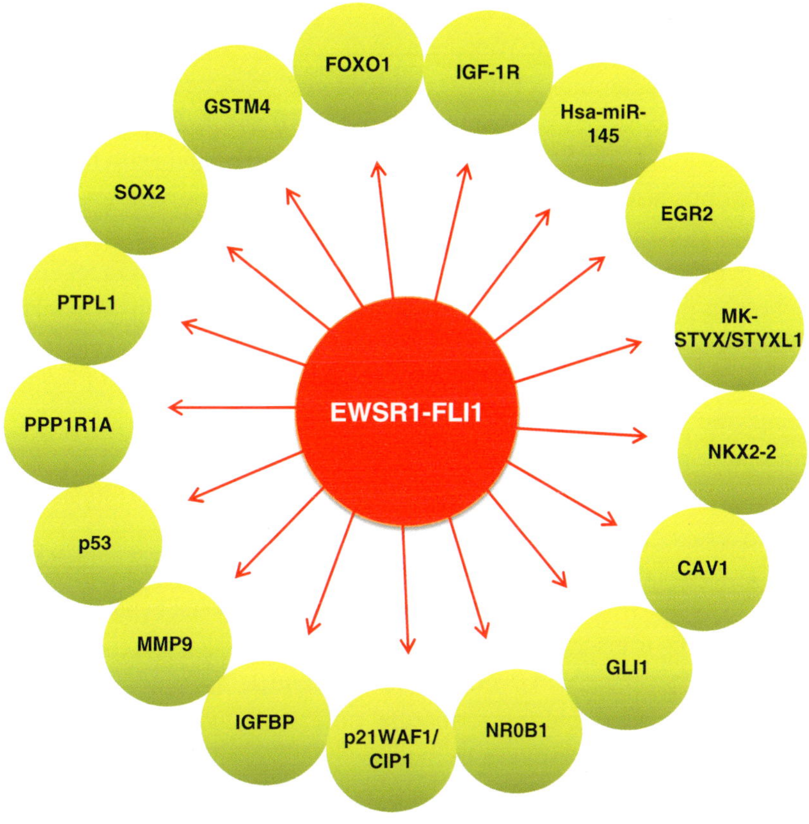

Figure 9.2: Molecular targets of EWSR1-FLI1.

et al., 2004; Siligan *et al.*, 2005; Bertolotti *et al.*, 1996, 1998; Li *et al.*, 2012; Scotlandi *et al.*,1996; Hancock *et al.*, 2008; Wai *et al.*, 2002; Yamamoto *et al.*, 2015; Kinsey *et al.*, 2006, 2009; Mendiola *et al.*, 2006; Smith *et al.*, 2006; Luo *et al.*, 2009; Grünewald *et al.*, 2015; Niedan *et al.*, 2014; Beauchamp *et al.*, 2009; García-Aragoncillo *et al.*, 2008; Tirado *et al.*, 2006; Abaan *et al.*, 2005; Nakatani *et al.*, 2003; Riggi *et al.*, 2010; France *et al.*, 2011). Moreover, it acts as a network hub for modulating alternative splicing process involved in oncogenesis (Selvanathan *et al.*, 2015; Yang *et al.*, 2000a).

In addition, EWSR1-FLI1 translocation resulted in the activation of E2F target genes by recruiting E2F3 to the target promotor sites and positively regulated the expression of mitotic kinases Aurora A and Aurora B thus contributing to the increased cell cycle progression in Ewing sarcoma (Schwentner *et al.*, 2015; Wakahara *et al.*, 2008). Moreover, it has been found to regulate the levels of critical cell cycle regulator proteins p57KIP2 and c-Myc (Dauphinot *et al.*, 2001). Besides, it also suppressed the expression of focal adhesion, extracellular matrix, and actin regulatory proteins. For instance, *in vivo* study using an orthotopic xenograft model proved that aberrant EWSR1-FLI1 activity downregulated α5 integrin and zyxin genes involved in cytoskeletal integrity and cell adhesion leading to anchorage-independent cell growth and tumor progression (Chaturvedi *et al.*, 2014). Further, it also increased the MMP9 levels by interacting with cofactor p300 and c-Jun and suppressed the levels of lysyl oxidase, an enzyme with tumor suppressing potential and the expression of let-7a tumor suppressor gene in ES cells (Fuchs *et al.*, 2003; Agra *et al.*, 2013; De Vito *et al.*, 2011). Additionally, EWSR1-FLI1 fusion also impaired the activity of a key tumor suppressor protein p53-via HDAC1-mediated deacetylation (Li *et al.*, 2010, 2012). Overexpression of this chimera was found to result in the aberrant activation of a neuronal repressor gene-RE1-silencing transcription factor (REST) that regulates the growth of ES cells (Zhou *et al.*, 2014). Further, EWSR1-FLI1 upregulated EYA3-a DNA repair protein and transcriptional cofactor activity by reducing the miR-708 levels thus resulting in increased cell survival and chemoresistance (Robin *et al.*, 2012). Moreover, EWS-FLI1-regulated miRNAs were shown to restore the activity of IGF pathway attributed to its oncogenic potential (McKinsey *et al.*, 2011). Similarly, Hsa-mir-145 microRNA was found to be the most commonly downregulated target miR of EWSR1-FLI1 indicating positive feedback mechanism as an essential component of EWS-FLI1-mediated ES (Ban *et al.*, 2011). The feedback regulation by EWS-FLI1 and MicroRNA 145 (miRNA145) reduced the expression of SRY-box 2 (SOX2) and mediated the process of mesenchymal stem cells (MSCs) to Ewing sarcoma cancer stem cells transformation (Riggi *et al.*, 2010). Further, it was shown to increase the disease progression by halting the expression of Wnt signaling inhibitor dickkopf WNT signaling pathway inhibitor 1 (DKK-1) and by reducing the β-catenin/TCF-dependent transcription and to inhibit senescence by downregulating retinoblastoma protein (Navarro *et al.*, 2010; Hu *et al.*, 2008). Besides the direct effects on transcription of targets, EWS-FLI1, were also proved to induce transcription of various genes via indirect mechanism of activating key transcription factors such as NF-κB (Lagirand-Cantaloube *et al.*, 2010). Interestingly, it has been reported that mice carrying ectopically expressed EWSR1-FLI1 developed no malignancy but extended cardiomyopathy and induced apoptosis of cardio myocytes (Tanaka *et al.*, 2015). Also, expression of this chimera in non-transformed primary cells led to the activation of caspase 3 and induced apoptosis (Sohn *et al.*, 2010).

EWSR1-ATF1 and EWSR1-CREB1

EWSR1-ATF1 and EWSR1-CREB1 gene fusions harboring respective t(12;22)(q13;q12) and t(2;22)(q34;q12) translocations have been consistently reported in five histopathologically different cancers, namely, angiomatoid fibrous histiocytoma, clear cell sarcoma-like tumor of the gastrointestinal tract, conventional clear cell sarcoma of tendons and aponeuroses, hyalinizing clear cell carcinoma of the salivary gland and primary pulmonary myxoid sarcoma (Figure 9.1) (Thway *et al.*, 2012; Wang *et al.*, 2009; Nakano *et al.*, 2015; Dunham *et al.*, 2008; Rossi *et al.*, 2007; Pacheco *et al.*, 2010; Tornóczky *et al.*, 2012; Antonescu *et al.*, 2006). The recurrent translocation t(12;22) drives the fusion of EWSR1 gene located on chromosome 22q12 to activating transcription factor-1 (ATF1) gene on chromosome 12q13 (Wang *et al.*, 2009). Till date, seven types of EWSR1-ATF1 fusion have been reported in clear cell sarcomas, of which four are in-frame mutations and encode functional proteins

(Tsukamoto *et al.*, 2013, Gineikiene *et al.*, 2012). Though the actual role of this chimera in the development of cancer remains elusive, Yamada *et al.* (2013) demonstrated that EWS-ATF1 directly activates fructooligosaccharides and increases the growth of EWS-ATF1-linked sarcomas (Yamada *et al.*, 2013). Another mechanism was proposed where phosphorylation of the EWS IQ domain by post-translational modifications may play a crucial role in the tumorigenesis (Olsen *et al.*, 2001). However, more studies are required to identify the molecular targets of these fusion genes and the driving mechanism.

EWSR1-DDIT3/(EWS-CHOP)

EWS-CHOP is a chimeric fusion of the N-terminal part of the EWS gene with CCAAT/enhancer binding protein (C/EBP) homologous protein (CHOP) generated by the MLS chromosomal translocation t(12;22)(q13;q12). However, frequency of occurrence was very less when compared to the more frequent t(12;16)(q13;p11) translocation resulting in TLS-CHOP or (FUS-CHOP) (Kubo *et al.*, 2010; Suzuki *et al.*, 2010, 2012a; Panagopoulos *et al.*, 1996; Matsui *et al.*, 2006). t(12;22) resulted in the in frame fusion of exon 13 of EWS to exon 2 of CHOP (Matsui *et al.*, 2006). However, the function of this fusion protein during oncogenic transformation is not clearly understood and remains to be elucidated. Two hypotheses have been proposed for the phenotypic selection of target cells by EWS-CHOP fusion protein during oncogenic transformation: repression of phenotype specific marker expression, (i) by binding to the C/EBP site within the promotor region through its DNA-binding domain consequently leading to inhibition of endogenous C/EBPβ function; or (ii) by epigenetic alterations such as enhanced histone deacetylation, DNA methylation and histone H3K9 trimethylation; yet the actual role remains elusive, needing extensive research (Suzuki *et al.*, 2012b).

EWSR1-NR4A3

Rearrangement between chromosomes 9 and 22 depicted as t(9;22)(q22;q12) was repeatedly detected in 75% of extraskeletal myxoid chondrosarcoma (EMC) and ligated the transactivation domain of EWS to the DNA binding domain of orphan nuclear receptor subfamily 4 group A member 3 (NR4A3) producing a chimeric transcriptional activator oncoprotein which deregulates various genes like serum- and glucocorticoid (GC)-regulated kinase 1 (SGK1) involved in cell proliferation and mediates oncogenic transformation of chondrogenic cells (Figure 9.1) (Labelle *et al.*, 1995; Ohkura *et al.*, 2002; Maltais *et al.*, 2002; Poulin *et al.*, 2006; Filion and Labelle, 2004). Intact AF2 domain of the NOR1 was found to be an essential factor for the EWS-NOR1 fusion-induced transactivation (Maltais *et al.*, 2002). Other than the transactivation potential, EWS-NOR1 also interacted with the splicing protein U1C and impaired the pre-mRNA splicing contributing to its oncogenic properties (Ohkura *et al.*, 2002). Six3, the homeotic protein despite being a coactivator of wild-type NOR1 acts as a corepressor of the chimeric EWS-NOR1 and was also found to be overexpressed in EMCs. Therefore, it was hypothesized to deregulate the NOR1 and EWS-NOR1 target genes by maintaining a balance between NOR1 and EWS-NOR1 leading to uncontrolled cell proliferation (Laflamme *et al.*, 2003). Further, the expression of PPARγ was also found to be elevated by the fused protein which may assist in tumorigenesis (Filion *et al.*, 2009).

EWS-WT1

A recurrent chromosomal rearrangement t(11;22)(p13;q12) resulted in the fusion of Wilms' tumor suppressor gene (WT1) and EWS gene and exclusively associated with desmoplastic small round cell tumors (DSRCT) (Rauscher *et al.*, 1994; Karnieli *et al.*, 1996; Benjamin *et al.*, 1996; Philippe-Chomette *et al.*, 2012). The resultant fusion protein was shown to have the N-terminal domain of EWS and DNA-binding domain of WT1 with ZnFs 2-4 and act as transcriptional activator of genes repressed by the intact WT1 gene (Lee *et al.*, 1997). For example, unlike the wild-type WT1, the EWS-WT1 chimera was proved to activate insulin-like growth factor I receptor (IGF-I-R) promoter thus contributing to tumor progression (Karnieli *et al.*, 1996; Werner *et al.*, 2007). DSRCT was characterized by tumor surrounding massive reactive fibrosis attributed to the fusion induced overexpression of fibroblast growth factor (FGF) and platelet-derived growth factor-A (PDGFA) (Lee *et al.*, 1997). Similarly, it was also shown to increase the promoter activity of a transcriptional regulator protein early growth response 1 (EGR-1) (Liu *et al.*, 2000). Additionally, another target of this fusion protein, namely, BAI1 associated protein 3 (BAIAP3) which is a potential regulator of exocytosis in cancer cell proliferation was found to be associated with EWS-WT1 induced tumorigenesis (Palmer *et al.*, 2002). Further, expression of EWS-WT1 in embryonic fibroblasts and DSRCT cells also induced the activation of several neural genes such as neuronal reprogramming factor achaete-scute family bHLH transcription factor 1 (ASCL1) therefore leading to partial neural differentiation (Kang *et al.*, 2014). Above all, the biological activities including transcriptional regulation of EWS-WT1 chimera were found to be controlled by its phosphorylation status through various cytoplasmic signaling pathways (Kim *et al.*, 1999, 2000).

OTHER FUSION GENES INVOLVING EWS

t(21;22)(q22;q12) producing EWS-ERG fusion protein was detected in 5–10% of EWS cases (Shibasaki *et al.*, 2013; Sorensen *et al.*, 1994). Rare fusions involving EWS gene, namely, EWS-ETV1, EWS-FEV and EWS-SP3 were found to be associated with undifferentiated small round cell sarcomas (Wang *et al.*, 2007). The EWS-ETV1, EWS-E1AF and EWS-FEV fusions present in very few cases of ES were produced by t(7;22)(p22;q12), t(17;22)(q12;q12) and t(2;22)(q33;q12) translocations, respectively (Wang *et al.*, 2007; Jeon *et al.*, 1995; Kaneko *et al.*, 1996; Peter *et al.*, 1997).

TAF15 GENE FUSIONS

The third member of the FET family TAF15 was also found to be involved in cancer inducible chromosomal translocations. For example, TAF15-ZNF384 fusion with t(12;17)(p13;q12) translocation was detected in ALL (Nyquist *et al.*, 2011). Likewise, t(9;17)(q22;q11.2) producing the fusion of NR4A3-CHN with TAF15 was also observed in leukemia (Attwooll *et al.*, 1999). Further, in extraskeletal myxoid chondrosarcoma, TAF15 was found to be fused with TEC gene (Sjögren *et al.*, 1999).

CONCLUSION

Altogether, FET family members have been found to be involved in several chromosomal translocations and frequently associated with cancer development. All these fusion proteins exert constitutive transcriptional regulatory effects and were shown to induce the expression of various oncogenes thus contributing to tumor initiation and progression. Besides, many of these fusion proteins serve as potential diagnostic markers as exclusively present in certain cancer types. Moreover, several studies reported that detection of these fusion transcripts could serve as both effective therapeutic targets and prognostic markers.

CONFLICT OF INTEREST

The authors express no conflict of interest.

REFERENCES

Abaan, O.D., A. Levenson, O. Khan, P.A. Furth, A. Uren, and J.A. Toretsky, PTPL1 is a direct transcriptional target of EWS-FLI1 and modulates Ewing's Sarcoma tumorigenesis, *Oncogene* **24**(16): 2715–2722 (2005).

Adelmant, G., J.D. Gilbert, and S.O. Freytag, Human translocation liposarcoma-CCAAT/enhancer binding protein (C/EBP) homologous protein (TLS-CHOP) oncoprotein prevents adipocyte differentiation by directly interfering with C/EBPbeta function, *J Biol Chem* **273**(25): 15574–15581 (1998).

Agra, N., F. Cidre, L. García-García, J. de la Parra, and J. Alonso, Lysyl oxidase is downregulated by the EWS/FLI1 oncoprotein and its propeptide domain displays tumor supressor activities in Ewing sarcoma cells, *PLoS One* **8**(6): e66281 (2013).

Åman, P., S. Dolatabadi, D. Svec, E. Jonasson, S. Safavi, D. Andersson, P. Grundevik, C. Thomsen, and A. Ståhlberg, Regulatory mechanisms, expression levels and proliferation effects of the FUS-DDIT3 fusion oncogene in liposarcoma. *J Pathol* **238**(5): 689–699 (2016).

Andersson, M.K., M. Göransson, A. Olofsson, C. Andersson, and P. Aman, Nuclear expression of FLT1 and its ligand PGF in FUS-DDIT3 carrying myxoid liposarcomas suggests the existence of an intracrine signaling loop, *BMC Canc* **10**: 249 (2010).

Antonescu, C.R., K. Nafa, N.H. Segal, P. Dal Cin, and M. Ladanyi, EWS-CREB1: a recurrent variant fusion in clear cell sarcoma — association with gastrointestinal location and absence of melanocytic differentiation, *Clin Canc Res* **12**(18): 5356–5362 (2006).

Attwooll, C., M. Tariq, M. Harris, J.D. Coyne, N. Telford, and J.M. Varley, Identification of a novel fusion gene involving hTAFII68 and CHN from a t(9;17)(q22;q11.2) translocation in an extraskeletal myxoid chondrosarcoma, *Oncogene* **18**(52): 7599–7601 (1999).

Baer, C., M. Nees, S. Breit, B. Selle, A.E. Kulozik, K.L. Schaefer, Y. Braun, D. Wai, and C. Poremba, Profiling and functional annotation of mRNA gene expression in pediatric rhabdomyosarcoma and Ewing's sarcoma, *Int J Canc* **110**(5): 687–694 (2004).

Ban. J., G. Jug, P. Mestdagh, R. Schwentner, M. Kauer, D.N. Aryee, K.L. Schaefer, F. Nakatani, K. Scotlandi, M. Reiter, D. Strunk, F. Speleman, J. Vandesompele, and H. Kovar, Hsa-mir-145 is the top EWS-FLI1-repressed microRNA involved in a positive feedback loop in Ewing's sarcoma, *Oncogene* **30**(18): 2173–2180 (2011).

Beauchamp, E., G. Bulut, O. Abaan, K. Chen, A. Merchant, W. Matsui, Y. Endo, J.S. Rubin, J. Toretsky, and A. Uren, GLI1 is a direct transcriptional target of EWS-FLI1 oncoprotein, *J Biol Chem* **284**(14): 9074–9082 (2009).

Benjamin, L.E., W.J. Fredericks, F.G. Barr, and F.J. Rauscher, 3rd. Fusion of the EWS1 and WT1 genes as a result of the t(11;22)(p13;q12) translocation in desmoplastic small round cell tumors, *Med Pediatr Oncol* **27**(5): 434–439 (1996).

Bento, C., M.K. Andersson, and P. Aman, DDIT3/CHOP and the sarcoma fusion oncoprotein FUS-DDIT3/TLS-CHOP bind cyclin-dependent kinase 2, *BMC Cell Biol* **10**: 89 (2009).

Berg, T., A.H. Kalsaas, J. Buechner, and L.T. Busund, Ewing sarcoma-peripheral neuroectodermal tumor of the kidney with a FUS-ERG fusion transcript, *Canc Genet Cytogenet* **194**(1): 53–57 (2009).

Bertolotti, A., Y. Lutz, D.J. Heard, P. Chambon, and L. Tora, hTAF(II)68, a novel RNA/ssDNA-binding protein with homology to the pro-oncoproteins TLS/FUS and EWS is associated with both TFIID and RNA polymerase II, *EMBO J* **15**(18): 5022–5031 (1996).

Bertolotti, A., T. Melot, J. Acker, M. Vigneron, O. Delattre, and L. Tora, EWS, but not EWS-FLI-1, is associated with both TFIID and RNA polymerase II: interactions between two members of the TET family, EWS and hTAFII68, and subunits of TFIID and RNA polymerase II complexes, *Mol Cell Biol* **18**(3): 1489–1497 (1998).

Borjigin, N., S. Ohno, W. Wu, M. Tanaka, R. Suzuki, K. Fujita, M. Takanashi, K. Oikawa, T. Goto, T. Motoi, T. Kosaka, K. Yamamoto, and M. Kuroda, TLS-CHOP represses miR-486 expression, inducing upregulation of a metastasis regulator PAI-1 in human myxoid liposarcoma, *Biochem Biophys Res Commun* **427**(2): 355–360 (2012).

Buchanan, J., and C.A. Tirado, A t(16;21)(p11;q22) in Acute myeloid leukemia (AML) resulting in fusion of the FUS/TLS and ERG genes: A review of the literature, *J Assoc Genet Technol* **42**(1): 24–33 (2016).

Chansky, H.A., M. Hu, D.D. Hickstein, and L. Yang, Oncogenic TLS/ERG and EWS/Fli-1 fusion proteins inhibit RNA splicing mediated by YB-1 protein, *Canc Res* **61**(9): 3586–3590 (2001).

Chaturvedi, A., L.M. Hoffman, C.C. Jensen, Y.C. Lin, A.H. Grossmann, R.L. Randall, S.L. Lessnick, A.L. Welm, and M.C. Beckerle, Molecular dissection of the mechanism by which EWS/FLI expression compromises actin cytoskeletal integrity and cell adhesion in Ewing sarcoma, *Mol Biol Cell* **25**(18): 2695–2709 (2014).

Chen, S., K. Deniz, Y.S. Sung, L. Zhang, S. Dry, and C.R. Antonescu, Ewing sarcoma with ERG gene rearrangements: A molecular study focusing on the prevalence of FUS-ERG and common pitfalls in detecting EWSR1-ERG fusions by FISH, *Genes Chromosomes Canc* **55**(4): 340–349 (2016).

Crozat, A., P. Aman, N. Mandahl, and D. Ron, Fusion of CHOP to a novel RNA-binding protein in human myxoid liposarcoma, *Nature* **363**(6430): 640–644 (1993).

Dauphinot, L., C. De Oliveira, T. Melot, N. Sevenet, V. Thomas, B.E. Weissman, and O. Delattre, Analysis of the expression of cell cycle regulators in Ewing cell lines: EWS-FLI-1 modulates p57KIP2and c-Myc expression, *Oncogene* **20**(25): 3258–3265 (2001).

De Vito, C., N. Riggi, M.L. Suvà, M. Janiszewska, J. Horlbeck, K. Baumer, P. Provero, and I. Stamenkovic, Let-7a is a direct EWS-FLI-1 target implicated in Ewing's sarcoma development, *PLoS One* **6**(8): e23592 (2011).

Deloulme, J.C., L. Prichard, O. Delattre, and D.R. Storm, The prooncoprotein EWS binds calmodulin and is phosphorylated by protein kinase C through an IQ domain, *J Biol Chem* **272**(43): 27369–27377 (1997).

Dunham, C., J. Hussong, M. Seiff, J. Pfeifer, and A. Perry, Primary intracerebral angiomatoid fibrous histiocytoma: report of a case with a t(12;22)(q13;q12) causing type 1 fusion of the EWS and ATF-1 genes, *Am J Surg Pathol* **32**(3): 478–484 (2008).

Felsch, J.S., W.S. Lane, and E.G. Peralta, Tyrosine kinase Pyk2 mediates G-protein-coupled receptor regulation of the Ewing sarcoma RNA-binding protein EWS, *Curr Biol* **9**(9): 485–488 (1999).

Filion, C., and Y. Labelle, The oncogenic fusion protein EWS/NOR-1 induces transformation of CFK2 chondrogenic cells, *Exp Cell Res* **297**(2): 585–592 (2004).

Filion, C., T. Motoi, A.B. Olshen, M. Laé, R.J. Emnett, D.H. Gutmann, A. Perry, M. Ladanyi, and Y. Labelle, The EWSR1/NR4A3 fusion protein of extraskeletal myxoid chondrosarcoma activates the PPARG nuclear receptor gene, *J Pathol* **217**(1): 83–93 (2009).

France, K.A., J.L. Anderson, A. Park, and C.T. Denny, Oncogenic fusion protein EWS/FLI1 down-regulates gene expression by both transcriptional and post-transcriptional mechanisms, *J Biol Chem* **286**(26): 22750–22757 (2011).

Fuchs, B., C.Y. Inwards, and R. Janknecht, Upregulation of the matrix metalloproteinase-1 gene by the Ewing's sarcoma associated EWS-ER81 and EWS-Fli-1 oncoproteins, c-Jun and p300, *FEBS Lett* **553**(1–2): 104–108 (2003).

García-Aragoncillo, E., J. Carrillo, E. Lalli, N. Agra, G. Gómez-López, A. Pestaña, and J. Alonso, DAX1, a direct target of EWS/FLI1 oncoprotein, is a principal regulator of cell-cycle progression in Ewing's tumor cells, *Oncogene* **27**(46): 6034–6043 (2008).

Gineikiene, E., D. Seinin, B. Brasiuniene, A. Brazaitis, L. Griskevicius, and A. Jakubauskas, Clear cell sarcoma expressing a novel chimerical transcript EWSR1 exon 7/ATF1 exon 6, *Virchows Arch* **461**(3): 339–343 (2012).

Göransson, M., M.K. Andersson, C. Forni, A. Ståhlberg, C. Andersson, A. Olofsson, R. Mantovani, and P. Aman, The myxoid liposarcoma FUS-DDIT3 fusion oncoprotein deregulates NF-kappaB target genes by interaction with NFKBIZ, *Oncogene* **28**(2): 270–278 (2009).

Göransson, M., E. Elias, A. Ståhlberg, A. Olofsson, C. Andersson, and P. Aman, Myxoid liposarcoma FUS-DDIT3 fusion oncogene induces C/EBP beta-mediated interleukin 6 expression, *Int J Canc* **115**(4): 556–560 (2005).

Grünewald, T.G., V. Bernard, P. Gilardi-Hebenstreit, V. Raynal, D. Surdez, M.M. Aynaud, O. Mirabeau, F. Cidre-Aranaz, F. Tirode, S. Zaidi, G. Perot, A.H. Jonker, C. Lucchesi, M.C. Le Deley, O. Oberlin, P. Marec-Bérard, A.S. Véron, S. Reynaud, E. Lapouble, V. Boeva, T. Rio Frio, J. Alonso,

S. Bhatia, G. Pierron, G. Cancel-Tassin, O. Cussenot, D.G. Cox, L.M. Morton, M.J. Machiela, S.J. Chanock, P. Charnay, and O. Delattre, Chimeric EWSR1-FLI1 regulates the Ewing sarcoma susceptibility gene EGR2 via a GGAA microsatellite, *Nat Genet* **47**(9): 1073–1078 (2015).

Hancock, J.D., and S.L. Lessnick, A transcriptional profiling meta-analysis reveals a core EWS-FLI gene expression signature, *Cell Cycle* **7**(2): 250–256 (2008). http://ghr.nlm.nih.gov/gene/EWSR1

Hu, H.M., A. Zielinska-Kwiatkowska, K. Munro, J. Wilcox, D.Y. Wu, L. Yang, and H.A. Chansky, EWS/FLI1 suppresses retinoblastoma protein function and senescence in Ewing's sarcoma cells, *J Orthop Res* **26**(6): 886–893 (2008).

Ichikawa, H., K. Shimizu, Y. Hayashi, and M. Ohki, An RNA-binding protein gene, TLS/FUS, is fused to ERG in human myeloid leukemia with t(16;21) chromosomal translocation, *Canc Res* **54**(11): 2865–2868 (1994).

Ichikawa, H., K. Shimizu, R. Katsu, and M. Ohki, Dual transforming activities of the FUS (TLS)-ERG leukemia fusion protein conferred by two N-terminal domains of FUS (TLS), *Mol Cell Biol* **19**(11): 7639–7650 (1999).

Jeon, I.S., J.N. Davis, B.S. Braun, J.E. Sublett, M.F. Roussel, C.T. Denny, and D.N. Shapiro, A variant Ewing's sarcoma translocation (7;22) fuses the EWS gene to the ETS gene ETV1, *Oncogene* **10**(6): 1229–1234 (1995).

Kanai, Y., N. Dohmae, and N. Hirokawa, Kinesin transports RNA: isolation and characterization of an RNA-transporting granule, *Neuron* **43**(4): 513–525 (2004).

Kanazawa, T., C. Ogawa, T. Taketani, T. Taki, Y. Hayashi, and A. Morikawa, TLS/FUS-ERG fusion gene in acute lymphoblastic leukemia with t(16;21)(p11;q22) and monitoring of minimal residual disease, *Leuk Lymphoma* **46**(12): 1833–1835 (2005).

Kaneko, Y., K. Yoshida, M. Handa, Y. Toyoda, H. Nishihira, Y. Tanaka, Y. Sasaki, S. Ishida, F. Higashino, and K. Fujinaga, Fusion of an ETS-family gene, EIAF, to EWS by t(17;22)(q12;q12) chromosome translocation in an undifferentiated sarcoma of infancy, *Genes Chromosomes Canc* **15**(2): 115–121 (1996).

Kang, H.J., J.H. Park, W. Chen, S.I. Kang, K. Moroz, M. Ladanyi, and S.B. Lee, EWS-WT1 oncoprotein activates neuronal reprogramming factor ASCL1 and promotes neural differentiation, *Canc Res* **74**(16): 4526–4535 (2014).

Karnieli, E., H. Werner, F.J. Rauscher, 3rd, L.E. Benjamin, and D. LeRoith, The IGF-I receptor gene promoter is a molecular target for the Ewing's sarcoma-Wilms' tumor 1 fusion protein, *J Biol Chem* **271**(32): 19304–19309 (1996).

Kim, J., J.M. Lee, P.E. Branton, and J. Pelletier, Modification of EWS/WT1 functional properties by phosphorylation, *Proc Natl Acad Sci USA* **96**(25): 14300–14305 (1999).

Kim, J., J.M. Lee, P.E. Branton, and J. Pelletier, Modulation of EWS/WT1 activity by the v-Src protein tyrosine kinase, *FEBS Lett* **474**(2–3): 121–128 (2000).

Kinsey, M., R. Smith, A.K. Iyer, E.R. McCabe, and S.L. Lessnick, EWS/FLI and its downstream target NR0B1 interact directly to modulate transcription and oncogenesis in Ewing's sarcoma, *Canc Res* **69**(23): 9047–9055 (2009).

Kinsey, M., R. Smith, and S.L. Lessnick, NR0B1 is required for the oncogenic phenotype mediated by EWS/FLI in Ewing's sarcoma, *Mol Canc Res* **4**(11): 851–859 (2006).

Kong, X.T., K. Ida, H. Ichikawa, K. Shimizu, M. Ohki, N. Maseki, Y. Kaneko, M. Sako, Y. Kobayashi, A. Tojou, I. Miura, H. Kakuda, T. Funabiki, K. Horibe, H. Hamaguchi, Y. Akiyama, F. Bessho, M. Yanagisawa, and Y. Hayashi, Consistent detection of TLS/FUS-ERG chimeric transcripts in acute myeloid leukemia with t(16;21)(p11;q22) and identification of a novel transcript, *Blood* **90**(3): 1192–1199 (1997).

Kubo, T., Y. Matsui, N. Naka, N. Araki, A. Myoui, K. Endo, N. Yasui, O. Ohtani, K. Suzuki, T. Kimura, H. Yoshikawa, and T. Ueda, Specificity of fusion genes in adipocytic tumors, *Anticancer Res* **30**(2): 661–664 (2010).

Labelle, Y., J. Zucman, G. Stenman, L.G. Kindblom, J. Knight, C. Turc-Carel, B. Dockhorn-Dworniczak, N. Mandahl, C. Desmaze, M. Peter, *et al.* Oncogenic conversion of a novel orphan nuclear receptor by chromosome translocation, *Hum Mol Genet* **4**(12): 2219–2226 (1995).

Laflamme, C., C. Filion, J.A. Bridge, M. Ladanyi, M.B. Goldring, and Y. Labelle, The homeotic protein Six3 is a coactivator of the nuclear receptor NOR-1 and a corepressor of the fusion protein EWS/NOR-1 in human extraskeletal myxoid chondrosarcomas, *Canc Res* **63**(2): 449–454 (2003).

Lagirand-Cantaloube, J., K. Laud, A. Lilienbaum, F. Tirode, O. Delattre, C. Auclair, and M.H. Kryszke, EWS-FLI1 inhibits TNFalpha-induced NFkappaB-dependent transcription in Ewing sarcoma cells, *Biochem Biophys Res Commun* **399**(4): 705–710 (2010).

Lee, S.B., K.A. Kolquist, K. Nichols, C. Englert, S. Maheswaran, M. Ladanyi, W.L. Gerald, and D.A. Haber, The EWS-WT1 translocation product induces PDGFA in desmoplastic small round-cell tumour, *Nat Genet* **17**(3): 309–313 (1997).

Li, Y., X. Li, G. Fan, J. Fukushi, Y. Matsumoto, Y. Iwamoto, and Y. Zhu, Impairment of p53 acetylation by EWS-Fli1 chimeric protein in Ewing family tumors, *Canc Lett* **320**(1): 14–22 (2012).

Li, Y., K. Tanaka, X. Fan, F. Nakatani, X. Li, T. Nakamura, M. Takasaki, S. Yamamoto, and Y. Iwamoto, Inhibition of the transcriptional function of p53 by EWS-Fli1 chimeric protein in Ewing Family Tumors, *Canc Lett* **294**(1): 57–65 (2010).

Liu, J., M.M. Nau, J.C. Yeh, C.J. Allegra, E. Chu, and J.J. Wright, Molecular heterogeneity and function of EWS-WT1 fusion transcripts in desmoplastic small round cell tumors, *Clin Canc Res* **6**(9): 3522–3529 (2000).

Luo, W., K. Gangwal, S. Sankar, K.M. Boucher, D. Thomas, and S.L. Lessnick, GSTM4 is a microsatellite-containing EWS/FLI target involved in Ewing's sarcoma oncogenesis and therapeutic resistance, *Oncogene* **28**(46): 4126–4132 (2009).

Maltais, A., C. Filion, and Y. Labelle, The AF2 domain of the orphan nuclear receptor TEC is essential for the transcriptional activity of the oncogenic fusion protein EWS/TEC, *Canc Lett* **183**(1): 87–94 (2002).

Matsui, Y., T. Ueda, T. Kubo, T. Hasegawa, Y. Tomita, M. Okamoto, A. Myoui, S. Kakunaga, N. Yasui, and H. Yoshikawa, A novel type of EWS-CHOP fusion gene in myxoid liposarcoma, *Biochem Biophys Res Commun* **348**(2): 437–440 (2006).

McKinsey, E.L., J.K. Parrish, A.E. Irwin, B.F. Niemeyer, H.B. Kern, D.K. Birks, and P. Jedlicka, A novel oncogenic mechanism in Ewing sarcoma involving IGF pathway targeting by EWS/Fli1-regulated microRNAs, *Oncogene* **30**(49): 4910–4920 (2011).

Mendiola, M., J. Carrillo, E. García, E. Lalli, T. Hernández, E. de Alava, F. Tirode, O. Delattre, P. García-Miguel, F. López-Barea, A. Pestaña, and J. Alonso, The orphan nuclear receptor DAX1 is up-regulated by the EWS/FLI1 oncoprotein and is highly expressed in Ewing tumors, *Int J Canc* **118**(6): 1381–1389 (2006).

Mertens, F., C.D. Fletcher, C.R. Antonescu, J.M. Coindre, M. Colecchia, H.A. Domanski, E. Downs-Kelly, C. Fisher, J.R. Goldblum, L. Guillou, R. Reid, J. Rosai, R. Sciot, N. Mandahl, and I. Panagopoulos, Clinicopathologic and molecular genetic characterization of low-grade fibromyxoid sarcoma, and cloning of a novel FUS/CREB3L1 fusion gene, *Lab Invest* **85**(3): 408–415 (2005).

Möller, E., J.L. Hornick, L. Magnusson, S. Veerla, H.A. Domanski, and F. Mertens, FUS-CREB3L2/L1-positive sarcomas show a specific gene expression profile with upregulation of CD24 and FOXL1, *Clin Canc Res* **17**(9): 2646–2656 (2011).

Nakano, T., H. Yamamoto, T. Nishijima, S. Tamiya, H. Shiratsuchi, T. Nakashima, S. Komune, and Y. Oda, Hyalinizing clear cell carcinoma with EWSR1-ATF1 fusion gene: report of three cases with molecular analyses, *Virchows Arch* **466**(1): 37–43 (2015).

Nakatani, F., K. Tanaka, R. Sakimura, Y. Matsumoto, T. Matsunobu, X. Li, M. Hanada, T. Okada, and Y. Iwamoto, Identification of p21WAF1/CIP1 as a direct target of EWS-Fli1 oncogenic fusion protein, *J Biol Chem* **278**(17): 15105–15115 (2003).

Navarro, D., N. Agra, A. Pestaña, J. Alonso, J.M. González-Sancho, The EWS/FLI1 oncogenic protein inhibits expression of the Wnt inhibitor DICKKOPF-1 gene and antagonizes beta-catenin/TCF-mediated transcription, *Carcinogenesis* **31**(3): 394–401 (2010).

Ng, T.L., O'M.J. Sullivan, C.J. Pallen, M. Hayes, P.W. Clarkson, M. Winstanley, P.H. Sorensen, T.O. Nielsen, Horsman D.E. Ewing sarcoma with novel translocation t(2;16) producing an in-frame fusion of FUS and FEV, *J Mol Diagn* **9**(4): 459–463 (2007).

Niedan, S., M. Kauer, D.N. Aryee, R. Kofler, R. Schwentner, A. Meier, U. Pötschger, U. Kontny, and H. Kovar, Suppression of FOXO1 is responsible for a growth regulatory repressive transcriptional sub-signature of EWS-FLI1 in Ewing sarcoma, *Oncogene* **33**(30): 3927–3938 (2014).

Nyquist, K.B., J. Thorsen, B. Zeller, A. Haaland, G. Trøen, S. Heim, and F. Micci, Identification of the TAF15-ZNF384 fusion gene in two new cases of acute lymphoblastic leukemia with a t(12;17)(p13;q12). *Canc Genet* **204**(3): 147–152 (2011).

Ohkura, N., H. Yaguchi, T. Tsukada, and K. Yamaguchi, The EWS/NOR1 fusion gene product gains a novel activity affecting pre-mRNA splicing, *J Biol Chem* **277**(1): 535–543 (2002).

Oikawa, K., M. Tanaka, S. Itoh, M. Takanashi, T. Ozaki, Y. Muragaki, and M. Kuroda, A novel oncogenic pathway by TLS-CHOP involving repression of MDA-7/IL-24 expression, *Br J Canc* **106**(12): 1976–1979 (2012).

Olofsson, A., H. Willén, M. Göransson, K. Engström, J.M. Meis-Kindblom, G. Stenman, L.G. Kindblom, and P. Aman, Abnormal expression of cell cycle regulators in FUS-CHOP carrying liposarcomas, *Int J Oncol* **25**(5): 1349–1355 (2004).

Olsen, R.J., Hinrichs S.H. Phosphorylation of the EWS IQ domain regulates transcriptional activity of the EWS/ATF1 and EWS/FLI1 fusion proteins, *Oncogene* **20**(14): 1756–1764 (2001).

Pacheco, M., D.E. Horsman, M.M. Hayes, P.W. Clarkson, H. Huwait, and T.O. Nielsen, Small blue round cell tumor of the interosseous membrane bearing a t(2;22)(q34;q12)/EWS-CREB1 translocation: a case report, *Mol Cytogenet* **3**:12 (2010).

Palmer, R.E., S.B. Lee, J.C. Wong, P.A. Reynolds, H. Zhang, V. Truong, J.D. Oliner, W.L. Gerald, and D.A. Haber, Induction of BAIAP3 by the EWS-WT1 chimeric fusion implicates regulated exocytosis in tumorigenesis, *Canc Cell* **2**(6): 497–505 (2002).

Pan, J., J. Zou, D.Y. Wu, R.S. Roberson, L.J. Hennings, X. Ma, M. Yared, M.L. Blackburn, H.A. Chansky, and L. Yang, TLS-ERG leukemia fusion protein deregulates cyclin-dependent kinase 1 and blocks terminal differentiation of myeloid progenitor cells, *Mol Canc Res* **6**(5): 862–872 (2008).

Panagopoulos, I., P. Aman, T. Fioretos, M. Höglund, B. Johansson, N. Mandahl, S. Heim, M. Behrendtz, and F. Mitelman, Fusion of the FUS gene with ERG in acute myeloid leukemia with t(16;21)(p11;q22), *Genes Chromosomes Canc* **11**(4): 256–262 (1994).

Panagopoulos, I., M. Höglund, F. Mertens, N. Mandahl, F. Mitelman, and P. Aman, Fusion of the EWS and CHOP genes in myxoid liposarcoma, *Oncogene* **12**(3): 489–494 (1996).

Panagopoulos, I., F. Mertens, M. Isaksson, and N. Mandahl, A novel FUS/CHOP chimera in myxoid liposarcoma, *Biochem Biophys Res Commun* **279**(3): 838–845 (2000).

Panagopoulos, I., E. Möller, A. Dahlén, M. Isaksson, N. Mandahl, A. Vlamis-Gardikas, and F. Mertens, Characterization of the native CREB3L2 transcription factor and the FUS/CREB3L2 chimera, *Genes Chromosomes Canc* **46**(2): 181–191 (2007).

Panagopoulos, I., C.T. Storlazzi, C.D. Fletcher, J.A. Fletcher, A. Nascimento, H.A. Domanski, J. Wejde, O. Brosjö, A. Rydholm, M. Isaksson, N. Mandahl, and F. Mertens, The chimeric FUS/CREB3l2 gene is specific for low-grade fibromyxoid sarcoma, *Genes Chromosomes Canc* **40**(3): 218–228 (2004).

Patil, N., S. Ahmed Kabeer, Rasheed, M. Abba, J. Hendrik Leupold, M. Schwarzbach, Allgayer H. A mechanistic study on the metastasis inducing function of FUS-CHOP fusion protein in liposarcoma, *Int J Canc* **134**(12): 2808–2819 (2014).

Pérez-Mancera, P.A., C. Bermejo-Rodríguez, M. Sánchez-Martín, F. Abollo-Jiménez, B. Pintado, and I. Sánchez-García, FUS-DDIT3 prevents the development of adipocytic precursors in liposarcoma by repressing PPARgamma and C/EBPalpha and activating eIF4E, *PLoS One* **3**(7): e2569 (2008).

Pérez-Mancera, P.A., C. Vicente-Dueñas, I. González-Herrero, M. Sánchez-Martín, T. Flores-Corral, and I. Sánchez-García, Fat-specific FUS-DDIT3-transgenic mice establish PPARgamma inactivation is required to liposarcoma development, *Carcinogenesis* **28**(10): 2069–2073 (2007).

Peter, M., J. Couturier, H. Pacquement, J. Michon, G. Thomas, H. Magdelenat, and O. Delattre O, A new member of the ETS family fused to EWS in Ewing tumors, *Oncogene* **14**(10): 1159–1164 (1997).

Philippe-Chomette, P., N. Kabbara, N. Andre, G. Pierron, A. Coulomb, V. Laurence, J.Y. Blay, O. Delattre, G. Schleiermacher, and D. Orbach, Desmoplastic small round cell tumors with EWS-WT1 fusion transcript in children and young adults, *Pediatr Blood Canc* **58**(6): 891–897 (2012).

Potikyan, G., R.O. Savene, J.M. Gaulden, K.A. France, Z. Zhou, E.S. Kleinerman, S.L. Lessnick, and C.T. Denny, EWS/FLI1 regulates tumor angiogenesis in Ewing's sarcoma via suppression of thrombospondins, *Canc Res* **67**(14): 6675–6684 (2007).

Poulin, H., C. Filion, M. Ladanyi, and Y. Labelle, Serum- and glucocorticoid-regulated kinase 1 (SGK1) induction by the EWS/NOR**1**(NR4A3) fusion protein, *Biochem Biophys Res Commun* **346**(1): 306–313 (2006).

Prasad, D.D., M. Ouchida, L. Lee, V.N. Rao, and E.S. Reddy, TLS/FUS fusion domain of TLS/FUS-ERG chimeric protein resulting from the t(16;21) chromosomal translocation in human myeloid leukemia functions as a transcriptional activation domain, *Oncogene* **9**(12): 3717–3729 (1994).

Prieur, A., F. Tirode, P. Cohen, and O. Delattre, EWS/FLI-1 silencing and gene profiling of Ewing cells reveal downstream oncogenic pathways and a crucial role for repression of insulin-like growth factor binding protein 3, *Mol Cell Biol* **24**(16): 7275–7283 (2004).

Rabbitts, T.H., A. Forster, R. Larson, and P. Nathan, Fusion of the dominant negative transcription regulator CHOP with a novel gene FUS by translocation t(12;16) in malignant liposarcoma, *Nat Genet* **4**(2): 175–180 (1993).

Raddaoui, E., L.R. Donner, and I. Panagopoulos, Fusion of the FUS and ATF1 genes in a large, deep-seated angiomatoid fibrous histiocytoma, *Diagn Mol Pathol* **11**(3): 157–162 (2002).

Rauscher, F.J. 3rd, L.E. Benjamin, W.J. Fredericks, Morris J.F. Novel oncogenic mutations in the WT1 Wilms' tumor suppressor gene: a t(11;22) fuses the Ewing's sarcoma gene, EWS1, to WT1 in desmoplastic small round cell tumor, *Cold Spring Harb Symp Quant Biol* **59**:137–146 (1994).

Riggi, N., M.L. Suvà, C. De Vito, P. Provero, J.C. Stehle, K. Baumer, L. Cironi, M. Janiszewska, T. Petricevic, D. Suvà, S. Tercier, J.M. Joseph, L. Guillou, and I. Stamenkovic, EWS-FLI-1 modulates miRNA145 and SOX2 expression to initiate mesenchymal stem cell reprogramming toward Ewing sarcoma cancer stem cells, *Genes Dev* **24**(9): 916–932 (2010).

Robin, T.P., A. Smith, E. McKinsey, L. Reaves, P. Jedlicka, and H.L. Ford, EWS/FLI1 regulates EYA3 in Ewing sarcoma via modulation of miRNA-708, resulting in increased cell survival and chemoresistance, *Mol Canc Res* **10**(8): 1098–1108 (2012).

Rodriguez, R., J. Tornin, C. Suarez, A. Astudillo, R. Rubio, C. Yauk, A. Williams, M. Rosu-Myles, J.M. Funes, C. Boshoff, and P. Menendez, Expression of FUS-CHOP fusion protein in immortalized/transformed human mesenchymal stem cells drives mixoid liposarcoma formation, *Stem Cells* **31**(10): 2061–2072 (2013).

Rossi, S., K. Szuhai, M. Ijszenga, H.J. Tanke, L. Zanatta, R. Sciot, C.D. Fletcher, A.P. Dei Tos, and P.C. Hogendoorn, EWSR1-CREB1 and EWSR1-ATF1 fusion genes in angiomatoid fibrous histiocytoma, *Clin Canc Res* **13**(24): 7322–7328 (2007).

Rossow, K.L. and R. Janknecht, The Ewing's sarcoma gene product functions as a transcriptional activator, *Canc Res* **61**(6): 2690–2695 (2001).

Schwartz, J.C., T.R. Cech, and R.R. Parker, Biochemical Properties and Biological Functions of FET Proteins, *Annu Rev Biochem* **84**:355–379 (2015).

Schwartz, J.C., X. Wang, E.R. Podell, and T.R. Cech, RNA seeds higher-order assembly of FUS protein, *Cell Rep* **5**(4): 918–925 (2013).

Schwentner, R., T. Papamarkou, M.O. Kauer, V. Stathopoulos, F. Yang, S. Bilke, P.S. Meltzer, M. Girolami, and H. Kovar, EWS-FLI1 employs an E2F switch to drive target gene expression, *Nucleic Acids Res* **43**(5): 2780–2789 (2015).

Scotlandi, K., S. Benini, M. Sarti, M. Serra, P.L. Lollini, D. Maurici, P. Picci, M.C. Manara, and N. Baldini, Insulin-like growth factor I receptor-mediated circuit in Ewing's sarcoma/peripheral neuroectodermal tumor: a possible therapeutic target, *Canc Res* **56**(20): 4570–4574 (1996).

Selvanathan, S.P., G.T. Graham, H.V. Erkizan, U. Dirksen, T.G. Natarajan, A. Dakic, S. Yu, X. Liu, M.T. Paulsen, M.E. Ljungman, C.H. Wu, E.R. Lawlor, A. Üren, and J.A. Toretsky, Oncogenic fusion protein EWS-FLI1 is a network hub that regulates alternative splicing, *Proc Natl Acad Sci USA* **112**(11): E1307–1316 (2015).

Shibasaki, M., T. Iwai, J. Maegawa, Y. Inayama, T. Yokosuka, S. Yokota, S. Ohta, Y. Matsui, K. Mitsudo, and I. Tohnai, Mandibular Ewing sarcoma with chromosomal translocation t(21;22)(q22;q12), *J Craniofac Surg* **24**(4): 1469–1472 (2013).

Siligan, C., J. Ban, R. Bachmaier, L. Spahn, M. Kreppel, K.L. Schaefer, C. Poremba, D.N. Aryee, and H. Kovar, EWS-FLI1 target genes recovered from Ewing's sarcoma chromatin, *Oncogene* **24**(15): 2512–2524 (2005).

Sjögren, H., J. Meis-Kindblom, L.G. Kindblom, P. Aman, and G. Stenman, Fusion of the EWS-related gene TAF2N to TEC in extraskeletal myxoid chondrosarcoma, *Canc Res* **59**(20): 5064–5067 (1999).

Smith, R., L.A. Owen, D.J. Trem, J.S. Wong, J.S. Whangbo, T.R. Golub, and S.L. Lessnick, Expression profiling of EWS/FLI identifies NKX2.2 as a critical target gene in Ewing's sarcoma, *Canc Cell* **9**(5): 405–416 (2006). Erratum in: *Cancer Cell* **11**(1): 97 (2007).

Sohn, E.J., H. Li, K. Reidy, L.F. Beers, B.L. Christensen, and S.B. Lee, EWS/FLI1 oncogene activates caspase 3 transcription and triggers apoptosis *in vivo*, *Canc Res* **70**(3): 1154–1163 (2010).

Sorensen, P.H., S.L. Lessnick, D. Lopez-Terrada, X.F. Liu, T.J. Triche, and C.T. Denny, A second Ewing's sarcoma translocation, t(21;22), fuses the EWS gene to another ETS-family transcription factor, ERG. *Nat Genet* **6**(2): 146–151 (1994).

Sotoca, A.M., K.H. Prange, B. Reijnders, A. Mandoli, L.N. Nguyen, H.G. Stunnenberg, and J.H. Martens, The oncofusion protein FUS-ERG targets key hematopoietic regulators and modulates the all-trans retinoic acid signaling pathway in t(16;21) acute myeloid leukemia, *Oncogene* **35**(15): 1965–1976 (2016).

Storlazzi, C.T., F. Mertens, A. Nascimento, M. Isaksson, J. Wejde, O. Brosjo, N. Mandahl, and I. Panagopoulos, Fusion of the FUS and BBF2H7 genes in low grade fibromyxoid sarcoma, *Hum Mol Genet* **12**(18): 2349–2358 (2003).

Suzuki, K., Y. Matsui, K. Endo, T. Kubo, T. Hasegawa, T. Kimura, O. Ohtani, and N. Yasui, Myxoid liposarcoma with EWS-CHOP type 1 fusion gene, *Anticancer Res* **30**(11): 4679–4683 (2010).

Suzuki, K., Y. Matsui, N. Hashimoto, N. Naka, N. Araki, T. Kimura, H. Yoshikawa, and T. Ueda, Variation in myxoid liposarcoma: Clinicopathological examination of four cases with detectable TLS-CHOP or EWS-CHOP fusion transcripts whose histopathological diagnosis was other than myxoid liposarcoma, *Oncol Lett* **3**(2): 293–296 (2012a).

Suzuki, K., Y. Matsui, M. Higashimoto, Y. Kawaguchi, S. Seki, H. Motomura, T. Hori, Y. Yahara, M. Kanamori, and T. Kimura, Myxoid liposarcoma-associated EWSR1-DDIT3 selectively represses osteoblastic and chondrocytic transcription in multipotent mesenchymal cells, *PLoS One* **7**(5): e36682 (2012b).

Tanaka, M., S. Yamaguchi, Y. Yamazaki, H. Kinoshita, K. Kuwahara, K. Nakao, P.Y. Jay, T. Noda, and T. Nakamura, Somatic chromosomal translocation between Ewsr1 and Fli1 loci leads to dilated cardiomyopathy in a mouse model, *Sci Rep* **5**: 7826 (2015).

Thway, K., and C. Fisher, Tumors with EWSR1-CREB1 and EWSR1-ATF1 fusions: the current status, *Am J Surg Pathol* **36**(7): e1–e11 (2012).

Tirado, O.M., S. Mateo-Lozano, J. Villar, L.E. Dettin, A. Llort, S. Gallego, J. Ban, H. Kovar, and V. Notario, Caveolin-1 (CAV1) is a target of EWS/FLI-1 and a key determinant of the oncogenic phenotype and tumorigenicity of Ewing's sarcoma cells, *Canc Res* **66**(20): 9937–9947 (2006).

Tornóczky, T., B. Bogner, T. Krausz, G. Ottóffy, and K. Szuhai, Angiomatoid fibrous histiocytoma: pleomorphic variant associated with multiplication of EWSR1-CREB1 fusion gene, *Pathol Oncol Res* **18**(2): 545–548 (2012).

Tsukamoto, Y., Y. Nakata, H. Futani, S. Fukunaga, K. Kajimoto, and S. Hirota, A rare case of clear cell sarcoma with 4 types of EWSR1-ATF1 fusions detected not in primary site but in metastatic site, *Pathol Res Pract* **209**(12): 803–807 (2013).

Turc-Carel, C., J. Limon, P. Dal Cin, U. Rao, C. Karakousis, A.A. Sandberg, Cytogenetic studies of adipose tissue tumors. II. Recurrent reciprocal translocation t(12;16)(q13;p11) in myxoid liposarcomas, *Canc Genet Cytogenet* **23**(4): 291–299 (1986).

Ueda, R., D. Maruyama, J. Nomoto, A.M. Maeshima, S. Fukuhara, H. Kitahara, K. Miyamoto, W. Munakata, T. Suzuki, H. Taniguchi, Y. Kobayashi, and K. Tobinai, FUS-ERG gene fusion in isolated myeloid sarcoma showing uncommon clinical features, *Oxf Med Case Reports* **2016**(1): 4–8 (2016).

Wai, D.H., K.L. Schaefer, A. Schramm, E. Korsching, F. Van Valen, T. Ozaki, W. Boecker, L. Schweigerer, B. Dockhorn-Dworniczak, and C. Poremba, Expression analysis of pediatric solid tumor cell lines using oligonucleotide microarrays, *Int J Oncol* **20**(3): 441–451 (2002).

Wakahara, K., T. Ohno, M. Kimura, T. Masuda, S. Nozawa, T. Dohjima, T. Yamamoto, A. Nagano, G. Kawai, A. Matsuhashi, M. Saitoh, I. Takigami, Y. Okano, and K. Shimizu, EWS-Fli1 up-regulates expression of the Aurora A and Aurora B kinases, *Mol Canc Res* **6**(12): 1937–1945 (2008).

Wang, L., R. Bhargava, T. Zheng, L. Wexler, M.H. Collins, D. Roulston, and M. Ladanyi, Undifferentiated small round cell sarcomas with rare EWS gene fusions: identification of a novel EWS-SP3 fusion and of additional cases with the EWS-ETV1 and EWS-FEV fusions, *J Mol Diagn* **9**(4): 498–509 (2007).

Wang, W.L., E. Mayordomo, W. Zhang, V.S. Hernandez, D. Tuvin, L. Garcia, D.C. Lev, A.J. Lazar, and D. López-Terrada, Detection and characterization of EWSR1/ATF1 and EWSR1/CREB1 chimeric transcripts in clear cell sarcoma (melanoma of soft parts), *Mod Pathol* **22**(9): 1201–1209 (2009).

Wang, X., S. Arai, X. Song, D. Reichart, K. Du, G. Pascual, P. Tempst, M.G. Rosenfeld, C.K. Glass, and R. Kurokawa, Induced ncRNAs allosterically modify RNA-binding proteins in cis to inhibit transcription, *Nature* **454**(7200): 126–130 (2008).

Werner, H., G. Idelman, M. Rubinstein, P. Pattee, S.R. Nagalla, and C.T. Roberts Jr., A novel EWS-WT1 gene fusion product in desmoplastic small round cell tumor is a potent transactivator of the insulin-like growth factor-I receptor (IGF-IR) gene, *Canc Lett* **247**(1): 84–90 (2007).

Yamada, K., T. Ohno, H. Aoki, K. Semi, A. Watanabe, H. Moritake, S. Shiozawa, T. Kunisada, Y. Kobayashi, J. Toguchida, K. Shimizu, A. Hara, and Y. Yamada, EWS/ATF1 expression induces sarcomas from neural crest-derived cells in mice, *J Clin Invest* **123**(2): 600–610 (2013).

Yamamoto, Y., K. Yamazaki, and Y. Ishida, Upregulation of NKX2.2, a target of EWSR1/FLI1 fusion transcript, in primary renal Ewing sarcoma, *J Cytol* **32**(1): 30–32 (2015).

Yang, L., H.A. Chansky, and D.D. Hickstein, EWS. Fli-1 fusion protein interacts with hyperphosphorylated RNA polymerase II and interferes with serine-arginine protein-mediated RNA splicing, *J Biol Chem* **275**(48): 37612–37618 (2000a).

Yang, L., L.J. Embree, and D.D. Hickstein, TLS-ERG leukemia fusion protein inhibits RNA splicing mediated by serine-arginine proteins, *Mol Cell Biol* **20**(10): 3345–3354 (2000b).

Zhou, Z., L. Yu, and E.S. Kleinerman, EWS-FLI-1 regulates the neuronal repressor gene REST, which controls Ewing sarcoma growth and vascular morphology, *Cancer* **120**(4): 579–588 (2014).

Zinszner, H., R. Albalat, and D. Ron, A novel effector domain from the RNA-binding protein TLS or EWS is required for oncogenic transformation by CHOP, *Genes Dev* **8**(21): 2513–2526 (1994).

Zinszner, H., J. Sok, D. Immanuel, Y. Yin, and D. Ron, TLS (FUS) binds RNA *in vivo* and engages in nucleo-cytoplasmic shuttling, *J Cell Sci* **110**(Pt 15): 1741–1750 (1997).

Zou, J., H. Ichikawa, M.L. Blackburn, H.M. Hu, A. Zielinska-Kwiatkowska, Q. Mei, G.J. Roth, H.A. Chansky, and L. Yang, The oncogenic TLS-ERG fusion protein exerts different effects in hematopoietic cells and fibroblasts, *Mol Cell Biol* **25**(14): 6235–6246 (2005).

10

Translocations of FGF and FGFR Proteins and Their Effect in Cancer

*Ganesan Padmavathi, Javadi Monisha, Choudhary Harsha and Ajaikumar B. Kunnumakkara**

INTRODUCTION

Fibroblast growth factor receptor (FGFR) is one of the most important classes of transmembrane tyrosine kinase receptors responsible for several normal cellular functions including proliferation and differentiation (Parish *et al.*, 2015). Also, FGFRs with the accompanying ligands (FGFs) are involved in the regulation of embryonic development, tissue homeostasis, inflammation, angiogenesis and wound healing, etc. (Parish *et al.*, 2015; Tiseo *et al.*, 2015). The FGFR family contains four tyrosine kinase

*Author for correspondence: Ajaikumar B. Kunnumakkara, Cancer Biology Laboratory, Department of Biosciences and Bioengineering, Indian Institute of Technology Guwahati, Assam 781039, India. kunnumakkara@iitg.ernet.in

receptors, namely, FGFR1-4 and their alternatively spliced isoforms that bind to 22 ligands with different binding affinities (Zhang *et al.*, 2006). As already mentioned, FGFRs are tyrosine kinase proteins with one transmembrane domain, one intracellular tyrosine kinase domain and one extracellular ligand binding domain (Zhang *et al.*, 2006; Tiseo *et al.*, 2015). Further, to facilitate and stabilize the receptor-ligand binding, most of the FGFs contain heparin sulfate proteoglycan (HSPG) binding site which shield the ligands from degradation and increase the FGF-FGFR binding stability when occupied with HSPG (Beenken and Mohammadi, 2009). In normal conditions, binding of FGFs and HSPG to specific FGFR induces receptor dimerization and phosphorylation activities which in turn recruit signaling molecules like phospholipase C-γ1 (PLC-γ1), fibroblast growth factor receptor substrate 2 (FRS2) and growth factor receptor bound protein 2 (GRB2) crucial for activating different signaling cascades such as RAS-MAPK and PI3K-Akt-mTOR, etc. Thus, the activated FGF-FGFR pathway drives the normal organ, vascular, and skeletal development (Parish *et al.*, 2015; Brooks *et al.*, 2012; Tiseo *et al.*, 2015; Beenken and Mohammadi, 2009; Dailey *et al.*, 2005).

IMPORTANCE OF FGF-FGFR SIGNALING

Initially thought to stimulate only the fibroblast growth, the FGF-FGFR was eventually proved to help in the proliferation and migration of variety of cells like osteoblasts, oligodendrocyte progenitors, endothelial cells and keratinocytes (Dailey *et al.*, 2005). In contrast, activation of FGFR signaling was found to suppress the proliferation of chondrocytes through induction of cell cycle arrest (Dailey *et al.*, 2005; Sahni *et al.*, 1999). It also stimulated the neuronal differentiation of PC12 cells; however, constitutive activation resulted in the inhibition of differentiation in osteoblasts, myoblasts and oligodendrocyte progenitors suggesting FGF signaling to be cell-type specific (Dailey *et al.*, 2005). Besides, FGF signaling was proved to induce apoptosis or inhibit apoptosis depending on the cell-type and maturational stage as well (Dailey *et al.*, 2005). Moreover, depending on the type of downstream signal transducers, FGF-FGFR was shown to induce different cellular processes including cytoskeletal organization, cell death regulation and transcriptional regulation, etc. (Dailey *et al.*, 2005).

FGF-FGFR SIGNALING IN CANCER

Despite the importance of FGF signaling pathway in the normal cellular functioning, deregulation of the same has been frequently implicated in the initiation and progression of different cancers like bladder cancer, breast cancer, endometrial cancer, haematological cancers, lung cancer and prostate cancer (Wesche *et al.*, 2011; Turner and Grose, 2010; Dienstmann *et al.*, 2014). Such deregulation was governed by oncogenic alterations of FGF and/or FGFR like mutations, amplifications and chromosomal translocations resulting in the constitutive activation (Wesche *et al.*, 2011; Brooks *et al.*, 2012). This constitutively active FGF-FGFR pathway was proved to induce uncontrolled cell proliferation, migration, invasion, EMT and angiogenesis contributing to the tumorigenesis (Tiseo *et al.*, 2015; Wesche *et al.*, 2011; Brooks *et al.*, 2012; Dienstmann *et al.*, 2014). In this chapter, we will discuss the role of translocation-mediated activation of FGF signaling in the development and progression of cancer.

Till date, several chromosomal translocations of FGF-FGFR have been identified including BAG4-FGFR1, BCR-FGFR1, FGFR1-PLAG1, FGFR1-TACC1, FGFR1-ZNF198, FGFR2-AFF3, FGFR2-AHCYL1, FGFR2-BICC1, FGFR2-KIAA1967, FGFR3-BAIAP2L1, FGFR3-TACC3 and SLC45A3-FGFR2, etc. in different cancers (Figures 10.1 and 10.2) (Wang *et al.*, 2014; Wu *et al.*, 2013; Tiseo *et al.*, 2015; Persson *et al.*, 2008; Nakanishi *et al.*, 2015; Arai *et al.*, 2014; Singh *et al.*, 2012).

FGFR3-TACC3

Translocation involving transforming acidic coiled-coil containing protein 3 (TACC3) and FGFR3 is frequently observed in variety of cancers including bladder cancer, cervical cancer, gallbladder cancer, glioblastoma, head and neck squamous cell carcinoma, lung cancer and oral cancer (Figure 10.2) (Nelson *et al.*, 2016; Yuan *et al.*, 2014; Williams *et al.*, 2013; Singh *et al.*, 2012). The partner genes are 48 kb apart in the chromosome 4p16 and the rearrangement occurred due to 70 kb tandem duplication leading to the fusion of the tyrosine kinase domain of the FGFR3, upstream to the coiled-coil domain of TACC3 (Parker *et al.*, 2013; Singh *et al.*, 2012). As seen in

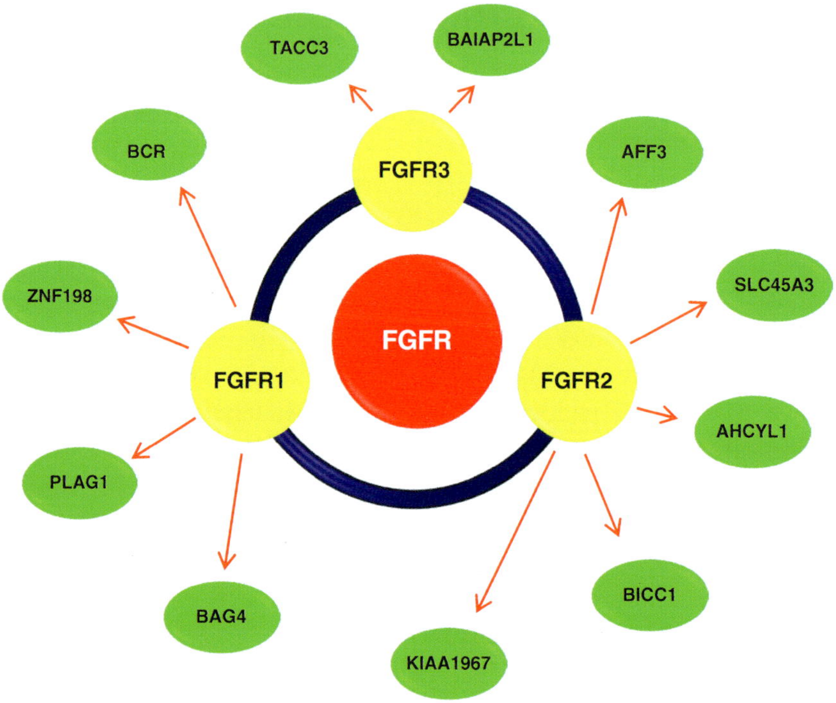

Figure 10.1: Fusion partners of FGFR proteins.

many other fusion kinases, FGFR3-TACC3 was also found to exert sustained kinase activity via coiled-coil oligomerization domain thus aberrantly activating FGF signaling cascade which in turn resulted in the activation of MAPK-ERK and PI3K-Akt pathways; nuclear localization and interleukin-3 (IL-3)-independent proliferation contributing to oncogenic transformation (Nelson *et al.*, 2016; Carneiro *et al.*, 2015; Williams *et al.*, 2013). Further, it has been confirmed to increase the cell proliferation, colony formation, and transforming ability *in vitro* through the enhanced FGFR kinase activity and activation of the signal transducer and activator of transcription 3 (STAT3), ERK and Akt signaling pathways in nasopharyngeal carcinoma (NPC) cells (Yuan *et al.*, 2014; Parker *et al.*, 2013). Moreover, loss of miRNA 99a (MiR-99a) binding site during chromosomal duplication resulted in uncontrolled activation of FGFR3 as MiR-99a binding was the regulator of wild-type FGFR3. Further, it also increased the mitotic and chromosomal segregation

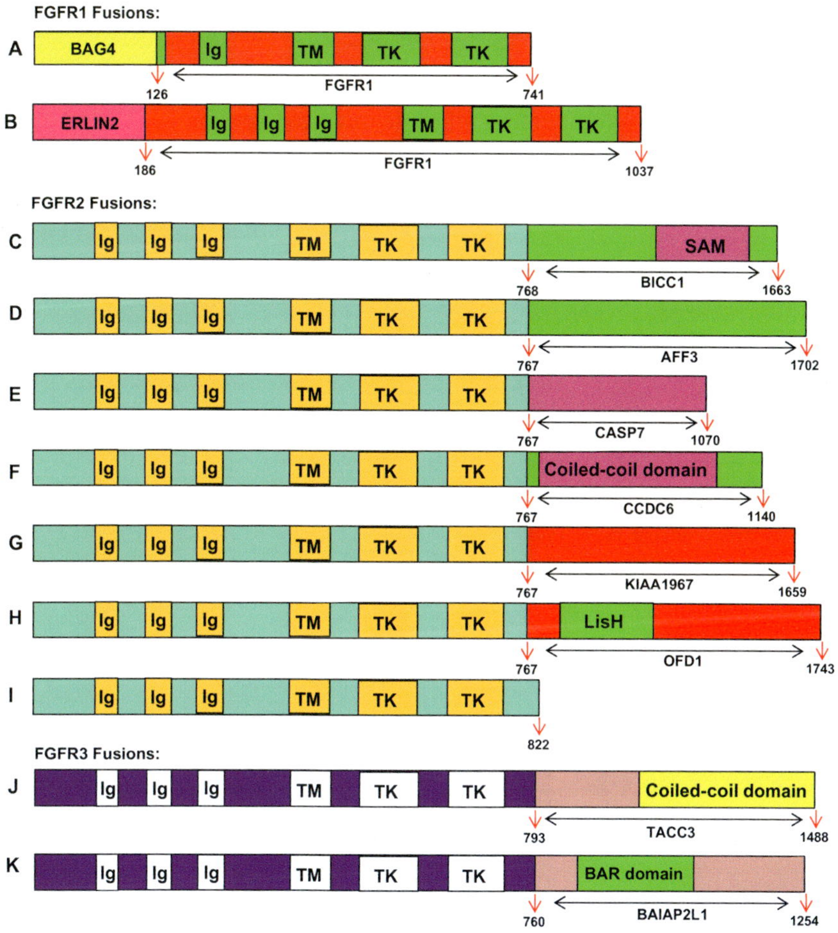

Figure 10.2: Schematic representations of the FGFR gene fusions. FGFR1 Fusions: (A) BAG4-FGFR1 (B) ERLIN 2-FGFR1; FGFR2 Fusions: (C) FGFR2-BICC1, (D) FGFR2-AFF3, (E) FGFR2-CASP7, (F) FGFR2-CCD6, (G) FGFR2-KIAA1967, (H) FGFR2-OFD1, (I) SLC45A3-FGFR2; FGFR3 Fusions: (J) FGFR3-TACC3, (K) FGFR3-BAIAP2L1 (Wu *et al*., 2013).

defects and induced aneuploidy in glioblastoma multiforme (GBM) (Singh *et al*., 2012). Therefore, as it was clear that constitutive activation of FGFR is the major driving factor for FGFR3-TACC3 carrying neoplasm and inhibitors of FGFR were believed to be potential therapeutic agents for this disease (Babic and Mischel, 2013; Parker *et al*., 2013).

BCR-FGFR1

BCR-ABL was thought to be the only BCR gene rearrangement associated with the development of chronic myeloid leukemia (CML) until another chromosomal translocation involving the BCR gene and the FGFR1 was identified. The translocation t(8;22)(p11;q11) produced a constitutively active fusion tyrosine kinase receptor BCR-FGFR1 (Demiroglu *et al.*, 2001; Fioretos *et al.*, 2001; Morishige *et al.*, 2013; Shimanuki *et al.*, 2013). The fusion protein induced CML development in mice models by binding to the GRB2 protein and also resulted in the increased activation of Src kinase and STAT5 (Roumiantsev *et al.*, 2004; Ren *et al.*, 2011; Baumann *et al.*, 2003). Unlike the other FGFR1 fusions associated with myeloid and T-cell proliferation, BCR-FGFR1 carrying myeloproliferative disorder (MPD) has a myeloid and B cell disease which indicated a new type of hematological malignancy (Murati *et al.*, 2005; Shimanuki *et al.*, 2013). Currently, allogeneic hematopoietic stem cell transplantation (HSCT) is the only therapy available to achieve long-term remission in BCR-FGFR1 carrying MPD patients (Haslam *et al.*, 2012; Dolan *et al.*, 2012).

FGFR1-ZNF198

t(8;13)(p11;q11-12) translocation resulted in the most common fusion of FGFR1 with ZnF gene, ZNF198 and associated with leukaemia/lymphoma or myeloproliferative syndrome presented with peripheral blood eosinophila and T- or B-cell leukemias (Xiao *et al.*, 1998; Reiter *et al.*, 1998; Kunapuli *et al.*, 2003). Resultant fusion protein which contains the intracellular tyrosine kinase domain and the ZnF domains of FGFR1 and ZNF198, respectively, induces the expression of constitutively active fusion tyrosine kinase through zinc finger domain-mediated homodimerization (Xiao *et al.*, 1998; Reiter *et al.*, 1998). Interestingly, heat shock protein family A member 1A (HSPA1A), a HSP70 family protein was shown to be involved in the stabilization of fusion kinase protecting it from the proteasomal degradation (Kasyapa *et al.*, 2007). Similar to other FGFR fusions, it was also proved to induce growth factor independence and to increase the phosphorylation of STAT 1, 3 and 5 proteins *in vitro* (Smedley *et al.*, 1999; Baumann *et al.*, 2003). This fusion gene activated STAT5 resulted in the increased expression of B-cell lymphoma-extra large (Bcl-xL) anti-apoptotic protein and Rad51 DNA repair protein; cell cycle progression and malignant transformation (Heath *et al.*, 2004). Moreover, this fusion also resulted in the elevated levels of plasminogen activator inhibitor-2 (PAI-2-SERPINB2) thus exhibiting resistance to apoptosis (Kasyapa *et al.*, 2006).

FGFR3-BAIAP2L1 (F3-B)

Fusion of FGFR3 with BAI1-associated protein 2-like 1 (BAIAP2L1) gene was detected in bladder and lung cancer patients and was generated by t(4;7) translocation (Figure 10.2). Both *in vitro* and *in vivo* analyses proved that F3-B fusion produced an aberrantly active FGFR3 tyrosine kinase thus resulting in the activation of MAPK pathway and inhibition of tumor suppressors like p53, retinoblastoma 1 (RB1), and cyclin-dependent kinase inhibitor 2A (CDKN2A) pathways ultimately leading to tumorigenesis. Moreover, the Bin-Amphiphysin-Rvs (BAR) dimerization domain of BAIAP2L1-mediated oligomerization was found to be the base for the activation of FGFR3 (Nakanishi *et al.*, 2015; Williams *et al.*, 2013).

CONCLUSION

Collectively, all the fusions have been shown to induce sustained activation of FGF-FGFR signaling and its downstream targets leading to increased cell proliferation, migration, invasion and most importantly angiogenesis ultimately resulting in oncogenic transformation. Therefore, it is evident that inhibition of FGF tyrosine kinase activity with the help of FGFR inhibitors would result in better prognosis.

CONFLICT OF INTEREST

The authors express no conflict of interest.

REFERENCES

Arai, Y., Y. Totoki, F. Hosoda, T. Shirota, N. Hama, H. Nakamura, H. Ojima, K. Furuta, K. Shimada, T. Okusaka, T. Kosuge, and T. Shibata, Fibroblast growth factor receptor 2 tyrosine kinase fusions define a unique molecular subtype of cholangiocarcinoma, *Hepatology* **59**: 1427–1434 (2014).

Babic, I. and P.S. Mischel, Multiple functions of a glioblastoma fusion oncogene, *J Clin Invest* **123**: 548–551 (2013).

Baumann, H., P. Kunapuli, E. Tracy, and J.K. Cowell, The oncogenic fusion protein-tyrosine kinase ZNF198/fibroblast growth factor receptor-1 has signaling function comparable with interleukin-6 cytokine receptors, *J Biol Chem* **278**: 16198–16208 (2003).

Beenken, A. and M. Mohammadi, The FGF family: biology, pathophysiology and therapy, *Nat Rev Drug Discov* **8**: 235–253 (2009).

Brooks, A.N., E. Kilgour, and P.D. Smith, Molecular pathways: fibroblast growth factor signaling: a new therapeutic opportunity in cancer, *Clin Canc Res* **18**: 1855–1862 (2012).

Carneiro, B.A., J.A., Elvin, S.D. Kamath, S.M. Ali, A.S. Paintal, A. Restrepo, E. Berry, F.J. Giles, and M.L Johnson, FGFR3-TACC3: A novel gene fusion in cervical cancer, *Gynecol Oncol Rep* **13**: 53–56 (2015).

Dailey, L., D. Ambrosetti, A. Mansukhani, and C. Basilico, Mechanisms underlying differential responses to FGF signaling, *Cytokine Growth Factor Rev* **16**: 233–247 (2005).

Demiroglu, A., E.J. Steer, C. Heath, K. Taylor, M. Bentley, S.L. Allen, P. Koduru, J.P. Brody, G. Hawson, R. Rodwell, M.L. Doody, F. Carnicero, A. Reiter, J.M. Goldman, J.V. Melo, and N.C. Cross, The t(8;22) in chronic myeloid leukemia fuses BCR to FGFR1: transforming activity and specific inhibition of FGFR1 fusion proteins, *Blood* **98**: 3778–3783 (2001).

Dienstmann, R., J. Rodon, A. Prat, J. Perez-Garcia, B. Adamo, E. Felip, J. Cortes, A.J. Iafrate, P. Nuciforo, and J. Tabernero, Genomic aberrations in the FGFR pathway: opportunities for targeted therapies in solid tumors, *Ann Oncol* **25**: 552–563 (2014).

Dolan, M., A. Cioc, N.C. Cross, J.P. Neglia, and J. Tolar, Favorable outcome of allogeneic hematopoietic cell transplantation for 8p11 myeloproliferative syndrome associated with BCR-FGFR1 gene fusion, *Pediatr Blood Canc* **59**: 194–196 (2012).

Fioretos, T., I. Panagopoulos, C. Lassen, A. Swedin, R. Billström, M. Isaksson, B. Strömbeck, T. Olofsson, F. Mitelman, and B. Johansson, Fusion of the BCR and the fibroblast growth factor receptor-1 (FGFR1) genes as a result of t(8;22)(p11;q11) in a myeloproliferative disorder: the first fusion gene involving BCR but not ABL, *Genes Chromosomes Canc* **32**: 302–310 (2001).

Haslam, K., S.E. Langabeer, J. Kelly, N. Coen, and N.M, O'Connell, and Conneally E. Allogeneic hematopoietic stem cell transplantation for a BCR-FGFR1 myeloproliferative neoplasm presenting as acute lymphoblastic Leukemia, *Case Rep Hematol* **2012**: 620967 (2012).

Heath, C., and N.C. Cross, Critical role of STAT5 activation in transformation mediated by ZNF198-FGFR1, *J Biol Chem* **279**: 6666–6673 (2004).

Kasyapa, C.S., P. Kunapuli, J.K. and Cowell, HSPA1A is an important regulator of the stability and function of ZNF198 and its oncogenic derivative, ZNF198-FGFR1, *J Cell Biochem* **102**: 1308–1317 (2007).

Kasyapa, C.S., P. Kunapuli, L. Hawthorn, and J.K. Cowell, Induction of the plasminogen activator inhibitor-2 in cells expressing the ZNF198/FGFR1 fusion kinase that is involved in atypical myeloproliferative disease, *Blood* **107**: 3693–3699 (2006).

Kunapuli, P., R. Somerville, I.H. Still, and J.K. Cowell, ZNF198 protein, involved in rearrangement in myeloproliferative disease, forms complexes with the DNA repair-associated HHR6A/6B and RAD18 proteins, *Oncogene* **22**: 3417–3423 (2003).

Morishige, S., E. Oku, Y. Takata, Y. Kimura, F. Arakawa, R. Seki, R. Imamura, K. Osaki, M. Hashiguchi, K. Yakushiji, S. Mizuno, K. Yoshimoto, K. Nagafuji, K. Ohshima, and T. Okamura, A case of 8p11 myeloproliferative syndrome with BCR-FGFR1 gene fusion presenting with trilineage acute leukemia/lymphoma, successfully treated by cord blood transplantation, *Acta Haematol* **129**: 83–89 (2013).

Murati, A., C. Arnoulet, M. Lafage-Pochitaloff, J. Adélaide, M. Derré, B. Slama, B. Delaval, C. Popovici, N. Vey, L. Xerri, M.J. Mozziconacci, O. Boulat, D. Sainty, D. Birnbaum, and M. Chaffanet, Dual lympho-myeloproliferative disorder in a patient with t(8;22) with BCR-FGFR1 gene fusion, *Int J Oncol* **26**: 1485–1492 (2005).

Nakanishi, Y., N. Akiyama, T. Tsukaguchi, T. Fujii, Y. Satoh, N. Ishii, and M. Aoki, Mechanism of Oncogenic Signal Activation by the Novel Fusion Kinase FGFR3-BAIAP2L1, *Mol Canc Ther* **14**: 704–712 (2015).

Nelson, K.N., A.N. Meyer, A. Siari, A.R. Campos, K. Motamedchaboki, and D.J. Donoghue, Oncogenic Gene Fusion FGFR3-TACC3 is Regulated by Tyrosine Phosphorylation, *Mol Canc Res* **14**: 458–469 (2016).

Parish, A., M. Schwaederle, G. Daniels, D. Piccioni, P. Fanta, R. Schwab, K. Shimabukuro, B.A. Parker, T. Helsten, and R. Kurzrock, Fibroblast growth factor family aberrations in cancers: clinical and molecular characteristics, *Cell Cycle* **14**: 2121–2128 (2015).

Parker, B.C., M.J. Annala, D.E. Cogdell, K.J. Granberg, Y. Sun, P. Ji, X. Li, J. Gumin, H. Zheng, L. Hu, O. Yli-Harja, H. Haapasalo, T. Visakorpi, X. Liu, C.G. Liu, R. Sawaya, G.N. Fuller, K. Chen, F.F. Lang, M. Nykter, and W. Zhang, The tumorigenic FGFR3-TACC3 gene fusion escapes miR-99a regulation in glioblastoma, *J Clin Invest* **123**: 855–865 (2013).

Persson, F., M. Winnes, Y. Andrén, B. Wedell, R. Dahlenfors, J. Asp, J. Mark, F. Enlund, and G. Stenman, High-resolution array CGH analysis of salivary gland tumors reveals fusion and amplification of the FGFR1 and PLAG1 genes in ring chromosomes, *Oncogene* **27**: 3072–3080 (2008).

Reiter, A., J. Sohal, S. Kulkarni, A. Chase, D.H. Macdonald, R.C. Aguiar, C. Gonçalves, J.M. Hernandez, B.A. Jennings, J.M. Goldman, and N.C. Cross, Consistent fusion of ZNF198 to the fibroblast growth factor receptor-1 in the t(8;13)(p11;q12) myeloproliferative syndrome, *Blood* **92**: 1735–1742 (1998).

Ren, M., H. Qin, R. Ren, J. Tidwell, and J.K Cowell, Src activation plays an important key role in lymphomagenesis induced by FGFR1 fusion kinases, *Canc Res* **71**: 7312–7322 (2011).

Roumiantsev, S., D.S. Krause, C.A. Neumann, C.A. Dimitri, F. Asiedu, N.C. Cross, and Van R.A. Etten, Distinct stem cell myeloproliferative/T lymphoma syndromes induced by ZNF198-FGFR1 and BCR-FGFR1 fusion genes from 8p11 translocations, *Cancer Cell* **5**: 287–298 (2004).

Sahni, M., D.C. Ambrosetti, A. Mansukhani, R. Gertner, D. Levy, and C. Basilico, FGF signaling inhibits chondrocyte proliferation and regulates bone development through the STAT-1 pathway, *Genes Dev* **13**: 1361–1366 (1999).

Shimanuki, M., T. Sonoki, H. Hosoi, J. Watanuki, S. Murata, T. Mushino, K. Kuriyama, S. Tamura, K. Hatanaka, N. Hanaoka, and H. Nakakuma, Acute leukemia showing t(8;22)(p11;q11), myelodysplasia, CD13/CD33/CD19 expression and immunoglobulin heavy chain gene rearrangement, *Acta Haematol* **129**: 238–242 (2013).

Singh, D., J.M. Chan, P. Zoppoli, F. Niola, R. Sullivan, A. Castano, E.M. Liu, J. Reichel, P. Porrati, S. Pellegatta, K. Qiu, Z. Gao, M. Ceccarelli, R. Riccardi, D.J. Brat, A. Guha, K. Aldape, J.G. Golfinos, D. Zagzag, T. Mikkelsen, G. Finocchiaro, A. Lasorella, R. Rabadan, and A. Iavarone, Transforming fusions of FGFR and TACC genes in human glioblastoma, *Science* **337**: 1231–1235 (2012).

Smedley, D., A. Demiroglu, M. Abdul-Rauf, C. Heath, C. Cooper, J. Shipley, and N.C. Cross, ZNF198-FGFR1 transforms Ba/F3 cells to growth factor independence and results in high level tyrosine phosphorylation of STATS 1 and 5, *Neoplasia* **1**: 349–355 (1999).

Tiseo, M., F. Gelsomino, R. Alfieri, A. Cavazzoni, C. Bozzetti, A.M. De Giorgi, and P.G. Petronini, A. Ardizzoni, FGFR as potential target in the treatment of squamous non-small cell lung cancer, *Cancer Treat Rev* **41**: 527–539 (2015).

Turner, N., and R. Grose, Fibroblast growth factor signaling: from development to cancer, *Nat Rev Canc* **10**: 116–129 (2010).

Wang, R., L. Wang, Y. Li, H. Hu, L. Shen, X. Shen, Y. Pan, T. Ye, Y. Zhang, X. Luo, Y. Zhang, B. Pan, B. Li, H. Li, J. Zhang, W. Pao, H. Ji, Y. Sun, and H. Chen, FGFR1/3 tyrosine kinase fusions define a unique molecular subtype of non-small cell lung cancer, *Clin Cancer Res* **20**: 4107–4114 (2014).

Wesche, J., K. Haglund, and E.M. Haugsten, Fibroblast growth factors and their receptors in cancer, *Biochem* **437**: 199–213 (2011).

Williams, S.V., C.D. Hurst, and M.A. Knowles, Oncogenic FGFR3 gene fusions in bladder cancer, *Hum Mol Genet* **22**: 795–803 (2013).

Wu, Y.M., F. Su, S. Kalyana-Sundaram, N. Khazanov, B. Ateeq, X. Cao, R.J. Lonigro, P. Vats, R. Wang, S.F. Lin, AJ. Cheng, L.P. Kunju, J. Siddiqui, S.A. Tomlins, P. Wyngaard, S. Sadis, S. Roychowdhury, MH. Hussain, F.Y. Feng, M.M. Zalupski, M. Talpaz, K.J. Pienta, D.R. Rhodes, and D.R. Robinson and A.M. Chinnaiyan, Identification of targetable FGFR gene fusions in diverse cancers, *Canc Discov* **3**: 636–647 (2013).

Xiao, S., S.R. Nalabolu, J.C. Aster, J. Ma, L. Abruzzo, E.S. Jaffe, R. Stone, S.M. Weissman, T.J. Hudson, and J.A. Fletcher, FGFR1 is fused with a novel zinc-finger gene, ZNF198, in the t(8;13) leukaemia/lymphoma syndrome, *Nat Genet* **18**: 84–87 (1998).

Yuan, L., Z.H. Liu, Z.R. Lin, L.H. Xu, Q. Zhong, and M.S. Zeng, Recurrent FGFR3-TACC3 fusion gene in nasopharyngeal carcinoma, *Canc Biol Ther* **15**: 1613–1621 (2014).

Zhang, X., O.A. Ibrahimi, S.K. Olsen, H. Umemori, M. Mohammadi, and D.M. Ornitz, Receptor specificity of the fibroblast growth factor family, The complete mammalian FGF family, *J Biol Chem* **281**: 15694–15700 (2006).

11

IG-MYC and Its Implication in Cancer

Ganesan Padmavathi, Kishore Banik,
*Krishan Kumar Thakur and Ajaikumar B. Kunnumakkara**

INTRODUCTION

v-Myc gene was first identified in avian retrovirus MC29 as a candidate gene for the development of myelocytomatosis (Sheiness *et al.*, 1978; Mellon *et al.*, 1978; Tansey, 2014). Further, identification of *c-Myc*- a cellular homolog of *v-myc* in chicken led to a series of crucial findings about the Myc induced tumorigenesis (Vennstrom *et al.*, 1982; Tansey, 2014). In mammals, the nuclear phosphoproteins called Myc proteins were found to be encoded by three distinct genes, namely, *c-Myc*, *N-Myc* and *L-Myc* grouped as Myc family of proteins (Tansey, 2014; Mukherjee *et al.*, 1992). All these proteins were shown to contain conserved structural

*Author for correspondence: Ajaikumar B. Kunnumakkara, Cancer Biology Laboratory, Department of Biosciences and Bioengineering, Indian Institute of Technology Guwahati, Assam 781039, India. kunnumakkara@iitg.ernet.in

motifs contributing to their transcriptional regulation and oncogenic transforming potentials (Barrett *et al.*, 1992). They were composed of an N-terminus transcriptional activation domain (TAD) and a C-terminus helix-loop-helix-leucine zipper (HLH-LZ) DNA-binding domain suggesting them to be DNA-binding transcriptional regulators (Kato *et al.*, 1990). Through these domains, Myc proteins were known to bind specific sequences of DNA and regulate the expression of various genes involved in cellular growth and differentiation (Mukherjee *et al.*, 1992). At physiological concentrations, Myc proteins were shown to heterodimerize with a small MYC associated factor X (MAX) protein through the HLH-LZ domain. This Myc-Max heterodimer specifically binds to E-boxes thus inducing the transcription of genes responsible for cell growth and proliferation (Dang, 2012; Grandori *et al.*, 1996). Wnt signalling, APC, β-catenin, RTKs induced ERK-MAPK signaling, Notch signaling and TGF-β signaling were found to be the potential upstream regulators of Myc gene amplification (Dang, 2012). Despite their similar structure and functionality, these three proteins were known to differ in potency and expression pattern (Tansey, 2014; Barrett *et al.*, 1992). For example, *c-Myc* overexpression increased the susceptibility to cytotoxic drugs, whereas elevated levels of *N-Myc*, and *L-Myc* reduced the susceptibility and induced resistance in hematopoietic cells (Nesbit *et al.*, 1998).

Increased expression levels of *c-Myc*, *N-Myc* and *L-Myc* oncoproteins have been frequently detected in 70% of all cancers including blood-borne cancers, solid tumors of neural origin and lung carcinomas (Tansey, 2014; Klapproth and Wirth, 2010). Unlike the other oncogenes like Ras, in all type of cancers except Burkitt's lymphoma (BL), Myc genes were reported to have no mutations in the coding sequence instead were activated by gene amplification, transcriptional induction or chromosomal translocations (Chakraborty and Tansey, 2015; Tansey, 2014). Moreover, this uncontrolled activation of Myc genes was proved to promote tumorigenesis through several mechanisms including transcriptional activation of proliferative genes; deregulation of cell cycle progression; increased growth and metabolism; deregulation of miRNAs network; induced genomic instability via DNA damage and replicative stress; promoted angiogenesis and metastasis, etc. (Tansey, 2014; Klapproth and Wirth, 2010; Dang, 2012). The most common translocation activating Myc genes is the IG-MYC translocation.

IG-MYC IN CANCER

Translocations depicted as t(8;14)(q24;q32), t(8;22)(q24;q11) and t(2;8)(p11;q24) produced the fusion of proto-oncogene *c-Myc* with any one of the three immunoglobulin (Ig) (IGH, IGK or IGL) loci forming IG-MYC fusion protein resulting in constitutively active Myc oncogene and most commonly detected in Epstein–Barr virus (EBV)-positive plasmablastic lymphoma (PBL), BL, mouse plasmacytomas (MPCs) and rat immunocytoma (Figure 11.1) (Boerma *et al.*, 2009; Valera *et al.*, 2010; Axelson *et al.*, 1994). Additionally, IG-MYC fusion was also observed in certain cases of multiple myeloma (MM) and plasma cell leukemia (PCL) (Fabris *et al.*, 2003). In general, the wild-type *c-Myc* was known to be switched

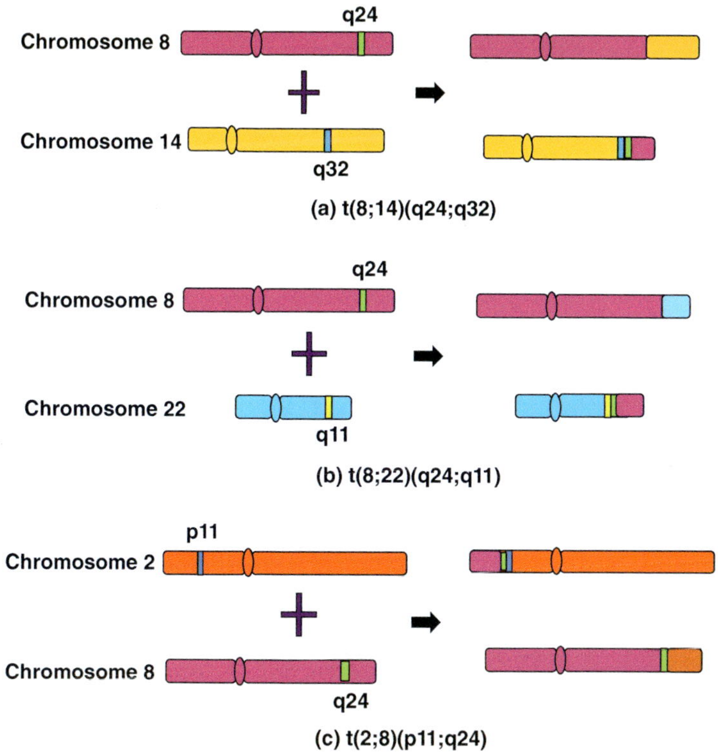

Figure 11.1: Schematic representation of MYC translocation to three different immunoglobulin (Ig) loci: (a) translocation of MYC to IGH; (b) translocation of MYC to IGK; and (c) translocation of MYC to IGL.

off when the cells enter terminal differentiation. However, translocated IG/MYC lost this control thus promoting the precursor cells of BL and MPS to escape growth control signals (Klein and Klein, 1985, 1986). Although the translocation was thought to be limited to *c-Myc*, an exception had been found in MPCs where the *N-Myc* not *c-Myc* was fused to Ig kappa through t(6;12)(CI;B) translocation (Axelson *et al.*, 1994). In addition, presence of IG-MYC fusion was found to be associated with poor survival in diffuse large B-cell lymphoma (DLBCL) patients (Copie-Bergman *et al.*, 2015; Pedersen *et al.*, 2014; Hummel *et al.*, 2006). Moreover, it was found to co-exist with BCL2-IgH, and IgL-BCL6 in DLBCL. However, co-existence did not affect the prognosis of the patient (Ueda *et al.*, 2004). Further, it was shown to induce malignant transformation of immature and/or mature B cells in MPCs (Ohno *et al.*, 1999). In addition, several *in vivo* experiments proved that activation-induced cytidine deaminase (AID) is an essential requirement for the immunoglobulin gene fusion with *c-Myc* (Kovalchuk *et al.*, 2007; Ramiro *et al.*, 2004; Robbiani *et al.*, 2008).

Effect of this translocation was well studied in BL and considered as a biological hallmark of BL as around 40% of the BL cases harbor IG-MYC as a sole disease initiating abnormality (Aukema *et al.*, 2014; Boerma *et al.*, 2009). Though IG-MYC was found responsible for the initiation of both *endemic* and *sporadic* BL, the breakpoint regions of *c-Myc* were different in both cases: in case of sporadic BLs, breakpoint occurred within exon 1-intron 1 which removed the 5′ regulatory elements, whereas in endemic BLs, it occurred upstream to Myc promoters leaving the regulatory elements intact (Kovalchuk *et al.*, 2012; Neri *et al.*, 1988). In addition, EBNA2 has been proved to induce growth arrest in t(8;14) carrying BL cells through the downregulation of Ig-mu and *c-Myc* (Jochner *et al.*, 1996). Further, this oncofusion gene was shown to protect the BL cells from host immune system by the preclusion of B cell resting stage through its non-immunological Myc portion and by the deregulation of human leukocyte antigen (HLA) class I polymorphic specificities, EBV encoded proteins and adhesion molecules through immunological Ig component (Klein, 1989, 1993). Moreover, secondary events like downregulation of tumor suppressors Rb and p53 were also found to induce the fusion-mediated tumorigenesis (Klein, 1993, 2009). Above all, generally, cells carrying the characteristic t(8;14) rearrangement were prone to apoptosis due to the presence of pro-apoptotic proteins like signaling lymphocytic activation molecule (SLAM)-associated protein (SAP). Supporting this, loss of SAP was found to be associated with EBV negative BL cells. However, in contrast, EBV positive BL cells were found to express SAP protein and to gain growth advantage through anti-apoptotic effect of EBNA1 leading to tumorigenesis (Nagy *et al.*, 2009; Nagy and Klein, 2010; Klein, 1994).

CONCLUSION

Taken together, it is apparent that Myc activating translocation, IG-MYC, plays a crucial role in the development of various cancers. However, extensive studies are required to elucidate the downstream effectors of this fusion protein and their role in cancer initiation and progression and to identify novel therapies targeting this fusion oncoprotein.

CONFLICT OF INTEREST

The authors express no conflict of interest.

REFERENCES

Aukema, S.M., M. Kreuz, C.W. Kohler, M. Rosolowski, D. Hasenclever, M. Hummel, R. Küppers, D. Lenze, G. Ott, C. Pott, J. Richter, A. Rosenwald, M. Szczepanowski, C. Schwaenen, H. Stein, H. Trautmann, S. Wessendorf, L. Trümper, M. Loeffler, R. Spang, P.M. Kluin, W. Klapper, and R. Siebert, Molecular mechanisms in malignant lymphomas network project. Biological characterization of adult MYC-translocation-positive mature B-cell lymphomas other than molecular Burkitt lymphoma, *Haematologica* **99**(4): 726–735 (2014).

Axelson, H., Y. Wang, S. Silva, M.G. Mattci, and G. Klein, Juxtaposition of N-myc and Ig kappa through a reciprocal t(6;12) translocation in a mouse plasmacytoma, *Genes Chromosomes Canc* **11**(2): 85–90 (1994).

Barrett, J., M.J. Birrer, G.J. Kato, H. Dosaka-Akita, and C.V. Dang, Activation domains of L-Myc and c-Myc determine their transforming potencies in rat embryo cells, *Mol Cell Biol* **12**(7): 3130–3137 (1992).

Boerma, E.G., R. Siebert, P.M. Kluin, and M. Baudis, Translocations involving 8q24 in Burkitt lymphoma and other malignant lymphomas: a historical review of cytogenetics in the light of today's knowledge, *Leukemia* **23**(2): 225–234 (2009).

Chakraborty, A.A. and W.P. Tansey, Do changes in the c-MYC coding sequence contribute to tumorigenesis? *Mol Cell Oncol* **2**(2): e965631 (2015).

Copie-Bergman, C., P. Cuillière-Dartigue, M. Baia, J. Briere, R. Delarue, D. Canioni, G. Salles, M. Parrens, K. Belhadj, B. Fabiani, C. Recher, T. Petrella, N. Ketterer, F. Peyrade, C. Haioun, I. Nagel, R. Siebert, F. Jardin, K. Leroy, J.P. Jais, H. Tilly, T.J. Molina, and P. Gaulard, MYC-IG rearrangements are negative predictors of survival in DLBCL patients treated with immunochemotherapy: a GELA/LYSA study, *Blood* **126**(22): 2466–2474 (2015).

Dang, C.V., MYC on the path to cancer, *Cell* **149**(1): 22–35 (2012).

Fabris, S., C.T. Storlazzi, L. Baldini, L. Nobili, L. Lombardi, A.T. Maiol, and M. Rocchi, A. Neri, Heterogeneous pattern of chromosomal breakpoints involving the MYC locus in multiple myeloma, *Genes Chromosomes Canc* **37**(3): 261–269 (2003).

Grandori, C., J. Mac, F. Siëbelt, D.E. Aye, and R.N. Eisenman, Myc-Max heterodimers activate a DEAD box gene and interact with multiple E box-related sites in vivo, *EMBO J* **15**(16): 4344–4357 (1996).

Hummel, M., S. Bentink, H. Berger, W. Klapper, S. Wessendorf, T.F. Barth, H.W. Bernd, S.B. Cogliatti, J. Dierlamm, A.C. Feller, M.L. Hansmann, E. Haralambieva, L. Harder, D. Hasenclever, M. Kühn, D. Lenze, P. Lichter, J.I. Martin-Subero, P. Möller, H.K. Müller-Hermelink, G. Ott, R.M. Parwaresch, C. Pott, A. Rosenwald, M. Rosolowski, C. Schwaenen, B. Stürzenhofecker, M. Szczepanowski, H. Trautmann, H.H. Wacker, R. Spang, M. Loeffler, L. Trümper, H. Stein, and R. Siebert. Molecular mechanisms in malignant lymphomas network project of the Deutsche krebshilfe, A biologic definition of Burkitt's lymphoma from transcriptional and genomic profiling, *N Engl J Med* **354**(23): 2419–2430 (2006).

Jochner, N., D. Eick, U. Zimber-Strobl, M. Pawlita, G.W. Bornkamm, and B. Kempkes, Epstein–Barr virus nuclear antigen 2 is a transcriptional suppressor of the immunoglobulin mu gene: implications for the expression of the translocated c-myc gene in Burkitt's lymphoma cells, *EMBO J* **15**(2): 375–382 (1996).

Kato, G.J., J. Barrett, M. Villa-Garcia, and C.V. Dang, An amino-terminal c-myc domain required for neoplastic transformation activates transcription, *Mol Cell Biol* **10**(11): 5914–5920 (1990).

Klapproth, K. and T. Wirth, Advances in the understanding of MYC-induced lymphomagenesis, *Br J Haematol* **149**(4): 484–497 (2010).

Klein, G. and E. Klein Conditioned tumorigenicity of activated oncogenes, *Cancer Res* **46**(7): 3211–3224 (1986).

Klein, G. and E. Klein, Myc/Ig juxtaposition by chromosomal translocations: some new insights, puzzles and paradoxes, *Immunol Today* **6**(7): 208–215 (1985).

Klein, G., Burkitt lymphoma — a stalking horse for cancer research? *Semin Canc Biol* **19**(6): 347–350 (2009).

Klein, G., Forward and reverse changes in Ig/myc translocation carrying tumors, *Princess Takamatsu Symp* **20**: 135–142 (1989).

Klein, G., Multistep evolution of B-cell-derived tumors in humans and rodents, *Gene* **135**(1–2): 189–196 (1993).

Klein, G., Role of EBV and Ig/myc translocation in Burkitt lymphoma, *Antibiot Chemother 1971* **46**: 110–116 (1994).

Kovalchuk, A.L., C. Ansarah-Sobrinho, O. Hakim, W. Resch, H. Tolarová, W. Dubois, A. Yamane, M. Takizawa, I. Klein, G.L. Hager, H.C. Morse, 3rd, M. Potter, M.C. Nussenzweig, and R. Casellas, Mouse model of endemic Burkitt translocations reveals the long-range boundaries of Ig-mediated oncogene deregulation, *Proc Natl Acad Sci USA* **109**(27): 10972–10977 (2012).

Kovalchuk, A.L., W. duBois, E. Mushinski, N.E. McNeil, C. Hirt, C.F. Qi, Z. Li, S. Janz, T. Honjo, M. Muramatsu, T. Ried, T. Behrens, and M. Potter, AID-deficient Bcl-xL transgenic mice develop delayed atypical plasma cell tumors with unusual Ig/Myc chromosomal rearrangements, *J Exp Med* **204**(12): 2989–3001 (2007).

Mellon, P., A. Pawson, K. Bister, G.S. Martin, and P.H. Duesberg, Specific RNA sequences and gene products of MC29 avian acute leukemia virus, *Proc Natl Acad Sci USA* **75**(12): 5874–5878 (1978).

Mukherjee, B., S.D. Morgenbesser, and R.A. DePinho, Myc family oncoproteins function through a common pathway to transform normal cells in culture: cross-interference by Max and trans-acting dominant mutants, *Genes Dev* **6**(8): 1480–1492 (1992).

Nagy, N. and E. Klein, Deficiency of the proapoptotic SAP function in X-linked lymphoproliferative disease aggravates Epstein–Barr virus (EBV) induced mononucleosis and promotes lymphoma development, *Immunol Lett* **130**(1–2): 13–18 (2010).

Nagy, N., G. Klei, and E. Klein, To the genesis of Burkitt lymphoma: regulation of apoptosis by EBNA-1 and SAP may determine the fate of Ig-myc translocation carrying B lymphocytes, *Semin Canc Biol* **19**(6): 407–410 (2009).

Neri, A., F. Barriga, D.M. Knowles, I.T. Magrath, and R. Dalla-Favera, Different regions of the immunoglobulin heavy-chain locus are involved in chromosomal translocations in distinct pathogenetic forms of Burkitt lymphoma, *Proc Natl Acad Sci USA* **85**(8): 2748–2752 (1988).

Nesbit, C.E., L.E. Grove, X. Yi, and E.V. Prochownik, Differential apoptotic behaviors of c-myc, N-myc, and L-myc oncoproteins, *Cell Growth Differ* **9**(9): 731–741 (1998).

Ohno, S., J. Hayakawa, N. Hashimoto, and F. Wiener, Murine plasmacytomas, carrier of the t(12;15) chromosomal translocation, develop from immature/mature B cells not from differentiated plasma cells, *Carcinogenesis* **20**(4): 529–538 (1999).

Pedersen, M.Ø., A.O. Gang, T.S. Poulsen, H. Knudsen, A.F. Lauritzen, S.L. Nielsen, T.W. Klausen, and P. Nørgaard, MYC translocation partner gene determines survival of patients with large B-cell lymphoma with MYC- or double-hit MYC/BCL2 translocations, *Eur J Haematol* **92**(1): 42–48 (2014).

Ramiro, A.R., M. Jankovic, T. Eisenreich, S. Difilippantonio, S. Chen-Kiang, M. Muramatsu, T. Honjo, A. Nussenzweig, and M.C. Nussenzweig, AID is required for c-myc/IgH chromosome translocations in vivo, *Cell* **118**(4): 431–438 (2004).

Robbiani, D.F., A. Bothmer, E. Callen, B. Reina-San-Martin, Y. Dorsett, S. Difilippantonio, D.J. Bolland, H.T. Chen, A.E. Corcoran, A. Nussenzweig, and M.C. Nussenzweig, AID is required for the chromosomal breaks in c-myc that lead to c-myc/IgH translocations, *Cell* **135**(6): 1028–1038 (2008).

Sheiness, D., L. Fanshier, and J.M. Bishop, Identification of nucleotide sequences which may encode the oncogenic capacity of avian retrovirus MC29, *J Virol* **28**(2): 600–610 (1978).

Tansey, W.P., Mammalian, MYC proteins and cancer, *New J Sci* **2013**: 1–27 (2014).

Ueda, C., M. Nishikori, T. Kitawaki, T. Uchiyama, and H. Ohno, Coexistent rearrangements of c-MYC, BCL2, and BCL6 genes in a diffuse large B-cell lymphoma, *Int J Hematol* **79**(1): 52–54 (2004).

Valera, A., O. Balagué, L. Colomo, A. Martínez, J. Delabie, L. Taddesse-Heath, E.S. Jaffe, E. Campo, IG/MYC rearrangements are the main cytogenetic alteration in plasmablastic lymphomas, *Am J Surg Pathol* **34**(11): 1686–1694 (2010).

Vennstrom, B., D. Sheiness, J. Zabielski, and J.M. Bishop, Isolation and characterization of c-myc, a cellular homolog of the oncogene (v-myc) of avian myelocytomatosis virus strain 29, *J Virol* **42**(3): 773–779 (1982).

12

Chimeric RAF Kinases in the Development of Cancer

*Ganesan Padmavathi, Kishore Banik, Devivasha Bordoloi, Choudhary Harsha and Ajaikumar B. Kunnumakkara**

INTRODUCTION

RAF, a serine-threonine-specific protein kinase, is an important component of RAS-RAF-MEK-ERK signaling pathway which is known to promote cell proliferation and malignant transformation (Dhomen and Marais, 2007). In general, RAF kinase is activated by its upstream regulator RAS which in turn is activated in response to growth factor signals. This activated RAF induced MAP kinase extracellular signal-regulated kinase (MEK) activation ultimately leading to the activation of extracellular signal-regulated kinases (ERK) (Dhomen and Marais, 2007). Till

*Author for correspondence: Ajaikumar B. Kunnumakkara, Cancer Biology Laboratory, Department of Biosciences and Bioengineering, Indian Institute of Technology Guwahati, Assam 781039, India. kunnumakkara@iitg.ernet.in

date, three major and highly conserved RAF genes, namely, ARAF, BRAF and CRAF (RAF-1) have been identified as potent oncogenes and reported to have different extent of kinase activity and distinct roles (Dhomen and Marais, 2007; Emuss *et al.*, 2005). Supporting this, Galabova-Kovacs *et al.* (2006) found BRAF lacking placentae to exhibit no ERK phosphorylation and impaired vascular development due to reduced levels of hypoxia-inducible factor 1-alpha (HIF-1α) and vascular endothelial growth factor (VEGF), whereas RAF-1 deficient placentae does not exert any such abnormalities (Galabova-Kovacs *et al.*, 2006; Mikula *et al.*, 2001; Hüser *et al.*, 2001). In addition, unlike BRAF, RAF-1 has been proved to induce anti-apoptotic signals rather proliferative signals (Mikula *et al.*, 2001; Hüser *et al.*, 2001). Moreover, while only a single mutation is sufficient for the oncogenic activation of BRAF kinase, other two RAF kinases required minimum of two somatic mutations explaining the rareness of ARAF and CRAF mutations (Dhomen and Marais, 2007; Emuss *et al.*, 2005). Thus, alterations of BRAF oncogene have been constantly reported in approximately 7% of neoplasms including colorectal cancers, lung cancers, melanoma and papillary thyroid cancers (Dhomen and Marais, 2007; Davies *et al.*, 2002; Lin *et al.*, 2014). BRAFV600E substitution mutation was the most common mutation that results in the constitutively activated BRAF kinase contributing to tumor initiation, maintenance and progression (Davies *et al.*, 2002; Dhomen and Marais, 2007). Though BRAF mutation is considered as a founder mutation of several cancers, it alone cannot promote complete tumorigenesis and required additional cooperating mutations (Dhomen and Marais, 2007). Further, several reports have shown that mutated BRAF can activate CRAF (RAF-1) which in turn activates ERK thus leading to uncontrolled MEK-ERK proliferative signals (Muhammad *et al.*, 2013).

Among numerous RAF mutations, this chapter focuses on the RAF kinase activating chromosomal rearrangements. As in other substitution mutations, rearrangements of BRAF gene were found to be frequently associated with various cancers. As already mentioned, all these translocations were resulted in the oncogenic activation of BRAF which in turn activates MEK-ERK-MAPK signaling cascade resulting in increased proliferation, survival and malignant transformation. Subsequent sections of this chapter explain the various RAF fusions, their implication in different cancers and the available treatment options.

KIAA1549-BRAF

KIAA1549-BRAF fusion with constitutive BRAF kinase activity is produced by tandem duplication of 7q34 and is the most common RAF fusion gene frequently seen in pilocytic astrocytoma (PA), a low-grade pediatric glioma (Figure 12.1) (Figarella-Branger *et al.*, 2013; Dimitriadis *et al.*, 2013; Tian *et al.*, 2011; Jeuken and Wesseling, 2010; Sievert *et al.*, 2009). The constitutive kinase activity was driven by the presence of kinase domain and removal of auto-inhibitory domain from BRAF by its fusion partner KIAA1549 (Sievert *et al.*, 2009). Though it is most common in PA (approximately 70%), it is rarely reported in pilomyxoid astrocytomas (PMA) as well (Ito *et al.*, 2015). Moreover, it was also reported to be restricted to PA and PMA among all other pediatric gliomas and correlated with age and infratentorial location of the brain (Gierke *et al.*, 2016). However, there are contradictory reports showing the presence of KIAA1549-BRAF fusion in non-PA tumors (Antonelli *et al.*, 2015; Kumar *et al.*, 2015; Lin *et al.*, 2012). For instance, it has

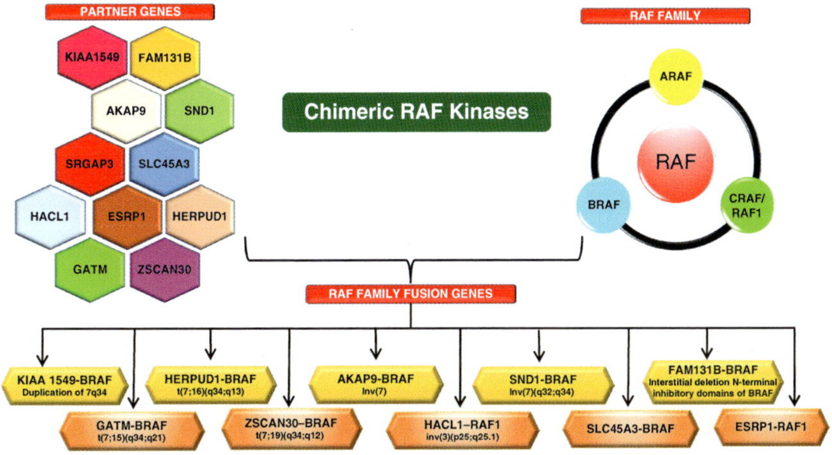

Figure 12.1: Different fusion partners of RAF kinases and the resulting fusion genes.

been detected in two cases of pediatric oligodendrogliomas (pODGs) and rosette-forming glioneuronal tumors (RGNT) with highly activated MAPK-ERK pathway (Kumar *et al.*, 2015; Dahiya *et al.*, 2012; Bidinotto *et al.*, 2015). Five variants of KIAA1549-BRAF fusion have been identified: variant 1 — fusion between KIAA1549 exon 16 and BRAF exon 9; variant 2 — fusion between KIAA1549 exon 15 and BRAF exon 9; variant 3 — fusion between KIAA1549 exon 16 and BRAF exon 11; variant 4 — fusion between KIAA1549 exon 18 and BRAF exon 10; variant 5 — fusion between KIAA1549 exon 19 and BRAF exon 9 (Forshew *et al.*, 2009).

Interestingly, KIAA1549-BRAF oncogene was proved to exhibit resistance to a first-generation BRAF inhibitor, PLX4720, and to act as homodimer thus activating the MEK-MAPK signaling cascade which can be reverted by destroying the dimer interface (Sievert *et al.*, 2013; Tatevossian *et al.*, 2010; Dasgupta *et al.*, 2013). Similarly, KIAA1549-BRAF integration was shown to exhibit a high affinity to kinase suppressor of RAS (KSR) and assists in the MEK phosphorylation which can also be reverted by breaking the BRAF kinase dimer interface (Sievert *et al.*, 2013; Jeuken and Wesseling, 2010). Further, it has been shown to regulate the proliferation of neural stem cell (NSC) through tuberin/Rheb-mediated hyperactivation of mTOR pathway and degradation of p27 (Kaul *et al.*, 2012). Hence, administration of MEK or mammalian target of rapamycin (mTOR) inhibitors is considered to be the promising treatment option for low-grade gliomas with KIAA1549-BRAF aberration (Dasgupta *et al.*, 2013). Supporting this, a combination therapy of sorafenib, temsirolimus, and bevazicumab in a phase I clinical trial was determined to target KIAA1549-BRAF fusion and to reduce the tumor size upto 25% (Subbiah *et al.*, 2014). Furthermore, it is expected that KIAA1549-BRAF fusion and BRAF (V600E) mutations would deregulate Ras-RAF-ERK signaling pathway and co-exist with additional genetic events like isocitrate dehydrogenase (IDH) mutations and 1p/19q co-deletion (Badiali *et al.*, 2012). Above all, the presence of KIAA1549-BRAF fusion has been found to be associated with better prognosis signifying it to be a prognostic biomarker for PAs (Becker *et al.*, 2015; Hawkins *et al.*, 2011).

FAM131B-BRAF

In addition to the KIAA1549-BRAF fusion gene, another oncogenic fusion as an alternative MAPK inducer has been discovered to be associated with the development of PA and dysembryoplastic neuroepithelial tumor (DNT) (Figure 12.1) (Cin *et al.*, 2011; Roth *et al.*, 2014, 2015). Family with sequence similarity 131 member B (FAM131B)-BRAF fusion was produced by an interstitial deletion which removed the N-terminal inhibitory domains of BRAF providing an aberrantly activated kinase (Cin *et al.*, 2011; Roth *et al.*, 2015).

AKAP9-BRAF

The first ever chromosomal rearrangement of RAF genes was described as a BRAF activating paracentric inversion of chromosome 7 in radiation-associated thyroid papillary carcinoma (Figure 12.1) (Fusco *et al.*, 2005; Ciampi *et al.*, 2005b). The resultant fusion protein contained the C-terminal kinase domain of BRAF and the N-terminus A-kinase anchor protein 9 (AKAP9). Like any other BRAF mutations, AKAP9-BRAF also lacked the N-terminal auto inhibitory domain of BRAF and exerted aberrant kinase activity thus resulting in the MAPK-mediated malignant transformation of NIH3T3 cells (Fusco *et al.*, 2005; Ciampi *et al.*, 2005a, 2005b). Further, it was proved that occurrence of AKAP9-BRAF fusion in sporadic papillary thyroid carcinomas (PTCs) may be a rare event (Lee *et al.*, 2006).

SND1-BRAF

SND1-BRAF was first identified as inversion of chromosome 7 leading to fusion of 7q32 and 7q34 in gastric cancer cells and was known to induce c-Met inhibition resistance through constitutive activation of MAPK pathway suggesting the requirement of treatment with both MET and RAF inhibitors (Figure 12.1) (Lee *et al.*, 2012; Chmielecki *et al.*, 2014). It was found to be expressed in castration-resistant prostate cancer (CRPC) biopsy specimens, pancreatic acinar cell carcinomas and lung adenocarcinomas (Sowalsky *et al.*, 2015; Chmielecki *et al.*, 2014; Jang *et al.*, 2015). Moreover, SND1-BRAF expressing cells were found to be susceptible for treatment with MEK inhibitors (Chmielecki *et al.*, 2014; Lee *et al.*, 2012).

OTHER RAF ACTIVATING FUSIONS

Apart from KIAA1549-BRAF, fusion between SLIT-ROBO Rho GTPase-activating protein 3 (SRGAP3) and RAF-1 was also identified in some cases of PA and similar to KIAA1549-BRAF, exons of SRGAP3 replaced the auto-inhibitory domain of RAF-1 resulting in a constitutive kinase activity thereby deregulating ERK-MAP kinase pathway (Figure 12.1) (Forshew *et al.*, 2009; Jones *et al.*, 2009). Likewise, SLC45A3-BRAF and ESRP1-RAF1 fusions have been detected in prostate cancers (Figure 12.1) (Palanisamy *et al.*, 2010). And three more BRAF fusions have been detected in preclinical Alzheimer cognitive composite (PACC). namely, HERPUD1-BRAF, ZSCAN30-BRAF and GATM-BRAF and denoted as t(7;16)(q34;q13), t(7;19)(q34;q12) and t(7;15)(q34;q21) respectively (Figure 12.1). Additionally, HACL1–RAF1 produced by an inversion of chromosome 3 inv(3)(p25;q25.1) was also identified in PACC (Figure 12.1) (Chmielecki *et al.*, 2014).

CONCLUSION

Collectively, RAF kinases, namely, ARAF, BRAF and CRAF being the important regulators of RAS-RAF-MEK-ERK pathway, induced uncontrolled growth when mutated. For instance, the BRAFV600E substitution mutation was found to be the major point mutation aberrantly activating the BRAF kinase activity leading to tumorigenesis of several cancers. Likewise, activating chromosomal translocations of RAF kinases were also found to be associated with various neoplasms including dysembryoplastic neuroepithelial tumor, gliomas, lung cancers, prostate cancers, RGNT, thyroid cancers, etc. The molecular base of all these fusion-mediated cancers was the activation of kinase oncoprotein which resulted in the aberrant activation of RAS-RAF-MEK-ERK signaling cascade and their downstream targets which in turn added growth advantage to the translocation carrying cells. In addition, the small molecule inhibitors like PLX4720 were found to pose a great potential in the management of RAF fusion-induced cancers. However, further studies are required to unravel the importance and role of various fusion RAF kinases in the development of cancer which would help to identify novel selective inhibitors for RAF fusion kinases with better efficacy.

CONFLICT OF INTEREST

The authors express no conflict of interest.

REFERENCES

Antonelli, M., M. Badiali, L. Moi, F.R. Buttarelli, C. Baldi, M. Massimino, M. Sanson, and F. Giangaspero, KIAA1549:BRAF fusion gene in pediatric brain tumors of various histogenesis, *Pediatr Blood Canc* **62**(4): 724–727 (2015).

Badiali, M., V. Gleize, S. Paris, L. Moi, S. Elhouadani, A. Arcella, R. Morace, M. Antonelli, F.R. Buttarelli, D. Figarella-Branger, Y.H. Kim, H. Ohgaki, K. Mokhtari, M. Sanson, and F. Giangaspero, KIAA1549-BRAF fusions and IDH mutations can coexist in diffuse gliomas of adults, *Brain Pathol* **22**(6): 841–847 (2012).

Becker, A.P., C. Scapulatempo-Neto, A.C. Carloni, A. Paulino, J. Sheren, D.L. Aisner, E. Musselwhite, C. Clara, H.R. Machado, R.S. Oliveira, L. Neder, M. Varella-Garcia, and R.M. Reis, KIAA1549: BRAF gene fusion and FGFR1 hotspot mutations are prognostic factors in pilocytic astrocytomas, *J Neuropathol Exp Neurol* **74**(7): 743–754 (2015).

Bidinotto, L.T., C. Scapulatempo-Neto, A. Mackay, G.C. de Almeida, B.W. Scheithauer, G.N. Berardinelli, R. Torrieri, C.A. Clara, L.T. Feltrin, M. Viana-Pereira, M. Varella-Garcia, C. Jones, and R. Reis. Molecular profiling of a rare rosette-forming glioneuronal tumor Arising in the Spinal Cord, *PLoS One* **10**(9): e0137690 (2015).

Chmielecki, J., K.E. Hutchinson, G.M. Frampton, Z.R. Chalmers, A. Johnson, C. Shi, J. Elvin, S.M. Ali, J.S. Ross, O. Basturk, S. Balasubramanian, D. Lipson, R. Yelensky, W. Pao, V.A. Miller, D.S. Klimstra, and P.J. Stephens, Comprehensive genomic profiling of pancreatic acinar cell carcinomas identifies recurrent RAF fusions and frequent inactivation of DNA repair genes, *Canc Discov* **4**(12): 1398–1405 (2014).

Ciampi, R., J.A. Knauf, R. Kerler, M. Gandhi, Z. Zhu, M.N. Nikiforova, H.M. Rabes, J.A. Fagin, and Y.E. Nikiforov, Oncogenic AKAP9-BRAF fusion is a novel mechanism of MAPK pathway activation in thyroid cancer, *J Clin Invest* **115**(1): 94–101 (2005a).

Ciampi, R., J.A. Knauf, H.M. Rabes, J.A. Fagin, and Y.E. Nikiforov, BRAF kinase activation via chromosomal rearrangement in radiation-induced and sporadic thyroid cancer, *Cell Cycle* **4**(4): 547–548 (2005b).

Cin, H., C. Meyer, R. Herr, W.G. Janzarik, S. Lambert, D.T. Jones, K. Jacob, A. Benner, H. Witt, M. Remke, S. Bender, F. Falkenstein, T.N. Van Anh, H. Olbrich, A. von Deimling, A. Pekrun, A.E. Kulozik, A. Gnekow, W. Scheurlen, O. Witt, H. Omran, N. Jabado, V.P. Collins, T. Brummer, R. Marschalek, P. Lichter, A. Korshunov, and S.M. Pfister, Oncogenic FAM131B-BRAF fusion resulting from 7q34 deletion comprises an alternative mechanism of MAPK pathway activation in pilocytic astrocytoma, *Acta Neuropathol* **121**(6): 763–774 (2011).

Dahiya, S., J. Yu, A. Kaul, J.R. Leonard, and D.H. Gutmann, Novel BRAF alteration in a sporadic pilocytic astrocytoma, *Case Rep Med* **2012**: 418672 (2012).

Dasgupta, T. and D.A. Haas-Kogan, The combination of novel targeted molecular agents and radiation in the treatment of pediatric gliomas, *Front Oncol* **3**:110 (2013).

Davies, H., G.R. Bignell, C. Cox, P. Stephens, S. Edkins, S. Clegg, J. Teague, H. Woffendin, M.J. Garnett, W. Bottomley, N. Davis, E. Dicks, R. Ewing, Y. Floyd, K. Gray, S. Hall, R. Hawes, J. Hughes, V. Kosmidou, A. Menzies, C. Mould, A. Parker, C. Stevens, S. Watt, S. Hooper, R. Wilson, H. Jayatilake, B.A. Gusterson, C. Cooper, J. Shipley, D. Hargrave, K. Pritchard-Jones, N. Maitland, G. Chenevix-Trench, G.J. Riggins, D.D. Bigner, G. Palmieri, A. Cossu, A. Flanagan, A. Nicholson, J.W. Ho, S.Y. Leung, S.T. Yuen, B.L. Weber, H.F. Seigler, T.L. Darrow, H. Paterson, R. Marais, C.J. Marshall, R. Wooster, M.R. Stratton, and P.A. Futreal, Mutations of the BRAF gene in human cancer, *Nature* **417**(6892): 949–954 (2002).

Dhomen, N. and R. Marais, New insight into BRAF mutations in cancer, *Curr Opin Genet Dev* **17**(1): 31–39 (2007).

Dimitriadis, E., G.A. Alexiou, P. Tsotsou, E. Simeonidi, K. Stefanaki, A. Patereli, N. Prodromou, and N. Pandis, BRAF alterations in pediatric low grade gliomas and mixed neuronal-glial tumors, *J Neurooncol* **113**(3): 353–358 (2013).

Emuss, V., M. Garnett, C. Mason, and R. Marais, Mutations of C-RAF are rare in human cancer because C-RAF has a low basal kinase activity compared with B-RAF, *Canc Res* **65**(21): 9719–9726 (2005).

Figarella-Branger, D., C. Chappe, L. Padovani, S. Mercurio, C. Colin, F. Forest, and C. Bouvier, Glial and glioneuronal tumors in adults and children: main genetic alterations and towards a histomolecular classification, *Bull Canc* **100**(7–8): 715–726 (2013) [in French].

Forshew, T., R.G. Tatevossian, A.R. Lawson, J. Ma, G. Neale, B.W. Ogunkolade, T.A. Jones, J. Aarum, J. Dalton, S. Bailey, T. Chaplin, R.L. Carter, A. Gajjar, A. Broniscer, B.D. Young, D.W. Ellison, and D. Sheer, Activation of the ERK/MAPK pathway: a signature genetic defect in posterior fossa pilocytic astrocytomas, *J Pathol* **218**(2): 172–181 (2009).

Fusco, A., G. Viglietto, and M. Santoro, A new mechanism of BRAF activation in human thyroid papillary carcinomas, *J Clin Invest* **115**(1): 20–23 (2005).

Galabova-Kovacs, G., D. Matzen, D. Piazzolla, K. Meissl, T. Plyushch, A.P. Chen, A. Silva, and M. Baccarini, Essential role of B-Raf in ERK activation during extraembryonic development, *Proc Natl Acad Sci USA* **103**(5): 1325–1330 (2006).

Gierke, M., J. Sperveslage, D. Schwab, R. Beschorner, M. Ebinger, M.U. Schuhmann, and J. Schittenhelm, Analysis of IDH1-R132 mutation, BRAF V600 mutation and KIAA1549-BRAF fusion transcript status in central nervous system tumors supports pediatric tumor classification, *J Canc Res Clin Oncol* **142**(1): 89–100 (2016).

Hawkins, C., E. Walker, N. Mohamed, C. Zhang, K. Jacob, M. Shirinian, N. Alon, D. Kahn, I. Fried, K. Scheinemann, E. Tsangaris, P. Dirks, R. Tressler, E. Bouffet, N. Jabado, and U. Tabori, BRAF-KIAA1549 fusion predicts better clinical outcome in pediatric low-grade astrocytoma, *Clin Canc Res* **17**(14): 4790–4798 (2011).

Hüser, M., J. Luckett, A. Chiloeches, K. Mercer, M. Iwobi, S. Giblett, X.M. Sun, J. Brown, R. Marais, and C. Pritchard, MEK kinase activity is not necessary for Raf-1 function, *EMBO J* **20**(8): 1940–1951 (2001).

Ito, T., K. Sato, M. Oikawa, H. Sugio, T. Asanome, Y. Ozaki, H. Nakamura, S. Tanaka, M. Tsuda, and K. Nagashima, [Clinicopathological Study of Pilomyxoid-Spectrum Astrocytomas: An Analysis of the BRAF Gene, Report of Two Cases] *No Shinkei Geka* **43**(9): 825–833 (2015).

Jang, J.S., A. Lee, J. Li, H. Liyanage, Y. Yang, L. Guo, Y.W. Asmann, P.W. Li, M. Erickson-Johnson, Y. Sakai, Z. Sun, H.S. Jeon, H. Hwang, A.O. Bungum, E.S. Edell, V.A. Simon, K.J. Kopp, B. Eckloff, A.M. Oliveira, E. Wieben, M.C. Aubry, E. Yi, D. Wigle, R.B. Diasio, P. Yang, and J. Jen, Common oncogene mutations and novel SND1-BRAF transcript fusion in lung adenocarcinoma from never smokers, *Sci Rep* **5**: 9755 (2015).

Jeuken, J.W. and P. Wesseling, MAPK pathway activation through BRAF gene fusion in pilocytic astrocytomas; a novel oncogenic fusion gene with diagnostic, prognostic, and therapeutic potential, *J Pathol* **222**(4): 324–328 (2010).

Jones, D.T., S. Kocialkowski, L. Liu, D.M. Pearson, K. Ichimura, and V.P. Collins, Oncogenic RAF1 rearrangement and a novel BRAF mutation as alternatives to KIAA1549:BRAF fusion in activating the MAPK pathway in pilocytic astrocytoma, *Oncogene* **28**(20): 2119–2123 (2009).

Kaul, A., Y.H. Chen, R.J. Emnett, S. Dahiya, and D.H. Gutmann, Pediatric glioma-associated KIAA1549:BRAF expression regulates neuroglial cell growth in a cell type-specific and mTOR-dependent manner, *Genes Dev* **26**(23): 2561–2566 (2012).

Kumar, A., P. Pathak, S. Purkait, M. Faruq, P. Jha, S. Mallick, V. Suri, M.C. Sharma, A. Suri, and C. Sarkar, Oncogenic KIAA1549-BRAF fusion with activation of the MAPK/ERK pathway in pediatric oligodendrogliomas, *Canc Genet* **208**(3): 91–95 (2015).

Lee, J.H., E.S. Lee, Y.S. Kim, N.H. Won, and Y.S. Chae, BRAF mutation and AKAP9 expression in sporadic papillary thyroid carcinomas, *Pathology* **38**(3): 201–204 (2006).

Lee, N.V., M.E. Lira, A. Pavlicek, J. Ye, D. Buckman, S. Bagrodia, S.P. Srinivasa, Y. Zhao, S. Aparicio, P.A. Rejto, J.G. Christensen, and K.A. Ching, A novel SND1-BRAF fusion confers resistance to c-Met inhibitor PF-04217903 in GTL16 cells through [corrected] MAPK activation, *PLoS One* **7**(6): e39653 (2012).

Lin, A., F.J. Rodriguez, M.A. Karajannis, S.C. Williams, G. Legault, D. Zagzag, P.C. Burger, J.C. Allen, C.G. Eberhart, and E.E. Bar, BRAF alterations in primary glial and glioneuronal neoplasms of the central nervous system with identification of 2 novel KIAA1549:BRAF fusion variants, *J Neuropathol Exp Neurol* **71**(1): 66–72 (2012).

Lin, L., S. Asthana, E. Chan, S. Bandyopadhyay, M.M. Martins, V. Olivas, J.J. Yan, L. Pham, M.M. Wang, G. Bollag, D.B. Solit, E.A. Collisson, C.M. Rudin, B.S. Taylor, and T.G. Bivona, Mapping the molecular determinants of BRAF oncogene dependence in human lung cancer, *Proc Natl Acad Sci USA* **111**(7): E748–E757 (2014).

Mikula, M., M. Schreiber, Z. Husak, L. Kucerova, J. Rüth, R. Wieser, K. Zatloukal, H. Beug, E.F. Wagner, and M. Baccarini, Embryonic lethality and fetal liver apoptosis in mice lacking the c-raf-1 gene, *EMBO J* **20**(8): 1952–1962 (2001).

Muhammad, S., Z. Jiang, Z. Liu, K. Kaur, and X. Wang, The role of EGFR monoclonal antibodies (MoABs) cetuximab/panitumab, and BRAF inhibitors in BRAF mutated colorectal cancer, *J Gastrointest Oncol* **4**(1): 72–81 (2013).

Palanisamy, N., B. Ateeq, S. Kalyana-Sundaram, D. Pflueger, K. Ramnarayanan, S. Shankar, B. Han, Q. Cao, X. Cao, K. Suleman, C. Kumar-Sinha, S.M. Dhanasekaran, Y.B. Chen, R. Esgueva, S. Banerjee, C.J. LaFargue, J. Siddiqui, F. Demichelis, P. Moeller, T.A. Bismar, R. Kuefer, D.R. Fullen, T.M. Johnson, J.K. Greenson, T.J. Giordano, P. Tan, S.A. Tomlins, S. Varambally, M.A. Rubin, C.A. Maher, and AM. Chinnaiyan, Rearrangements of the RAF kinase pathway in prostate cancer, gastric cancer and melanoma, *Nat Med* **16**(7): 793–798 (2010).

Roth, J.J., M. Santi, A.N. Pollock, B.N. Harding, L.B. Rorke-Adams, L.S. Tooke, and JA. Biegel, Chromosome band 7q34 deletions resulting in KIAA1549-BRAF and FAM131B-BRAF fusions in pediatric low-grade Gliomas, *Brain Pathol* **25**(2): 182–192 (2015).

Roth, J.J., M. Santi, L.B. Rorke-Adams, B.N. Harding, T.M. Busse, L.S. Tooke, and JA. Biegel, Diagnostic application of high resolution single nucleotide polymorphism array analysis for children with brain tumors, *Canc Genet* **207**(4): 111–123 (2014).

Sievert, A.J., E.M. Jackson, X. Gai, H. Hakonarson, A.R. Judkins, A.C. Resnick, L.N. Sutton, P.B. Storm, T.H. Shaikh, and J.A. Biegel, Duplication of 7q34 in pediatric low-grade astrocytomas detected by high-density single-nucleotide polymorphism-based genotype arrays results in a novel BRAF fusion gene, *Brain Pathol* **19**(3): 449–458 (2009).

Sievert, A.J., S.S. Lang, K.L. Boucher, P.J. Madsen, E. Slaunwhite, N. Choudhari, M. Kellet, P.B. Storm, and A.C. Resnick, Paradoxical activation and RAF inhibitor resistance of BRAF protein kinase fusions characterizing pediatric astrocytomas, *Proc Natl Acad Sci USA* **110**(15): 5957–5962 (2013).

Sowalsky, A.G., Z. Xia, L. Wang, H. Zhao, S. Chen, G.J. Bubley, S.P. Balk, and W. Li, Whole transcriptome sequencing reveals extensive unspliced mRNA in metastatic castration-resistant prostate cancer, *Mol Canc Res* **13**(1): 98–106 (2015).

Subbiah, V., S.N. Westin, K. Wang, D. Araujo, W.L. Wang, V.A. Miller, J.S. Ross, P.J. Stephens, G.A. Palmer, and S.M. Ali, Targeted therapy by combined inhibition of the RAF and mTOR kinases in malignant spindle cell neoplasm harboring the KIAA1549-BRAF fusion protein, *J Hematol Oncol* **7**:8 (2014).

Tatevossian, R.G., A.R. Lawson, T. Forshew, G.F. Hindley, D.W. Ellison, and D. Sheer, MAPK pathway activation and the origins of pediatric low-grade astrocytomas, *J Cell Physiol* **222**(3): 509–514 (2010).

Tian, Y., B.E. Rich, N. Vena, J.M. Craig, L.E. Macconaill, V. Rajaram, S. Goldman, H. Taha, M. Mahmoud, M. Ozek, A. Sav, J.A. Longtine, N.I. Lindeman, L.A. Garraway, A.H. Ligon, C.D. Stiles, S. Santagata, J.A. Chan, M.W. Kieran, and K.L. Ligon, Detection of KIAA1549-BRAF fusion transcripts in formalin-fixed paraffin-embedded pediatric low-grade gliomas, *J Mol Diagn* **13**(6): 669–677 (2011).

13

Mucoepidermoid Carcinoma (MEC) and Associated MAML2 Fusion Genes

*Ganesan Padmavathi, Choudhary Harsha, Devivasha Bordoloi, Kishore Banik and Ajaikumar B. Kunnumakkara**

INTRODUCTION

Mucoepidermoid carcinoma (MEC) is described as cancer arising from the salivary-type mucous glands of aerodigestive tract and other organs like breast, cervix, esophagus, lung, pancreas, skin and thyroid and also classified as low, intermediate and high grade tumors (Saade *et al.*, 2016; Yokouchi *et al.*, 2015; Seethala, 2009; Chen *et al.*, 2015). In addition, the 5 year survival rate of MEC patients was highly correlated with the grade of the disease. For instance, low grade tumor was associated with

*Author for correspondence: Ajaikumar B. Kunnumakkara, Cancer Biology Laboratory, Department of Biosciences and Bioengineering, Indian Institute of Technology Guwahati, Assam 781039, India. kunnumakkara@iitg.ernet.in

92–100%, intermediate grade tumor with 62–92% and high grade tumor with 0–43% of 5 year survival (Seethala, 2009). Advanced stage MEC tumors were often found to be associated with angiolymphatic invasion, perineural invasion, infiltrative growth, anaplasia and coagulative necrosis, etc. (Saade *et al.*, 2016; Seethala, 2009). Interestingly, translocation of chromosomes 11 and 19 was found to be the characteristic feature of MEC which remains unique to MEC and was mostly associated with intermediate grade tumors (Saade *et al.*, 2016; Fujinaga *et al.*, 2016; Seethala *et al.*, 2010). Translocation denoted as t(11;19)(q21;p13.1) was resulted in the juxtaposition of a cAMP response element binding protein (CREB)-regulated transcriptional coactivator (CRTC1) and Notch coactivator mastermind-like 2 (MAML2) producing CRTC1-MAML2 fusion gene (Conkright *et al.*, 2003).

CREB-regulated transcriptional coactivator is a family of CREB cofactors comprising three proteins, namely, CRTC1, CRTC2 and CRTC3. CRTC proteins were also known as transducer of regulated CREB activity (TORCs) or mucoepidermoid carcinoma translocated protein (MECTs) (Conkright *et al.*, 2003; Iourgenko *et al.*, 2003; Luo *et al.*, 2012; Chen *et al.*, 2015). These proteins were shown to regulate cAMP response element (CRE)-mediated expression of various genes involved in metabolism, aging, memory, and cancer (Iourgenko *et al.*, 2003; Conkright *et al.*, 2003). Under resting conditions, CRTCs were known to be restricted to cytoplasm by forming complexes with 14-3-3 proteins which was induced by phosphorylation of CRTCs. However, they are dephosphorylated, detached from 14-3-3 proteins and translocated to nucleus where they bind with bZip domain of CREB and activate CREB-mediated gene expression upon induction with calcium or cAMP (Luo *et al.*, 2012; Screaton *et al.*, 2004).

Mastermind-like proteins (MAMLs) were also a family of transcriptional coactivators for Notch receptors containing three members known as MAML1, MAML2 and MAML3. Unlike CRTC proteins, the MAML proteins were packed into nuclear bodies (NBs), bound to Notch receptors and induced the expression of Notch target genes critically regulating the Notch signaling cascade (Wu *et al.*, 2002; Chen *et al.*, 2015). Being a key regulator of Notch signaling, MAML proteins contribute to both normal biological processes and human diseases. Moreover, these proteins were also shown to regulate various other signaling components like MEF2C, p53 and beta-catenin essential for normal cellular functioning (McElhinny *et al.*, 2008). Therefore, t(11;19) governed the fusion of CREB binding domain (CBD) of CRTC1 and transcriptional activation domain (TAD) of MAML2 generating an aberrant transcriptional coactivator constitutively localized to the nucleus, mediating the development of MECs (Clark *et al.*, 2015). Moreover, being expressed in more than 50% of MECs, MECT1-MAML2 translocation is successfully used as a diagnostic biomarker for MECs (Bell *et al.*, 2013; Clauditz *et al.*, 2012).

MECT1-MAML2 OR CRTC1-MAML2

As already mentioned, MECT1-MAML2 or CRTC1-MAML2 is the fusion of CREB coactivator-mucoepidermoid carcinoma translocated-1 (MECT1) and Notch coactivator-mastermind-like 2 (MAML2) genes resulted from t(11;19) (q21;p13.1) and associated with MEC of various origin, particularly with the low-grade and intermediate-grade tumors (Figure 13.1) (Cazorla *et al.*, 2014; Bell *et al.*, 2013; Argyris *et al.*, 2015; Clauditz *et al.*, 2012; Behboudi *et al.*, 2006; Tonon *et al.*, 2003). Apart from MECs, few cases of Warthin's tumor and around 50% of skin hidradenomas were also detected positive for t(11;19) translocation suggesting it to be associated with tumors of diverse exocrine glands (Kazakov *et al.*, 2007; Tirado *et al.*, 2007; Winnes *et al.*, 2007). Additionally, this fusion protein was proved to contain both CREB-binding and transactivation domains of MECT1 or CRTC1 and transcriptional activation domain of MAML2 thus activating the target genes of both cAMP-CREB and Notch signaling resulting in deregulation of cell cycle and cellular differentiation (Argyris *et al.*, 2015; Amelio *et al.*, 2014). Supporting this, it was also demonstrated to activate CREB-dependent transcription of target genes such as amphiregulin (AREG), IL6, MMP10, NR4A2, NR4A3 and PEPCK1 thereby mimicking cAMP signaling activation (Komiya *et al.*, 2006; Wu *et al.*, 2005; Coxon *et al.*, 2005; Stenman, 2013). The nuclear nature of this fusion protein was proved to impart constitutive recruitment of CBP/p300 complex to CREB-regulated genes which can tremendously increase their expression (Figure 13.2) (Clark *et al.*, 2015). Moreover, besides CREB targets, it also induced the expression of Notch target gene

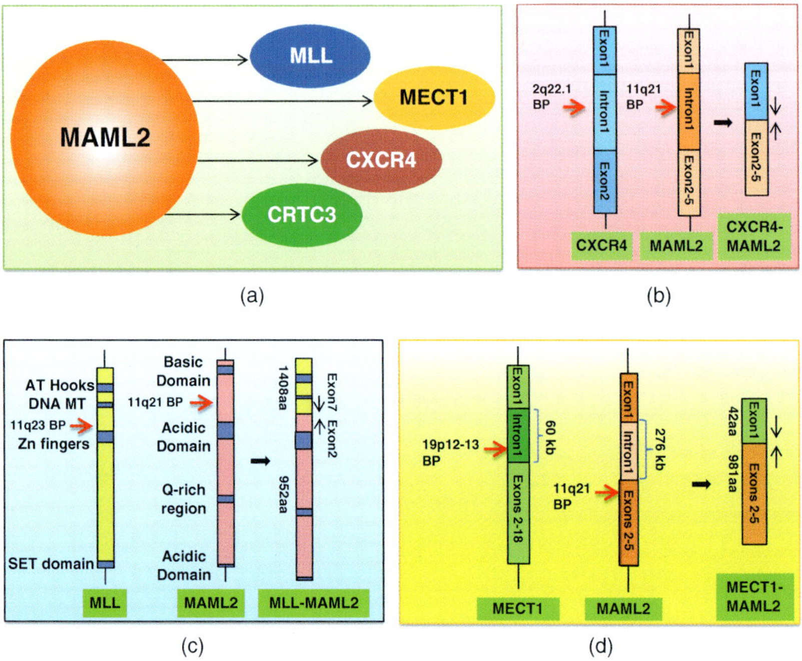

Figure 13.1: (A) Fusion partners of MAML2; (B) CXCR4-MAML2 translocation; (C) MLL-MAML2 translocation; (D) MECT1-MAML2 or CRTC1-MAML2 translocation (BP- breakpoint).

HES1 and deregulated the Notch signaling pathway (Röser *et al.*, 2005; Enlund *et al.*, 2004; Argyris *et al.*, 2015). Further, it was shown to stimulate the MYC related genes by creating a CRTC1-MAML2-MYC interface (Figure 13.2) (Amelio *et al.*, 2014). In addition, recently CRTC1-MAML2 fusion protein has been shown to deregulate the expression of several genes involved in cell growth, proliferation, survival, migration, and metabolism and to induce tumorigenesis via both CREB-dependent and independent manners (Chen *et al.*, 2015). Furthermore, CRTC1-MAML2 fusion protein was shown to increase the CREB-mediated expression of AREG, an epidermal growth factor receptor (EGFR) ligand thereby activating the EGFR signaling cascade. Thus, it is proved to be involved in the regulation of EGFR signaling ultimately leading to uncontrolled growth and proliferation of MEC cells (Figure 13.2)

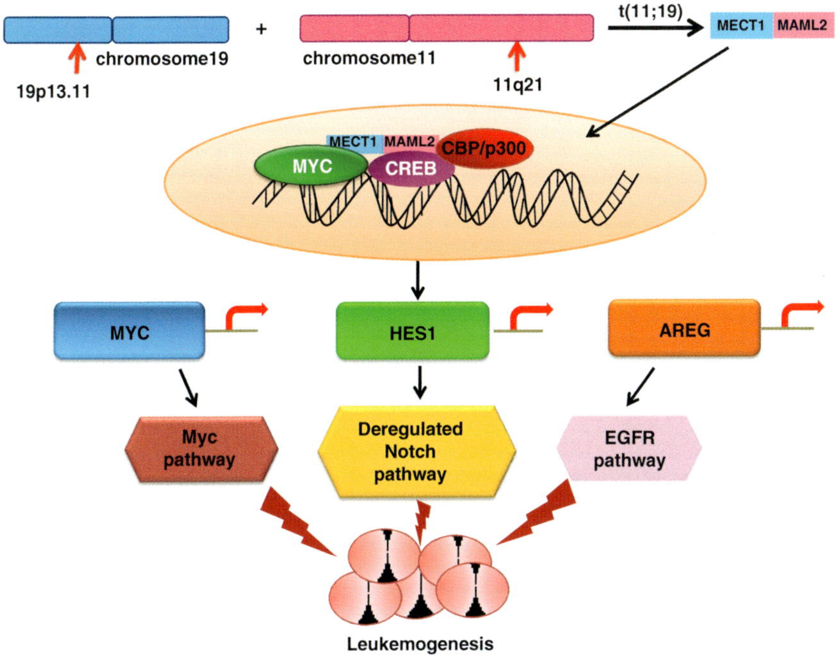

Figure 13.2: Mechanism of MECT1-MAML2 induced leukemogenesis.

(Chen *et al.*, 2014). Therefore, EGFR-TKI therapy was found to be effective against t(11;19) harboring MECs as it suppressed the fusion-mediated proliferation through increased amphiregulin expression (Yokouchi *et al.*, 2015; O'Neill, 2009).

Above all, presence of this fusion gene was regarded as better prognostic marker as it was associated with better prognosis than fusion negative MEC (Anzick *et al.*, 2010). Supporting this fact, expression of HMGA2, a stem cell marker expressed in cancer stem cells, was found to be upregulated in case of fusion negative MEC tissues over the fusion positive MEC tissues (Fehr *et al.*, 2009). Likewise, this fusion was shown to be associated with stable genome and better clinical outcome than the fusion negative MECs proving it to be a potential prognostic marker (Bell *et al.*, 2013; Bhaijee *et al.*, 2011; Miyabe *et al.*, 2009; Okabe *et al.*, 2006). However, contrastingly, recent studies have reported that the presence of CRTC1-MAML2 fusion has no correlation with better prognosis (Saade *et al.*, 2016).

Other than CRTC1, three more fusion partners of MAML2 namely, CRTC3, CXCR4 and MLL had also been identified (Figure 13.1) (Fehr *et al.*, 2008; Prieto-Granada *et al., 2015;* Chan *et al.*, 2013; Nemoto *et al.*, 2007; Tang *et al.*, 2014; Acunzo *et al.*, 2014). Similar to CRTC1-MAML2, CRTC3-MAML2 was produced by the translocation of chromosomes 11 and 15 denoted as t(11;15)(q21;q26) and associated with MECs (Prieto-Granada *et al.*, 2015; Chan *et al.*, 2013; Nakayama *et al.*, 2009; Fehr *et al.*, 2008). While, MLL-MAML2 is a product of chromosomal inversion inv(11)(q21q23) and involved in the tumorigenesis of AML and T-cell ALL through the dysregulation of Notch signaling (Nemoto *et al.*, 2007; Metzler *et al.*, 2008). CXCR4-MAML2 was identified as a product of t(2;11)(q22.1;q21) translocation in chronic lymphocytic leukemia (CLL) cells (Acunzo *et al.*, 2014). Further studies are required to elucidate the exact roles of these fusions in the development of cancer.

CONFLICT OF INTEREST

The authors express no conflict of interest.

REFERENCES

Acunzo, M., G. Romano, D. Wernicke, V. Balatti, L.Z. Rassenti, dell'M. Aquila, T.J. Kipps, Y. Pekarsky, and C.M. Croce, Translocation t(2;11) in CLL cells results in CXCR4/MAML2 fusion oncogene, *Blood* **124**(2): 259–262 (2014).

Amelio, A.L., M. Fallahi, F.X. Schaub, M. Zhang, M.B. Lawani, A.S. Alperstein, M.R. Southern, B.M. Young, L. Wu, M. Zajac-Kaye, F.J. Kaye, J.L. Cleveland, and M.D. Conkright, CRTC1/MAML2 gain-of-function interactions with MYC create a gene signature predictive of cancers with CREB-MYC involvement, *Proc Natl Acad Sci USA* **111**(32): E3260–E3268 (2014).

Anzick, S.L., W.D. Chen, Y. Park, P. Meltzer, D. Bell, A.K. El-Naggar, and F.J. Kaye, Unfavorable prognosis of CRTC1-MAML2 positive mucoepidermoidtumors with CDKN2A deletions, *Genes Chromosomes Canc* **49**(1): 59–69 (2010).

Argyris, P.P., R.N. Wehrs, J.J. García, and I.G. Koutlas, Fluorescence *in situ* hybridization identifies Mastermind-like 2 (MAML2) rearrangement in odontogenic cysts with mucous prosoplasia: a pilot study, *Histopathology* **66**(6): 791–797 (2015).

Behboudi, A., F. Enlund, M. Winnes, Y. Andrén, A. Nordkvist, I. Leivo, E. Flaberg, L. Szekely, A. Mäkitie, R. Grenman, J. Mark, and G. Stenman, Molecular classification of mucoepidermoid carcinomas-prognostic significance of the MECT1-MAML2 fusion oncogene, *Genes Chromosomes Canc* **45**(5): 470–481 (2006).

Bell, D., and A.K. El-Naggar, Molecular heterogeneity in mucoepidermoid carcinoma: conceptual and practical implications, *Head Neck Pathol* **7**(1): 23–27 (2013).

Bhaijee, F., D.J. Pepper, K.T. Pitman, and D. Bell, New developments in the molecular pathogenesis of head and neck tumors: a review of tumor-specific fusion oncogenes in mucoepidermoid carcinoma, adenoid cystic carcinoma, and NUT midline carcinoma, *Ann DiagnPathol* **15**(1): 69–77 (2011).

Cazorla, A., G. Viennet, E. Uro-Coste, and S. Valmary-Degano, Mucoepidermoid carcinoma: A yet unreported cancer associated with familial adenomatous polyposis, *J Craniomaxillofac Surg* **42**(3): 262–264 (2014).

Chan, E.S., J.H. Tong, and K.F. To, CRTC3-MAML2 fusion transcript in a bronchial mucoepidermoid carcinoma, *Pathology* **45**(7): 698–701 (2013).

Chen, J., J.L. Li, Z. Chen, J.D. Griffin, and L. Wu, Gene expression profiling analysis of CRTC1-MAML2 fusion oncogene-induced transcriptional program in human mucoepidermoid carcinoma cells, *BMC Cancer* **15**: 803 (2015).

Chen, Z., J. Chen, Y. Gu, C. Hu, J.L. Li, S. Lin, H. Shen, C. Cao, R. Gao, J. Li, P.K. Ha, F.J. Kaye, J.D. Griffin, and L. Wu, Aberrantly activated AREG-EGFR signaling is required for the growth and survival of CRTC1-MAML2 fusion-positive mucoepidermoid carcinoma cells, *Oncogene* **33**(29): 3869–3877 (2014).

Clark, M.D., G.S. Kumar, R. Marcum, Q. Luo, Y. Zhang, and I. Radhakrishnan, Molecular Basis for the Mechanism of Constitutive CBP/p300 Coactivator Recruitment by CRTC1-MAML2 and Its Implications in cAMPSignaling, *Biochemistry* **54**(35): 5439–5446 (2015).

Clauditz, T.S., A. Gontarewicz, C.J. Wang, A. Münscher, S. Laban, M.C. Tsourlakis, R. Knecht, G. Sauter, and W. Wilczak, 11q21 rearrangement is a frequent and highly specific genetic alteration in mucoepidermoid carcinoma, *Diagn Mol Pathol* **21**(3): 134–137 (2012).

Conkright, M.D., G. Canettieri, R. Screaton, E. Guzman, L. Miraglia, J.B. Hogenesch, and M. Montminy, TORCs: transducers of regulated CREB activity, *Mol Cell* **12**(2): 413–423 (2003).

Coxon, A., E. Rozenblum, Y.S. Park, N. Joshi, J. Tsurutani, P.A. Dennis, I.R. Kirsch, and F.J. Kaye, Mect1-Maml2 fusion oncogene linked to the aberrant activation of cyclic AMP/CREB regulated genes, *Cancer Res* **65**(16): 7137–7144 (2005).

Enlund, F., A. Behboudi, Y. Andrén, C. Oberg, U. Lendahl, J. Mark, and G. Stenman, Altered Notch signaling resulting from expression of a WAMTP1-MAML2 gene fusion in mucoepidermoid carcinomas and benign Warthin's tumors, *Exp Cell Res* **292**(1): 21–28 (2004).

Fehr, A., A. Meyer, K. Heidorn, K. Röser, T. Löning, and J. Bullerdiek, A link between the expression of the stem cell marker HMGA2 grading, and the fusion CRTC1-MAML2 in mucoepidermoid carcinoma, *Genes Chromosomes Canc* **48**(9): 777–785 (2009).

Fehr, A., K. Röser, K. Heidorn, C. Hallas, T. Löning, and J. Bullerdiek, A new type of MAML2 fusion in mucoepidermoid carcinoma, *Genes Chromosomes Canc* **47**(3): 203–206 (2008).

Fujinaga, M., H. Hirose, T. Saito-Shono, K. Ishikawa, H. Shimada, Y. Hatano, S. Fujiwara, F. Shimizu, H. Nishida, K. Kawamura, T. Daa, and S. Yokoyama, CRTC1-MAML2 gene fusion in G-CSF-secreting mucoepidermoid carcinoma: an indicator of favourable prognosis? *Eur J Dermatol* **26**(4): 402–403 (2016).

Iourgenko, V., W. Zhang, C. Mickanin, I. Daly, C. Jiang, J.M. Hexham, A.P. Orth, L. Miraglia, J. Meltzer, D. Garza, G.W. Chirn, E. McWhinnie, D. Cohen, J. Skelton, R. Terry, Y. Yu, D. Bodian, F.P. Buxton, J. Zhu, C. Song, and M.A. Labow, Identification of a family of cAMP response element-binding protein coactivators by genome-scale functional analysis in mammalian cells, *Proc Natl Acad Sci USA* **100**(21): 12147–12152 (2003).

Kazakov, D.V., T. Vanecek, I.E. Belousova, P. Mukensnabl, D. Kollertova, and M. Michal, Skin-type hidradenoma of the breast parenchyma with t(11;19) translocation: hidradenoma of the breast, *Am J Dermatopathol* **29**(5): 457–461 (2007).

Komiya, T., Y. Park, S. Modi, A.B. Coxon, H. Oh, and F.J. Kaye, Sustained expression of Mect1-Maml2 is essential for tumor cell growth in salivary gland cancers carrying the t(11;19) translocation, *Oncogene* **25**(45): 6128–6132 (2006).

Luo, Q., K. Viste, J.C. Urday-Zaa, G. Senthil, Kumar, W.W. Tsai, A. Talai, K.E. Mayo, M. Montminy, and I. Radhakrishnan, Mechanism of CREB recognition and coactivation by the CREB-regulated transcriptional coactivator CRTC2, *Proc Natl Acad Sci USA* **109**(51): 20865–20870 (2012).

McElhinny, A.S., J.L. Li, and L. Wu, Mastermind-like transcriptional co-activators: emerging roles in regulating cross talk among multiple signaling pathways, *Oncogene* **27**(38): 5138–5147 (2008).

Metzler, M., M.S. Staege, L. Harder, D. Mendelova, J. Zuna, E. Fronkova, C. Meyer, T. Flohr, D. Bednarova, J. Harbott, T. Langer, S. Gesk, J. Trka, R. Siebert, T. Dingermann, R. Marschalek, C. Niemeyer, and W. Rascher, Inv(11)(q21q23) fuses MLL to the Notch co-activator mastermind-like 2 in secondary T-cell acute lymphoblastic leukemia, *Leukemia* **22**(9): 1807–1811 (2008).

Miyabe, S., M. Okabe, H. Nagatsuka, Y. Hasegawa, A. Inagaki, K. Ijichi, N. Nagai, T. Eimoto, M. Yokoi, K. Shimozato, and H. Inagaki, Prognostic significance of p27Kip1, Ki-67, and CRTC1-MAML2 fusion transcript in mucoepidermoid carcinoma: a molecular and clinicopathologic study of 101 cases, *J Oral Maxillofac Surg* **67**(7): 1432–1441 (2009).

Nakayama, T., S. Miyabe, M. Okabe, H. Sakuma, K. Ijichi, Y. Hasegawa, H. Nagatsuka, K. Shimozato, and H. Inagaki, Clinicopathological significance of the CRTC3-MAML2 fusion transcript in mucoepidermoid carcinoma, *Mod Pathol* **22**(12): 1575–1581 (2009).

Nemoto, N., K. Suzukawa, S. Shimizu, A. Shinagawa, N. Takei, T. Taki, Y. Hayashi, H. Kojima, Y. Kawakami, and T. Nagasawa, Identification of a novel fusion gene MLL-MAML2 in secondary acute myelogenous leukemia and myelodysplastic syndrome with inv(11)(q21q23), *Genes Chromosomes Canc* **46**(9): 813–819 (2007).

Okabe, M., S. Miyabe, H. Nagatsuka, A. Terada, N. Hanai, M. Yokoi, K. Shimozato, T. Eimoto, S. Nakamura, N. Nagai, Y. Hasegawa, and H. Inagaki, MECT1-MAML2 fusion transcript defines a favorable subset of mucoepidermoid carcinoma, *Clin Cancer Res* **12**(13): 3902–3907 (2006).

O'Neill, I.D., Gefitinib as targeted therapy for mucoepidermoid carcinoma of the lung: possible significance of CRTC1-MAML2 oncogene, *Lung Cancer* **64**(1): 129–130 (2009).

Prieto-Granada, C.N., H. Inagaki, and J. Mueller, Thymic mucoepidermoid carcinoma: Report of a case with CTRC1/3-MALM2 molecular studies, *Int J SurgPathol* **23**(4): 277–283 (2015).

Röser, K., K.T. Jäkel, J. Bullerdiek, and T. Löning, [Significance of molecular-cytogenetic findings in mucoepidermoid carcinoma as an example of salivary gland tumors], *Pathologe* **26**(5): 359–366 (2005).

Saade, R.E., D. Bell, J. Garcia, D. Roberts, and R. Weber, Role of CRTC1/MAML2 translocation in the prognosis and clinical outcomes of mucoepidermoid carcinoma, *JAMA Otolaryngol Head Neck Surg* **142**(3): 234–240 (2016).

Screaton, R.A., M.D. Conkright, Y. Katoh, J.L. Best, G. Canettieri, S. Jeffries, E. Guzman, S. Niessen, Yates JR 3rd, H. Takemori, M. Okamoto, and

M. Montminy, The CREB coactivator TORC2 functions as a calcium- and cAMP-sensitive coincidence detector, *Cell* **119**(1): 61–74 (2004).

Seethala, R.R., S. Dacic, K. Cieply, L.M. Kelly, and M.N. Nikiforova, A reappraisal of the MECT1/MAML2 translocation in salivary mucoepidermoid carcinomas, *Am J SurgPathol* **34**(8): 1106–1121 (2010).

Seethala, R.R., An update on grading of salivary gland carcinomas, *Head Neck Pathol* **3**(1): 69–77 (2009).

Stenman, G., Fusion oncogenes in salivary gland tumors: molecular and clinical consequences, *Head Neck Pathol* (Suppl 1): S12–S19 (2013).

Tang, G., X. Lu, S.A. Wang, E.K. Roney, L. Zhang, S. Hu, G. Lu, L.J. Medeiros, and A. Patel, Homozygous inv(11)(q21q23) and MLL gene rearrangement in two patients with myeloid neoplasms, *Int J ClinExpPathol* **7**(6): 3196–3201 (2014).

Tirado, Y., M.D. Williams, E.Y. Hanna, F.J. Kaye, J.G. Batsakis, A.K. El-Naggar, CRTC1/MAML2 fusion transcript in high grade mucoepidermoid carcinomas of salivary and thyroid glands and Warthin's tumors: implications for histogenesis and biologic behavior, *Genes Chromosomes Canc* **46**(7): 708–715 (2007).

Tonon, G., S. Modi, L. Wu, A. Kubo, A.B. Coxon, T. Komiya, O'K. Neil, K. Stover, A. El-Naggar, J.D. Griffin, I.R. Kirsch, and F.J. Kaye, t(11;19)(q21;p13) translocation in mucoepidermoid carcinoma creates a novel fusion product that disrupts a Notch signaling pathway, *Nat Genet* **33**(2): 208–213 (2003).

Winnes, M., L. Mölne, M. Suurküla, Y. Andrén, F. Persson, F. Enlund, and G. Stenman, Frequent fusion of the CRTC1 and MAML2 genes in clear cell variants of cutaneous hidradenomas, *Genes Chromosomes Cancer* **46**(6): 559–563 (2007).

Wu, L., J. Liu, P. Gao, M. Nakamura, Y. Cao, H. Shen, and J.D. Griffin, Transforming activity of MECT1-MAML2 fusion oncoprotein is mediated by constitutive CREB activation, *EMBO J* **24**(13): 2391–2402 (2005).

Wu, L., T. Sun, K. Kobayashi, P. Gao, and J.D. Griffin, Identification of a family of mastermind-like transcriptional coactivators for mammalian notch receptors, *Mol Cell Biol* **22**(21): 7688–7700 (2002).

Yokouchi, H., M. Miyazaki, T. Miyamoto, T. Minami, F. Tsuji, K. Murata, and K. Ohishi, [Pulmonary mucoepidermoid carcinoma — A case report], *Gan To Kagaku Ryoho* **42**(12): 1830–1832 (2015).

14

Mixed Lineage Leukemia/AF9 Fusion and Associated Leukemia

*Ganesan Padmavathi, Choudhary Harsha and Ajaikumar B. Kunnumakkara**

INTRODUCTION

Around 2–5% of acute myeloid leukemia (AML) and 25% of pediatric de novo acute monocytic leukemia (AML-M5a) were reported to possess MLL-AF9 abnormality (Wu *et al.*, 2014). One of the fusion partners mixed lineage leukemia (MLL), also known as ALL1, HTRX or HRX, highly homologous to *Drosophila* trithorax (Trx) gene, and is a nuclear protein which plays essential roles in hematopoiesis and known to be involved in more than 80 chromosomal translocations leading to the development of acute leukemia (Popovic and Zeleznik-Le, 2005; Rowley, 1993; Thirman *et al.*, 1993; Balgobind *et al.*, 2009; Marschalek, 2015).

*Author for correspondence: Ajaikumar B. Kunnumakkara, Cancer Biology Laboratory, Department of Biosciences and Bioengineering, Indian Institute of Technology Guwahati, Assam 781039, India. kunnumakkara@iitg.ernet.in

All these translocations are governed by deletions, duplications, inversions and reciprocal translocations and have been shown to hamper the regular histone methyltransferase (HMT) activity of MLL (Slany, 2009; Chowdhury and Brady, 2008). Wild-type MLL was found to be crucial for embryogenesis and proper hematopoietic development and known to positively regulate the expression of homeobox (HOX) genes by binding to their regulatory elements such as promoters and to other transcriptional regulators thus critically controlling the segment specificity and cell fate in the developing embryo (Popovic and Zeleznik-Le, 2005; Rowley, 1998; Yu *et al.*, 1995). However, the chimeric genes were proved to lack several important functional domains of wild-type MLL thus hampering its proper function. Further, fusion-mediated gain of function was confirmed to be a deciding factor for the development of MLL associated leukemia (Popovic and Zeleznik-Le, 2005). Moreover, MLL fusion genes have been shown to activate the transcription of several target genes which was mediated by either of two mechanisms: acting as chromatin modifiers by histone acetylation or recruiting HMTs (Slany, 2009).

MLL contains three AT hooks which can bind to adenosine triphosphate (ATP) and minor groove of DNA in a sequence-independent manner and believed to assist in chromatin structural organization being a HMT (Rowley, 1998; Slany, 2009). In addition to the AT hooks, MLL also contains a zinc finger motif similar to plant homology domain (PHD), a transcriptional repression domain, a transactivation domain and a SET domain (Rowley, 1998). As MLL has both transcription repressor and activator domains, it was found to exert transcriptional repressor activity through the recruitment of repressor complexes such as histone deacetylases (HDAC) and polycomb proteins and to induce transcriptional activation by facilitating the interaction of CREB-binding protein (CBP) and cAMP response element-binding (CREB) protein (Xia *et al.*, 2003; Ernst *et al.*, 2001; Eguchi *et al.*, 2003). During proteolytic cleavage, the MLL protein was divided into N-terminal and C-terminal portions and the interaction of these two portions was proved to impart stability to the MLL protein. But, MLL fusion proteins lacked this interaction domain leaving the N-terminal MLL instable. However, the incoming partner genes were shown to replace the function of C-terminal MLL and impart stability through a common feature (Eguchi *et al.*, 2003).

Notably, treatment of primary leukemia with topoisomerase II inhibitors resulted in several DSBs which mediated the rearrangement of non-homologous chromosomes producing several fusion oncogenes including MLL fusion genes leading to the development of secondary/therapy related leukemia (Rowley, 1998; Eguchi *et al.*, 2003). BCR of translocation was often observed within or just upstream to the PHD of MLL (Rowley, 1998). Some of the partner genes of MLL include AF4, AF6, AF9, AF10, ELL and ENL and their rearrangements denoted as t(4;11)(q21;q23), t(6;11)(q27;q23), t(9;11)(p22;q23), t(10;11)(p12;q23), t(11;19)(q23;p13.1), and t(11;19)(q23;p13.3) are the most common MLL translocations associated with AML (Figure 14.1) (Rowley, 1998; Balgobind *et al.*, 2009; Eguchi *et al.*, 2003; Marschalek, 2015; Barretto *et al.*, 2014). Apart from this, several other fusion partners have been identified and rarely reported in leukemia including various transcription factors, transcriptional activators, elongation factors, Rho GTPases activators, RTKs regulators and chromatin structure modifying factors, etc. namely: ABI1, ABI2, AF15q14, AF17, AF17q25, AF1p, AF1q, AF22, AF3p21, AF5q31,

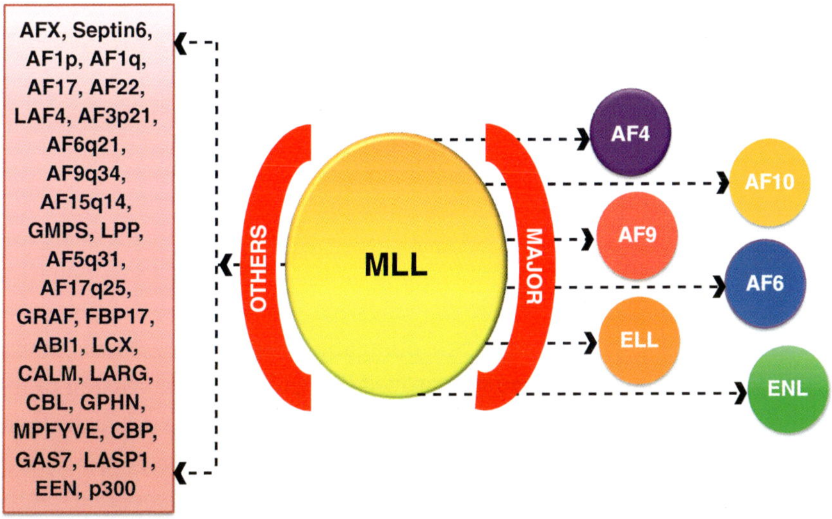

Figure 14.1: Fusion partners of MLL gene.

AF6q21, AF9q34, AFX, CALM, CBL, CBP, EEN, FBP17, GAS7, GMPS, GPHN, GRAF, LAF4, LARG, LASP1, LCX, LPP, MPFYVE, p300, septin 2, 5 and 6, etc. (Figure 14.1) (Eguchi *et al.*, 2003; Coenen *et al.*, 2012; Cerveira *et al.*, 2006; Megonigal *et al.*, 1998). Further, the resulting fusion proteins were determined to contain the N-terminal AT hooks, nuclear localization signals (NLSs) and transcriptional repression domains of MLL and the C-terminal region of the fusion partners and lack C-terminal transactivation and SET domains of MLL (Chowdhury and Brady, 2008). Additionally, MLL fusion genes have been reported to be involved in the development of ALL, AML and myelodysplastic syndrome (MDS), etc. and most often associated with poor treatment outcome (Eguchi *et al.*, 2003; Marschalek, 2015). Further in this chapter, we will discuss in detail about the MLL-AF9 fusion gene.

MLL-AF9 OR MLL-MLLT3

MLL-AF9 chimeric oncoprotein produced by the recurrent t(9;11) (p22;q23) translocation was frequently observed in infant and monoblastic AML, therapy- related leukemia (t-AML), and rarely in ALL, and was associated with poor prognosis (Super *et al.*, 1997; Strissel *et al.*, 2000; Fleischmann *et al.*, 2016; Chowdhury and Brady, 2008; Balgobind *et al.*, 2009). In a patient with AML, this fusion had been detected; however, it was produced by a cryptic insertion of the MLL gene into the 9p22 locus and not by the t(9;11) translocation indicating that the chimeric genes can be produced by various cytogenetically undetectable mechanisms as well (Shago *et al.*, 2004). In addition, the fusion protein was thought to elevate the levels of target genes through transcriptional initiation and elongation properties as the wild-type partner genes MLL and AF9 were known to control transcriptional initiation and elongation respectively (Fleischmann *et al.*, 2016). This fusion gene was proved to regulate the expression of the homeobox genes HOXA7 and -A10 and to escape the leukemic cells from apoptotic cell death (Kawagoe *et al.*, 2001). It also increased the activation of HOXA9 by interacting with the polymerase associated factor complex (PAFc) and by increasing the expression of dachshund family transcription factor 1 (DACH1) which was essential for the induction and maintenance of leukemogenesis (Figure 14.2) (Muntean *et al.*, 2010; Lee *et al.*, 2012). Further, regulation of these homeobox genes was found to be mediated by the interaction of MLL-AF9 with the polycomb group protein chromobox homolog 8 (CBX8) and further the co-existence of polycomb repressive complex 2 (PRC2) was required for the fusion-mediated leukemogenesis (Tan *et al.*, 2011; Neff *et al.*, 2012; Shi *et al.*, 2013; Danis *et al.*, 2015). Besides, the Rac signaling cascade was determined as one of the potential downstream targets of the MLL-AF9 fusion (Muntean *et al.*, 2008; Wei *et al.*, 2008).

Interestingly, the expression of the fusion gene was known to induce cell growth but does not play any significant role in the regulation of differentiation which is mainly mediated by the secondary mutations associated with this fusion gene and moreover the co-expression of wild-type

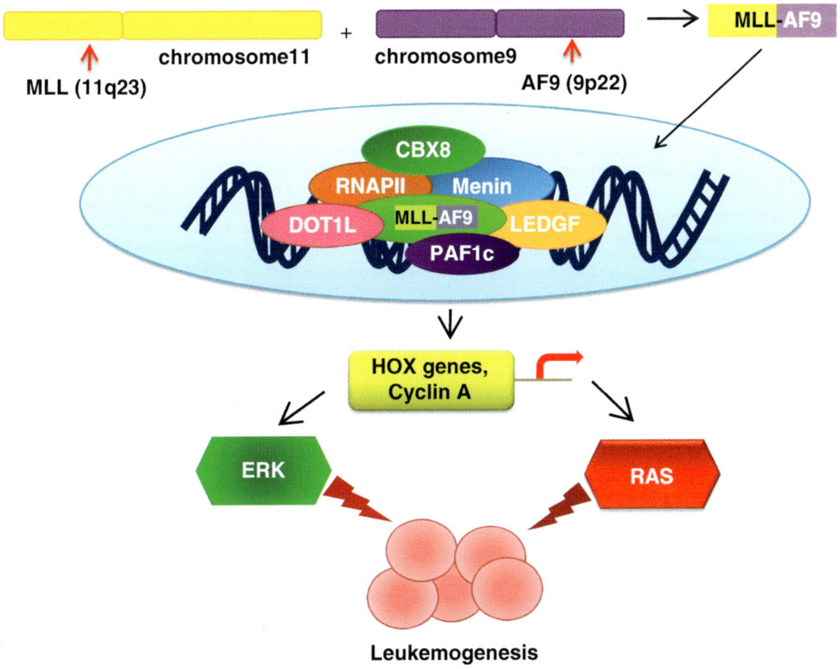

Figure 14.2: Mechanism of MLL-AF9 mediated leukemogenesis.

MLL and DOT1 like histone lysine methyltransferase (DOT1L) genes were also found to be required for the fusion-mediated leukemogenesis (Figure 14.2) (Pession *et al.*, 2003; Thiel *et al.*, 2010; Jo *et al.*, 2011; Nguyen *et al.*, 2011; Kuntimaddi *et al.*, 2015). Further, the leukemogenic effect of MLL-AF9 was found to be mainly dependent on the DNA-binding CXXC domain of MLL gene which protects it from DNA methylation-mediated deactivation (Cierpicki *et al.*, 2010). However, inhibition of tumor suppressing activity of PRDM16 by DNA methylation which otherwise can prevent the fusion-induced leukemic transformation was constantly observed in MLL-AF9 presenting leukemia (Zhou *et al.*, 2016). In addition, it has been confirmed that MLL fusions driven tumorigenesis to be mediated by altered gene expression profile which in turn achieved through aberrant chromatin remodelling by several epigenetic modulators such as HDAC, HMTs, bromodomain-containing proteins, and transcription elongation factors Therefore, inhibitors of such epigenetic modulators were expected to exert potent antitumor effect against MLL-rearranged AML which are resistant to other conventional therapies (Baker *et al.*, 2016). Moreover, it has been confirmed that the malignant transformation induced by the fusion gene was mediated by deregulation of insulin-like growth factor (IGF) signaling (Jenkins *et al.*, 2012). It was also shown to deregulate the microRNAs like miR-511 resulting in blockade of monoblastic differentiation (Fleischmann *et al.*, 2016). In addition, co-occurrence of activating mutations of non-receptor protein-tyrosine phosphatase Shp2 and MLL-AF9 fusion was resulted in increased rate of leukemogenesis through the upregulation of anti-apoptotic proteins B-cell lymphoma 2 (Bcl2), B-cell lymphoma-extra-large (Bcl-xL) and induced Mcl1 (Chen *et al.*, 2015). Contrastingly, co-expression of MLL-AF9 with the ubiquitination related genes in particular brain and reproductive organ-expressed (BRE) gene was highly correlated with better prognosis (Noordermeer *et al.*, 2011). Above all, as reported in several studies, MLL-AF9 drives leukemogenesis through one of its target genes, Meis homeobox 1 (MEIS1) which belongs to a three-amino-acid loop extension (TALE) transcription factor family (Li *et al.*, 2016). Interestingly, another member of the same family was shown to negatively regulate the fusion-mediated leukemogenesis through a competitive manner suggesting

MEIS1: TGIF1 ratio to be an essential factor for deciding the fate of leukemogenesis and associated clinical outcome (Willer *et al.*, 2015). Further, effective inhibition of PI3K/mTOR signaling cascade, which plays a significant role in AML was found to exert anti-leukemic activity against MLL-AF9 positive AML through reduced tumor progression and prolonged survival *in vivo* (Sandhöfer *et al.*, 2015).

Like MLL-AF9, the MLL-AF4 fusion protein produced by t(4;11) was also found to be associated with leukemia. It has been revealed to alter the expression of cyclin-dependent kinase inhibitor CDKN1B (p27kip1) depending on the cell type (Xia *et al.*, 2005; Nakanishi *et al.*, 2007). It also enhanced the expression of protein tyrosine kinase Eph receptor A7 (EphA7) thus increased the phosphorylation activation of extracellular signal-regulated kinases (ERK) giving growth advantage to the leukemic cells (Figure 14.2) (Nakanishi *et al.*, 2007). The other frequently observed MLL fusion genes including, MLL-AF10, MLL-ELL and MLL-ENL were shown to downregulate functions of the important tumor suppressor p53 thereby deregulating its downstream pathways like stress induced p21, mouse double minute 2 (MDM2) homolog, and Bcl-2-associated X protein (Bax) activities which could be a major driving factor for leukemia (Wiederschain *et al.*, 2005). Adding to their leukemogenic potential, MLL fusions were also known to prevent the disassociation of elongation assisting proteins (EAPs) from its target sites which is essential during the differentiation process (Monroe *et al.*, 2011).

CONCLUSION

On the whole, it is obvious that the fusion of other genes with MLL results in the gain of function mutation of MLL gene. Supporting this fact, overexpression of MLL target genes HOXA-MEIS1-PBX3 was frequently detected and regarded as hallmark of MLL-rearranged AML and the upregulation of HOX genes resulted from elevated levels and interaction of PBX3 and MEIS1 is found to be responsible for leukemic transformation. Additionally, it is also apparent that the epigenetic modulators have a significant role in the MLL fusion induced leukemogenesis. Moreover, inhibitors of such epigenetic modulators like dinaciclib have been shown to be effective in preclinical studies. Moreover, agents which can induce oxidative metabolism are also believed to have potent therapeutic effect against MLL rearranged leukemia as the MEIS1 mediates leukemogenesis through hypoxia or hepatic leukemia factor (HLF) expression. However, it is essential to have detailed preclinical and clinical studies to find the safe and effective therapy for this disease.

CONFLICT OF INTEREST

The authors express no conflict of interest.

REFERENCES

Baker, A., G.P. Gregory, I. Verbrugge, L. Kats, J.J. Hilton, E. Vidacs, E.M. Lee, R.B. Lock, J. Zuber, J. Shortt, and R.W. Johnstone, The CDK9 inhibitor Dinaciclib exerts potent apoptotic and antitumor effects in preclinical models of MLL-rearranged Acute Myeloid Leukemia, *Cancer Res* **76**(5): 1158–1169 (2016).

Balgobind, B.V., S.C. Raimondi, J. Harbott, M. Zimmermann, T.A. Alonzo, A. Auvrignon, H.B. Beverloo, M. Chang, U. Creutzig, M.N. Dworzak, E. Forestier, B. Gibson, H. Hasle, C.J. Harrison, N.A. Heerema, G.J. Kaspers, A. Leszl, N. Litvinko, L.L. Nigro, A. Morimoto, C. Perot, R. Pieters, D. Reinhardt, J.E. Rubnitz, F.O. Smith, J. Stary, I. Stasevich, S. Strehl, T. Taga, D. Tomizawa, D. Webb, Z. Zemanova, C.M. Zwaan, and M.M. van den Heuvel-Eibrink, Novel prognostic subgroups in childhood 11q23/MLL-rearranged acute myeloid leukemia: results of an international retrospective study, *Blood* **114**(12): 2489–2496 (2009).

Barretto, N.N., D.S. Karahalios, D. You, and C.S. Hemenway, An AF9/ENL-targeted peptide with therapeutic potential in mixed lineage leukemias, *J Exp Ther Oncol* **10**(4): 293–300 (2014).

Cerveira, N., C. Correia, S. Bizarro, C. Pinto, S. Lisboa, J.M. Mariz, M. Marques, and M.R. Teixeira, SEPT2 is a new fusion partner of MLL in acute myeloid leukemia with t(2;11)(q37;q23), *Oncogene* **25**(45): 6147–6152 (2006).

Chen, L., W. Chen, M. Mysliwski, J. Serio, J. Ropa, F.A. Abulwerdi, R.J. Chan, J.P. Patel, M.S. Tallman, E. Paietta, A. Melnick, R.L. Levine, O. Abdel-Wahab, Z. Nikolovska-Coleska, and A.G. Muntean, Mutated Ptpn11 alters leukemic stem cell frequency and reduces the sensitivity of acute myeloid leukemia cells to Mcl1 inhibition, *Leukemia* **29**(6): 1290–1300 (2015).

Chowdhury, T., and H.J. Brady, Insights from clinical studies into the role of the MLL gene in infant and childhood leukemia, *Blood Cells Mol Dis* **40**(2): 192–199 (2008).

Cierpicki, T., L.E. Risner, J. Grembecka, S.M. Lukasik, R. Popovic, M. Omonkowska, D.D. Shultis, N.J. Zeleznik-Le, and J.H. Bushweller, Structure of the MLL CXXC domain-DNA complex and its functional role in MLL-AF9 leukemia, *Nat Struct Mol Biol* **17**(1): 62–68 (2010).

Coenen, E.A., C.M. Zwaan, C. Meyer, R. Marschalek, U. Creutzig, R. Pieters, J. Bradtke, M.M. van den Heuvel-Eibrink, Abl-interactor 2 (ABI2): a novel MLL translocation partner in acute myeloid leukemia, *Leuk Res* **36**(5): e113–115 (2012).

Danis, E., T. Yamauchi, K. Echanique, J. Haladyna, R. Kalkur, S. Riedel, N. Zhu, H. Xie, K.M. Bernt, S.H. Orkin, S.A. Armstrong, and T. Neff, Inactivation of Eed impedes MLL-AF9-mediated leukemogenesis through Cdkn2a-dependent and Cdkn2a-independent mechanisms in a murine model, *Exp Hematol* **43**(11): 930–935.e6 (2015).

Eguchi, M., M. Eguchi-Ishimae, and M. Greaves, The role of the MLL gene in infantleukemia, *Int J Hematol* **78**(5): 390–401 (2003).

Ernst, P., J. Wang, M. Huang, R.H. Goodman, and S.J. Korsmeyer, MLL and CREB bind cooperatively to the nuclear coactivator CREB-binding protein, *Mol Cell Biol* **21**(7): 2249–2258 (2001).

Fleischmann, K.K., P. Pagel, J. von, Frowein, T. Magg, A.A. Roscher, and I. Schmid, The leukemogenic fusion gene MLL-AF9 alters microRNA expression pattern and inhibits monoblastic differentiation via miR-511 repression, *J Exp Clin Canc Res* **35**(1): 9 (2016).

Jenkins, C.R., O.O. Shevchuk, V. Giambra, S.H. Lam, J.M. Carboni, M.M. Gottardis, M. Holzenberger, M. Pollak, R.K. Humphries, and A.P. Weng, IGF signaling contributes to malignant transformation of hematopoietic progenitors by the MLL-AF9 oncoprotein, *Exp Hematol* **40**(9): 715–723.e6 (2012).

Jo, S.Y., E.M. Granowicz, I. Maillard, D. Thomas, and J.L. Hess, Requirement for Dot1l in murine postnatal hematopoiesis and leukemogenesis by MLL translocation, *Blood* **117**(18): 4759–4768 (2011).

Kawagoe, H., R. Kawagoe, and K. Sano, Targeted down-regulation of MLL-AF9 with antisense oligodeoxyribonucleotide reduces the expression of the HOXA7 and -A10 genes and induces apoptosis in a human leukemia cell line, THP-1, *Leukemia* **15**(11): 1743–1749 (2001).

Kuntimaddi, A., N.J. Achille, J. Thorpe, A.A. Lokken, R. Singh, C.S. Hemenway, M. Adli, N.J. Zeleznik-Le, and J.H. Bushweller, Degree of recruitment of DOT1L to MLL-AF9 defines level of H3K79 Di- and tri-methylation on target genes and transformation potential, *Cell Rep* **11**(5): 808–820 (2015).

Lee, J.W., H.S. Kim, J. Hwang, Y.H. Kim, G.Y. Lim, W.J. Sohn, S.R. Yoon, J.Y. Kim, T.S. Park, S.H. Oh, K.M. Park, S.U. Choi, Z.Y. Ryoo, and S. Lee, Regulation of HOXA9 activity by predominant expression of DACH1 against C/EBPα and GATA-1 in myeloid leukemia with MLL-AF9, *Biochem Biophys Res Commun* **426**(3): 299–305 (2012).

Li, Z., P. Chen, R. Su, C. Hu, Y. Li, A.G. Elkahloun, Z. Zuo, S. Gurbuxani, S. Arnovitz, H. Weng, Y. Wang, S. Li, H. Huang, M.B. Neilly, G.G. Wang, X. Jiang, P.P. Liu, J. Jin, and J. Chen, PBX3 and MEIS1 cooperate in hematopoietic cells to drive Acute Myeloid Leukemias characterized by a core transcriptome of the MLL-rearranged disease, *Canc Res* **76**(3): 619–629 (2016).

Marschalek, R., MLL leukemia and future treatment strategies, *Arch Pharm* (Weinheim) **348**(4): 221–228 (2015).

Megonigal, M.D., E.F. Rappaport, D.H. Jones, T.M. Williams, B.D. Lovett, K.M. Kelly, P.H. Lerou, T. Moulton, M.L. Budarf, and C.A. Felix, t(11;22)(q23;q11.2) in acute myeloid leukemia of infant twins fuses MLL with hCDCrel, a cell division cycle gene in the genomic region of deletion in DiGeorge and velocardiofacial syndromes, *Proc Natl Acad Sci USA* **95**(11): 6413–6418 (1998).

Monroe, S.C., S.Y. Jo, D.S. Sanders, V. Basrur, K.S. Elenitoba-Johnson, R.K. Slany, and J.L. Hess, MLL-AF9 and MLL-ENL alter the dynamic association of transcriptional regulators with genes critical for leukemia, *Exp Hematol* **39**(1): 77–86.e1-5 (2011).

Muntean, A.G. and J.L. Hess, MLL-AF9 leukemia stem cells: hardwired or taking cues from the microenvironment? *Cancer Cell* **13**(6): 465–467 (2008).

Muntean, A.G., J. Tan, K. Sitwala, Y. Huang, J. Bronstein, J.A. Connelly, V. Basrur, K.S. Elenitoba-Johnson, and J.L. Hess, The PAF complex synergizes with MLL fusion proteins at HOX loci to promote leukemogenesis, *Cancer Cell* **17**(6): 609–621 (2010).

Nakanishi, H., T. Nakamura, E. Canaani, and C.M. Croce, ALL1 fusion proteins induce deregulation of EphA7 and ERK phosphorylation in human acute leukemias, *Proc Natl Acad Sci USA* **104**(36): 14442–14447 (2007).

Neff, T., A.U. Sinha, M.J. Kluk, N. Zhu, M.H. Khattab, L. Stein, H. Xie, S.H. Orkin, and S.A. Armstrong, Polycomb repressive complex 2 is required for MLL-AF9 leukemia, *Proc Natl Acad Sci USA* **109**(13): 5028–5033 (2012).

Nguyen, A.T., O. Taranova, J. He, and Y. Zhang, DOT1L, the H3K79 methyltransferase, is required for MLL-AF9-mediated leukemogenesis, *Blood* **117**(25): 6912–6922 (2011).

Noordermeer, S.M., M.A. Sanders, C. Gilissen, E. Tönnissen, A. van der Heijden, K. Döhner, L. Bullinger, J.H. Jansen, P.J. Valk, and B.A. van der Reijden, High BRE expression predicts favorable outcome in adult acute myeloid leukemia, in particular among MLL-AF9-positive patients, *Blood* **118**(20): 5613–5621 (2011).

Pession, A., V. Martino, R. Tonelli, C. Beltramini, F. Locatelli, G. Biserni, M. Franzoni, F. Freccero, L. Montemurro, L. Pattacini, and G. Paolucci, MLL-AF9 oncogene expression affects cell growth but not terminal differentiation and is downregulated during monocyte-macrophage maturation in AML-M5 THP-1 cells, *Oncogene* **22**(54): 8671–8676 (2003).

Popovic, R., and N.J. Zeleznik-Le, MLL: how complex does it get? *J Cell Biochem* **95**(2): 234–242 (2005).

Rowley, J.D., Rearrangements involving chromosome band 11Q23 in acute leukaemia, *Semin Cancer Biol* **4**(6): 377–385 (1993).

Rowley, J.D., The critical role of chromosome translocations in human leukemias, *Annu Rev Genet* **32**: 495–519 (1998).

Sandhöfer, N., K.H. Metzeler, M. Rothenberg, T. Herold, S. Tiedt, V. Groiß, M. Carlet, G. Walter, T. Hinrichsen, O. Wachter, M. Grunert, S. Schneider, M. Subklewe, A. Dufour, S. Fröhling, H.G. Klein, W. Hiddemann, I. Jeremias, and K. Spiekermann, Dual PI3K/mTOR inhibition shows antileukemic activity in MLL-rearranged acute myeloid leukemia, *Leukemia* **29**(4): 828–838 (2015).

Shago, M., D. Bouman, S. Kamel-Reid, M. Minden, and K. Chun, Cryptic insertion of MLL gene into 9p22 leads to MLL-MLLT3 (AF9) fusion in a case of acute myelogenous leukemia, *Genes Chromosomes Cancer* **40**(4): 349–354 (2004).

Shi, J., E. Wang, J. Zuber, A. Rappaport, M. Taylor, C. Johns, S.W. Lowe, and C.R. Vakoc, The Polycomb complex PRC2 supports aberrant self-renewal in a mouse model of MLL-AF9;Nras(G12D) acute myeloid leukemia, *Oncogene* **32**(7): 930–938 (2013).

Slany, R.K., The molecular biology of mixed lineage leukemia, *Haematologica* **94**(7): 984–993 (2009).

Strissel, P.L., R. Strick, R.J. Tomek, B.A. Roe, J.D. Rowley, and N.J. Zeleznik-Le, DNA structural properties of AF9 are similar to MLL and could act as recombination hot spots resulting in MLL/AF9 translocations and leukemogenesis, *Hum Mol Genet* **9**(11): 1671–1679 (2000).

Super, H.G., P.L. Strissel, O.M. Sobulo, D. Burian, S.C. Reshmi, B. Roe, N.J. Zeleznik-Le, M.O. Diaz, and J.D. Rowley, Identification of complex genomic breakpoint junctions in the t(9;11) MLL-AF9 fusion gene in acute leukemia, *Genes Chromosomes Canc* **20**(2): 185–195 (1997).

Tan, J., M. Jones, H. Koseki, M. Nakayama, A.G. Muntean, I. Maillard, and J.L. Hess, CBX8 a polycomb group protein, is essential for MLL-AF9-induced leukemogenesis, *Canc Cell* **20**(5): 563–575 (2011).

Thiel, A.T., P. Blessington, T. Zou, D. Feather, X. Wu, J. Yan, H. Zhang, Z. Liu, P. Ernst, G.A. Koretzky, and X. Hua, MLL-AF9-induced leukemogenesis requires coexpression of the wild-type Mll allele, *Canc Cell* **17**(2): 148–159 (2010).

Thirman, M.J., H.J. Gill, R.C. Burnett, D. Mbangkollo, N.R. McCabe, H. Kobayashi, S. Ziemin-van der Poel, Y. Kaneko, R. Morgan, and A.A. Sandberg, *et al.*, Rearrangement of the MLL gene in acute lymphoblastic and acute myeloid leukemias with 11q23 chromosomal translocations, *N Engl J Med* **329**(13): 909–914 (1993).

Wei, J., M. Wunderlich, C. Fox, S. Alvarez, J.C. Cigudosa, J.S. Wilhelm, Y. Zheng, J.A. Cancelas, Y. Gu, M. Jansen, J.F. Dimartino, and J.C. Mulloy, Microenvironment determines lineage fate in a human model of MLL-AF9 leukemia, *Canc Cell* **13**(6): 483–495 (2008).

Wiederschain, D., H. Kawai, A. Shilatifard, and Z.M. Yuan, Multiple mixed lineage leukemia (MLL) fusion proteins suppress p53-mediated response to DNA damage, *J Biol Chem* **280**(26): 24315–24321 (2005).

Willer, A., J.S. Jakobsen, E. Ohlsson, N. Rapin, J. Waage, M. Billing, L. Bullinger, S. Karlsson, and B.T. Porse, TGIF1 is a negative regulator of MLL-rearranged acute myeloid leukemia, *Leukemia* **29**(5): 1018–1031 (2015).

Wu, B., F. Li, and S. Zou, MLL-AF9 rearrangement in myeloid sarcomas involving the breast, *Ann Hematol* **93**(4): 709–710 (2014).

Xia, Z.B., M. Anderson, M.O. Diaz, and N.J. Zeleznik-Le, MLL repression domain interacts with histone deacetylases, the polycomb group proteins HPC2 and BMI-1, and the corepressor C-terminal-binding protein, *Proc Natl Acad Sci USA* **100**(14): 8342–8347 (2003).

Xia, Z.B., R. Popovic, J. Chen, C. Theisler, T. Stuart, D.A. Santillan, F. Erfurth, M.O. Diaz, and N.J. Zeleznik-Le, The MLL fusion gene, MLL-A.F, regulates cyclin-dependent kinase inhibitor CDKN1B (p27kip1) expression, *Proc Natl Acad Sci USA* **102**(39): 14028–14033 (2005).

Yu, B.D., J.L. Hess, S.E. Horning, G.A. Brown, and S.J. Korsmeyer, Altered Hox expression and segmental identity in Mll-mutant mice, *Nature* **378**(6556): 505–508 (1995).

Zhou, B., J. Wang, S.Y. Lee, J. Xiong, N. Bhanu, Q. Guo, P. Ma, Y. Sun, R.C. Rao, B.A. Garcia, J.L. Hess, and Y. Dou, PRDM16 suppresses MLL1r leukemia via intrinsic histone methyltransferase activity, *Mol Cell* pii: S1097-2765(16)00188-X (2016).

15

MYB-NFIB Fusion Gene — Hallmark of Adenoid Cystic Carcinoma (ACC)

*Ganesan Padmavathi, Krishan Kumar Thakur and Ajaikumar B. Kunnumakkara**

INTRODUCTION

v-myb avian myelobastosis viral oncogene homolog (c-MYB) is a proto-oncogene identified as an integration site of retroviruses causing oncogenic transformation and leukemogenesis (Mikse *et al.*, 2016). It is regarded as member of a transcription factor family which also possess two closely related family members viz. MYBL1 and MYBL2 also known as AMYB and BMYB, respectively (Ramsay and Gonda, 2008;

*Author for correspondence: Ajaikumar B. Kunnumakkara, Cancer Biology Laboratory, Department of Biosciences and Bioengineering, Indian Institute of Technology Guwahati, Assam 781039, India. kunnumakkara@iitg.ernet.in

Stenman *et al.*, 2010; Oh and Reddy, 1999). These nuclear transcription factor proteins were confirmed to have three important functional domains contributing to their transcriptional regulatory function: (i) a highly homologous N-terminal DNA-binding domain which can specifically recognize and bind to PyAACG/TG nucleotide sequence; (ii) a transcription activation domain responsible for transcriptional activation; and (iii) a C-terminal negative regulatory domain (NRD) responsible for transcriptional repression (Stenman *et al.*, 2010; Ramsay and Gonda, 2008; Oh and Reddy, 1999). Being a transcription factor, MYB gene was known to regulate the expression of various genes responsible for cell differentiation, proliferation, survival, apoptosis and oncogenesis (Ramsay and Gonda, 2008). In addition, it has been found to play essential roles in the regulation of haematopoiesis, renewal of colonic crypts and brain neurogenesis (Ramsay and Gonda, 2008). Moreover, the transcriptional regulatory functions of MYB proteins were firmly monitored and regulated by its C-terminal leucine zipper and EVES-motifs. Consequently, as interaction of C-terminal portion with N-terminal DNA binding domain was proved vital to critically control the transactivation function of MYB, truncation of these terminal domains was believed to stimulate aberrant expression of MYB and transactivation leading to transformation and tumorigenesis (Dash *et al.*, 1996; Stenman *et al.*, 2010). However, despite the homology, the C-terminal regulatory domains of AMYB and c-MYB were shown to negatively regulate the function of transactivation domain in contrast to that of BMYB which positively regulates the transactivation function (Oh and Reddy, 1999).

According to several preclinical studies, elevated levels of the leucine zipper transcription factor MYB were frequently associated with proliferating endothelial, epithelial, and hematopoietic cells, haematological malignancies including leukemia and lymphoma, and solid tumors including breast cancer, colon cancer, and pancreatic cancer (Mikse *et al.*, 2016; Ramsay and Gonda, 2008; Stenman *et al.*, 2010). As already mentioned, this elevated expression of MYB oncogene might be driven by the truncation through several mechanisms including gene fusions. Such MYB activating fusion was first discovered in adenoid cystic carcinomas (ACC) of breast and head and neck by Persson *et al.* (2009) where the exons of MYB gene were connected to another transcription factor nuclear factor I/B-type (NFIB) through a previously identified reciprocal t(6;9) translocation (Persson *et al.*, 2009; Nordkvist *et al.*, 1994; Dillon *et al.*, 2016). Further, they also reported that fusion breakpoint occurred at the target sites of negatively regulating micro-RNAs leaving the chimera unregulated therefore driving the overexpression of highly active MYB-NFIB fusion protein (Persson *et al.*, 2009; Mikse *et al.*, 2016; Stenman *et al.*, 2010; Dillon *et al.*, 2016). The chimeric protein was associated with the overexpression of several MYB target genes involved in cell cycle regulation such as *CCNB1*, *CDC2* and *MAD1L1*; apoptosis such as *API5*, *BCL2*, *BIRC3*, *HSPA8* and *SET*; and growth and angiogenesis such *CD53*, *FGF2*, *KIT*, *MYC*, *VEGFA,* etc. (Figure 15.1) (Stenman *et al.*, 2010; Dillon *et al.*, 2016). The next part of this chapter deals with the association of MYB-NFIB fusion transcript and the role of its downstream targets in the development of different cancers.

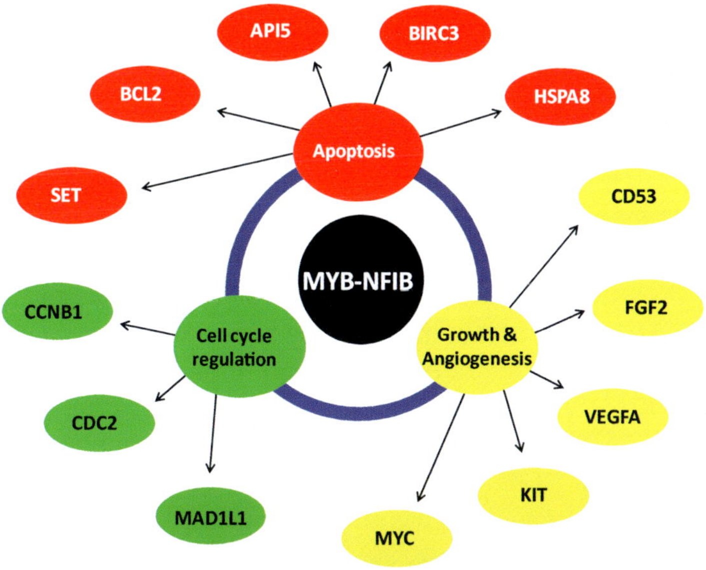

Figure 15.1: Molecular targets of MYB-NFIB fusion gene.

MYB-NFIB

MYB oncogene is fused to NFIB, a transcription factor gene, through t(6;9)(q22–23;p23–24) translocation specifically found in ACC of the breast and head and neck (Persson *et al.*, 2009; von Holstein *et al.*, 2013; Fehr *et al.*, 2011; Stenman, 2013). ACC is defined as a basaloid tumor of myoepithelial and ductal cells organized in a cribriform pattern (Bishop *et al.*, 2015). In addition, prostatic basal cell carcinoma (PBCC), a prostate carcinoma with ACC-like features was also found to possess MYB-NFIB attributing to its ACC-like features (Bishop *et al.*, 2015). Strikingly, ACCs of the breast were found to be triple negative breast cancers (TNBCs); however, they seem to have an indolent disease course unusual to the other aggressive TNBCs (Miyai *et al.*, 2014). In a study for chromosomal aberrations in ACC, around 86% of ACC tumor samples were shown positive to MYB-NFIB juxtaposition and 97% overexpressed MYB mRNA. Thus, MYB-NFIB remains a hallmark of ACC as expression of this fusion protein has been observed in ACCs of any origin (Persson *et al.*, 2009, 2012; Chae *et al.*, 2015; Dillon *et al.*, 2016). In addition, it also plays a remarkable role in the development of dermal cylindroma, a benign adnexal tumor (Fehr *et al.*, 2011; Rajan *et al.*, 2016).

The wild-type MYB gene expression is known to control cell proliferation, angiogenesis, cell adhesion and apoptosis, and negatively regulated by MYB targeting microRNAs (miRNAs) such as miR-15a/16 and miR-150. t(6;9)(q22–23;p23–24) rearrangement resulted in deletion of miRNA binding sites of MYB gene which gives it a gain of function mutation responsible for tumorigenesis (Stenman, 2013; Stenman *et al.*, 2010; Persson *et al.*, 2009). In contrast to this, recent studies showed no correlation between the miR-16 and -150 levels and fusion status of MYB-NFIB. However, overexpression of miR-17-92 cluster was found to be associated with aggressive disease course (Mitani *et al.*, 2013). Moreover, MYB-NFIB fusion enhanced the transcriptional regulatory activity of MYB protein and increased the chromatin structure modifications (Frierson and Moskaluk, 2013; Fehr *et al.*, 2011). However, the prognosis of treatment depends on the expression level of MYB and its downstream effectors regardless of MYB-NFIB status of the tumor (Brill *et al.*, 2011; Mitani *et al.*, 2010, 2011; Rettig *et al.*, 2015). In conclusion, all these findings suggested that MYB-NFIB could be a promising target for the diagnosis and treatment of ACC and adnexal tumors.

CONFLICT OF INTEREST

The authors express no conflict of interest.

REFERENCES

Bishop, J.A., R. Yonescu, J.I. Epstein, and W.H. Westra, A subset of prostatic basal cell carcinomas harbor the MYB rearrangement of adenoid cystic carcinoma, *Hum Pathol* **46**(8): 1204–1208 (2015).

Brill, L.B., W.A. Kanner, A. Fehr, Y. Andrén, C.A. Moskaluk, T. Löning, G. Stenman, and H.F. Frierson Jr, Analysis of MYB expression and MYB-NFIB gene fusions in adenoid cystic carcinoma and other salivary neoplasms, *Mod Pathol* **24**(9): 1169–1176 (2011).

Chae, Y.K., S.Y. Chung, A.A. Davis, B.A. Carneiro, S. Chandra, J. Kaplan, A. Kalyan, and F.J. Giles, Adenoid cystic carcinoma: current therapy and potential therapeutic advances based on genomic profiling, *Oncotarget* **6**(35): 37117–37134 (2015).

Dash, A.B., F.C. Orrico, and S.A. Ness, The EVES motif mediates both intermolecular and intramolecular regulation of c-MYB, *Genes Dev* **10**(15): 1858–1869 (1996).

Dillon, P.M., S. Chakraborty, C.A. Moskaluk, P.J. Joshi, and C.Y. Thomas, Adenoid cystic carcinoma: A review of recent advances, molecular targets, and clinical trials, *Head Neck* **38**(4): 620–627 (2016).

Fehr, A., A. Kovács, T. Löning, H. Frierson, Jr, J. van den Oord, and G. Stenman, The MYB-NFIB gene fusion-a novel genetic link between adenoid cystic carcinoma and dermal cylindroma, *J Pathol* **224**(3): 322–327 (2011).

Frierson, H.F., Jr. and C.A. Moskaluk, Mutation signature of adenoid cystic carcinoma: evidence for transcriptional and epigenetic reprogramming, *J Clin Invest* **123**(7): 2783–2785 (2013).

Mikse, O.R., J.H. Tchaicha, E.A. Akbay, L. Chen, R.T. Bronson, P.S. Hammerman, and K.K. Wong, The impact of the MYB-NFIB fusion protooncogene in vivo, *Oncotarget* **7**(22): 31681–31688 (2016).

Mitani, Y., J. Li, P.H. Rao, Y.J. Zhao, D. Bell, S.M. Lippman, R.S. Weber, C. Caulin, and A.K. El-Naggar, Comprehensive analysis of the MYB-NFIB gene fusion in salivary adenoid cystic carcinoma: Incidence, variability, and clinicopathologic significance, *Clin Cancer Res* **16**(19): 4722–4731 (2010).

Mitani, Y., P.H. Rao, P.A. Futreal, D.B. Roberts, P.J. Stephens, Y.J. Zhao, L. Zhang, M. Mitani, Weber, R.S., S.M. Lippman, C. Caulin, and A.K. El-Naggar, Novel chromosomal rearrangements and break points at the t(6;9) in salivary adenoid cystic carcinoma: association with MYB-NFIB chimeric fusion, MYB expression, and clinical outcome, *Clin Cancer Res* **17**(22): 7003–7014 (2011).

Mitani, Y., D.B. Roberts, H. Fatani, R.S. Weber, M.S. Kies, S.M. Lippman, and A.K. El-Naggar, MicroRNA profiling of salivary adenoid cystic carcinoma: association of miR-17-92 upregulation with poor outcome, *PLoS One* **8**(6): e66778 (2013).

Miyai, K., M.R. Schwartz, M.K., Divatia, R.C. Anton, Y.W. Park, A.G. Ayala, and J.Y. Ro, Adenoid cystic carcinoma of breast: Recent advances, *World J Clin Cases* **2**(12): 732–741 (2014).

Nordkvist, A., J. Mark, H. Gustafsson, G. Bang, and G. Stenman, Non-random chromosome rearrangements in adenoid cystic carcinoma of the salivary glands, *Genes Chromosomes Cancer* **10**(2): 115–121 (1994).

Oh, I.H. and E.P. Reddy, The MYB gene family in cell growth, differentiation and apoptosis, *Oncogene* **18**(19): 3017–3033 (1999).

Persson, M., Y. Andrén, J. Mark, H.M. Horlings, F. Persson, and G. Stenman, Recurrent fusion of MYB and NFIB transcription factor genes in carcinomas of the breast and head and neck, *Proc Natl Acad Sci* **106**(44): 18740–18744 (2009).

Persson, M., Y. Andrén, C.A. Moskaluk, H.F. Frierson Jr., S.L. Cooke, P.A. Futreal, T. Kling, S., Nelander, A. Nordkvist, F. Persson, and G. Stenman, Clinically significant copy number alterations and complex rearrangements of MYB and NFIB in head and neck adenoid cystic carcinoma, *Genes Chromosomes Cancer* **51**(8): 805–817 (2012).

Rajan, N., M.K. Andersson, N. Sinclair, A. Fehr, K. Hodgson, C.J. Lord, D.V. Kazakov, T. Vanecek, A. Ashworth, and G. Stenman, Overexpression of MYB drives proliferation of CYLD-defective cylindroma cells, *J Pathol* **239**(2): 197–205 (2016).

Ramsay, R.G. and T.J. Gonda, MYB function in normal and cancer cells, *Nat Rev Cancer* **8**(7): 523–534 (2008).

Rettig, E.M., M. Tan, S. Ling, R. Yonescu, J.A. Bishop, C. Fakhry, and P.K. Ha, MYB rearrangement and clinicopathologic characteristics in head and neck adenoid cystic carcinoma, *Laryngoscope* **125**(9): E292–E299 (2015).

Stenman, G., M.K. Andersson, and Y. Andrén, New tricks from an old oncogene: gene fusion and copy number alterations of MYB in human cancer, *Cell Cycle* **9**(15): 2986–2995 (2010).

Stenman, G., Fusion oncogenes in salivary gland tumors: molecular and clinical consequences, *Head Neck Pathol* **7**(Suppl 1): S12–S19 (2013).

von Holstein, S.L., A. Fehr, M. Persson, M.H. Therkildsen, J.U. Prause, S. Heegaard, and G. Stenman, Adenoid cystic carcinoma of the lacrimal gland: MYB gene activation, genomic imbalances, and clinical characteristics, *Ophthalmology* **120**(10): 2130–2138 (2013).

16

Translocations Involving PAX Family Genes and Their Effect in Cancer

*Ganesan Padmavathi, Krishan Kumar Thakur and Ajaikumar B. Kunnumakkara**

INTRODUCTION

Paired box, shortly known as PAX, is a transcription factor protein family containing nine members, namely, PAX 1–9 divided into four groups. All these proteins share some of the common structural features including a highly conserved paired box DNA binding domain, an octapeptide and a homeobox DNA binding domain (Barr, 1997; Dahl *et al.*, 1997). It is based on the presence of these additional octapeptide and homeobox domains that the proteins were divided, i.e. PAX 1 and 9 with octapeptide

*Author for correspondence: Ajaikumar B. Kunnumakkara, Cancer Biology Laboratory, Department of Biosciences and Bioengineering, Indian Institute of Technology Guwahati, Assam 781039, India. kunnumakkara@iitg.ernet.in

and without homeodomain were encompassed in group I; PAX 2, 5 and 8 with octapeptide and incomplete homeodomain were regarded as group II; PAX 3 and 7 with both octapeptide and complete homeodomain were clustered into group III; and finally PAX 4 and 6 with complete homeodomain and without octapeptide comprised the group IV (Barr, 1997; Stuart and Gruss, 1996; Underhill, 2012; Blake and Ziman, 2014; Sharma *et al.*, 2015). Both paired box and homeodomains together contributed to the sequence specific DNA binding activity of these proteins and octapeptide portion was found crucial for protein–protein interaction (Sharma *et al.*, 2015). Besides, PAX proteins were also shown to have a transactivation domain within their C-terminal region which drives the transcriptional activation of target genes (Blake and Ziman, 2014; Sharma *et al.*, 2015).

Above all, these proteins were considered as nuclear transcription factors regulating the expression of genes involved in embryogenesis and organ development by binding to their regulatory elements (Stuart and Gruss, 1996; Epstein *et al.*, 1994; Dahl *et al.*, 1997; Mansouri *et al.*, 1999; Wang *et al.*, 2008). Proving this, several mutational and genomic analyses revealed specific PAX proteins involved in the development of different organs. In that way, it was determined that PAX1 is associated with vertebrae and thymus organogenesis; PAX2 with ear, kidney and central nervous system (CNS) development; PAX3 with cardiac blood vessels, skeletal muscle, melanocytes, Schwann cells, central and enteric nervous system development; PAX4 with pancreas development; PAX5 with CNS, and B-lymphocytes development; PAX6 with CNS, pancreas and eye development; PAX7 with thymus, skeletal muscle, teeth, central and enteric nervous system development; PAX8 with ear, CNS development; and finally PAX9 with teeth development (Blake and Ziman, 2014; Lang *et al.*, 2007). Likewise, PAX8 protein was proved to play an essential role in thyroid cell differentiation, deletion of which can badly impair thyroid development in mice; PAX3 and PAX7 were both known to play an essential role in the nervous system and the skeletal muscle development (Pasca di Magliano *et al.*, 2000; Blake and Ziman, 2014; Mercado and Barr, 2007; Goulding *et al.*, 1991). In addition, PAX5 expression was found to be limited to B-lymphoid cell lines which faded during the terminal differentiation of mature B-cells to plasma cells, unregulated constitutive expression of which could result in the malignant transformation (Barr, 1997).

Interestingly, all the paired box proteins were proved to bind similar DNA sequences; to acquire a structural change upon binding and also believed to regulate critical cellular processes including proliferation, differentiation, apoptosis, and motility (Barr, 1997; Epstein *et al.*, 1994; Wang *et al.*, 2008). Also, they play an essential role in maintaining cell fate specification (Underhill, 2012). Despite their similarity, these proteins exhibited diverse roles depending on their ability to produce transcript variants. Further, it has been confirmed that except PAX 4, 5 and 9, all other PAX proteins produce transcript variants through alternative splicing resulting in structural and functional diversity. Moreover, the known transcript variants have been listed as PAX1 (variants 1 and 2), PAX2 (variants a–e), PAX3 (variants a, b, c, d, e, g and h), PAX6 (variants 1–7), PAX7 (variants 1–3) and PAX8 (variants a, b, d and e) (Blake and Ziman, 2014). These genes were considered as proto-oncogene as their expression was proved to transform normal cells into tumor forming cells in mice and also to be deregulated in numerous cancers (Stuart and Gruss, 1996; Maulbecker and Gruss, 1993; Wang *et al.*, 2008). Moreover, these proteins were also known to suppress apoptosis and terminal differentiation thus increasing the levels of stem cell or progenitor cell populations in specific malignancies (Lang *et al.*, 2007). They were also shown to alter the epigenetic status of certain target genes thus either activating or repressing their expression. Therefore, uncontrolled expression of PAX genes would result in irregular epigenetic changes and chromatin remodeling ultimately leading to cancer (Blake and Ziman, 2014; Sharma *et al.*, 2015). Further proving their tumorigenic potential, one of the PAX genes, PAX5 was shown to downregulate the expression of a crucial tumor suppressor p53 thus adding growth advantage to the cells similar to other loss of function mutations of p53. Therefore, the PAX transcription factors were proved to have several target genes and to exert both transcriptional activation and inhibitory effect on their target genes depending on the molecular complex they are interacting with (Stuart and Gruss, 1996; Sharma *et al.*, 2015). Moreover, these genes were important in maintaining the balance between proliferation and differentiation of progenitor cells and deregulation of PAX proteins resulted in defective transcription networks leading to uncontrolled cell proliferation and survival which was regularly observed in various disease pathologies such as Aniridia, Peter's anomaly, bilateral congenital optic nerve head pits, cancers, congenital anomalies of the kidney and urinary tract (CAKUT), diabetes, hypothyroidism, optic-nerve malformations, polycystic kidney disease, renal anomalies, renal coloboma syndrome, renal hypoplasia, vesicoureteral reflux and Waardenburg syndrome, etc. (Blake and Ziman, 2014; Sharma *et al.*, 2015; Jonas and Freisler, 1997; Hornby *et al.*, 2000; Azuma *et al.*, 2003; Tekin *et al.*, 2001; Wollnik *et al.*, 2003; Sanyanusin *et al.*, 1995; Hwang *et al.*, 2014; Dahl *et al.*, 1997; Lang *et al.*, 2007; Epstein *et al.*, 1994; Wang *et al.*, 2008).

Among several other mechanisms of deregulation, chromosomal translocation of PAX genes was found to be frequently associated with development of various neoplasms. For example, translocations of PAX3 and PAX7 genes were found to be involved in the development of ARMS (Barr, 1997). Similarly, translocations of PAX5 and PAX8 were involved in the initiation and progression of haematological cancers and thyroid carcinomas, respectively (Barr, 1997; Vu-Phan *et al.*, 2013; Bousquet *et al.*, 2007; Nebral *et al.*, 2007). Therefore, further in this chapter, we will review the generation of different PAX chromosomal translocations, their partner genes and role in the development of associated neoplasms.

PAX-FOXO1 OR PAX-FKHR

Rearrangement of PAX family of genes (PAX3 or PAX7) on chromosomes 2 or 1 to the forkhead box O1 (FOXO1) gene on chromosome 13 was frequently observed in alveolar rhabdomyosarcoma (ARMS), a subtype of rhabdomyosarcoma affecting the children, adolescents, and young adults (Skapek *et al.*, 2013; Chang *et al.*, 2009; Ren *et al.*, 2008; Gao *et al.*, 2007; Fredericks *et al.*, 1995). In addition to rhabdomyosarcoma, the PAX3-FOXO1 fusion gene was reported in biphenotypic sinonasal sarcoma (BSNS) as well (Wong *et al.*, 2016). The chromosomal translocations producing these rearrangements were denoted as t(2;13)(q35;q14) and (1:13)(p36;q14) for PAX3-FOXO1 and PAX7-FOXO1, respectively (Chang *et al.*, 2009; Fredericks *et al.*, 1995; Rengaswamy *et al.*, 2016). Further, translocation of PAX3 gene was found to be more frequent than the PAX7 rearrangement with occurrence of 60% and 20%, respectively (Rengaswamy *et al.*, 2016). Juxtaposition of the DNA binding domain of PAX to the transactivation domain of FOXO1 resulted in the oncogenic fusion transcription factor which is resistant to the N-terminal PAX3/PAX7 inhibitory domains thus drives the uncontrolled expression of various PAX target genes involved in cell growth, apoptosis, differentiation and motility, etc. Moreover, it is hypothesized that PAX-FOXO1 induced the tumorigenesis by altering several functions of wild-type PAX genes such as protein function, regulation of gene expression, and subcellular localization (Barr, 2001; Sublett *et al.*, 1995; Fredericks *et al.*, 1995). In addition, PAX3 fusion hampered the normal functioning of FOXO by decreasing the tumor suppressor effect of FOXO proteins and FOXO-dependent TGF-β pathways (Schmitt-Ney and Camussi, 2015). Ectopic expression of this fusion protein in MSCs, progenitor cells for most of the sarcomas, increased the transactivation of MyoD and myogenin leading to myogenesis, yet failed to form tumors *in vivo* as sole mutation. Therefore, it was proposed that the expression of PAX-FOXO1 and secondary additional mutations are required to initiate ARMS tumorigenesis and the MSCs to be the progenitor for the same (Ren *et al.*, 2008). Besides MyoD, it also increased the activation of Met signaling through the ligand-independent overexpression of c-met and led to myogenesis (Relaix *et al.*, 2003). In contrast to the previous studies, the PAX fusion was shown to inhibit myogenesis through reduced myogenin expression and increased NF-κB activity (Charytonowicz *et al.*, 2012; Calhabeu *et al.*, 2013). In addition, it also increased the activity of glycogen synthase kinase 3β (GSK3β) resulting in unregulated myogenic pathway producing an undifferentiated and proliferative phenotype (Dionyssiou *et al.*, 2014). Further, PAX-FOXO1 fusion with accompanying loss of function mutation of Ink4a-ARF was found to be crucial for malignant transformation *in vitro* and tumor initiation *in vivo*. Moreover, cyclin-dependent kinase 4 (Cdk4) was found to phosphorylate PAX fusion protein contributing to its oncogenic potential (Liu *et al.*, 2013). It was also shown to interact with the insulin-like growth factor II which may play a crucial role in the fusion-induced tumorigenesis (Wang *et al.*, 1998). In addition, a recent study identified an upstream regulator of PAX3-FOXO1 fusion gene, polo like kinase 1 (PLK1). PLK1 is a kinase protein that was shown to stabilize the activity of PAX3-FOXO1 fusion through phosphorylation. Remarkably, inhibition of PLK1 kinase resulted in proteasomal degradation of the PAX3-FOXO1 chimera and tumor regression *in vivo* (Thalhammer *et al.*, 2015). Other than this, the chimeric protein was also observed to be associated with upregulation of RASSF4 adaptor protein, a core component of Hippo tumor suppressor pathway, which in turn associated with increased cell proliferation and senescence evasion suggesting deregulation of Hippo pathway to be an underlying mechanism of fusion-mediated tumorigenesis (Cross *et al.*, 2014). Similarly, Ahn *et al.* (2013) identified several other downstream targets of PAX-FOXO fusion protein including cell death-related and development-related genes such as GREM1, DAPK1, MYOD1 and HEY1, etc. (Ahn *et al.*, 2013; Ahn, 2013). Quite interestingly, PAX-FOXO fusion was shown to induce the expression of pro-apoptotic Noxa in a p53-independent manner thus favoring chemotherapy induced apoptosis of fusion positive cells (Marshall *et al.*, 2013). Further, analysis of the effect of PAX fusion genes on the prognosis of ARMS patients for the standard therapy showed that PAX3-FOXO1 fusion positive ARMS is associated with poorer clinical outcome than the PAX7-FOXO1 positive and fusion negative ARMS with the overall 5-year survival rates of 64%, 87% and 89%, respectively, making it essential to know the PAX-FOXO1 status of the patients before the proper treatment allocation (Skapek *et al.*, 2013; Sorensen *et al.*, 2002; Rengaswamy *et al.*, 2016; Kubo *et al.*, 2015). In addition, expressed exclusively in ARMS, PAX-FOXO1 fusion gene also acts as a potent biomarker for the more specific and early diagnosis (Sorensen *et al.*, 2002).

Apart from FOXO1, MAML3 and NCOA1 were the other fusion partners of PAX3 juxtaposed by the t(2;4)(q35;q31.1) and inv(2)(q35p23), respectively; and BSNS and ARMS were the corresponding neoplasms (Huang *et al.*, 2016; Wang *et al.*, 2014).

PAX8-PPARγ

Paired box 8-peroxisome proliferator-activated receptor gamma (PAX8-PPARG) fusion protein (PPFP) is the product of t(2;3)(q13;p25) chromosomal translocation found in approximately 35% of follicular thyroid carcinomas (FTCs) and in a subset of follicular variant of papillary thyroid carcinoma (Vu-Phan *et al.*, 2013; Klemke *et al.*, 2012; Castro *et al.*, 2005; Dwight *et al.*, 2003; Eberhardt *et al.*, 2010). However, a recent report from Japan showed the frequency of this fusion in Japanese FTCs to be very low as 4% which attributed to the intake of iodine rich diet (Mochizuki *et al.*, 2015; Hibi *et al.*, 2004). Even though PAX8-PPARG fusion is prevalent in follicular carcinomas, very few cases reported in adenomas as well (Klemke *et al.*, 2011; Eberhardt *et al.*, 2010). PPFP, product of t(2;3) rearrangement resulting in the fusion of PAX8 DNA binding domains and PPARG A to F domains, was confirmed as an oncoprotein yet the exact mode of tumorigenesis has not been identified thus far. Fusion-mediated increase in cell cycle kinetics and reduction in apoptosis were thought to be responsible for high growth rate. Further, it is believed to act as an inhibitor of wild-type PPARγ and an activator or inhibitor of PAX8 and PPARγ responsive genes involved in signal transduction, cell growth and translation control (Raman and Koenig, 2014; McIver *et al.*, 2004; Kroll *et al.*, 2000; Dwight *et al.*, 2003; Lui *et al.*, 2005; Gregory Powell *et al.*, 2004; Reddi *et al.*, 2007; Placzkowski *et al.*, 2008; Eberhardt *et al.*, 2010). It was evidenced that PPFP activates Wnt-TCF pathway through PPARG DNA binding domain and elevates the invasiveness and anchorage-independent growth of tumor cells (Vu-Phan *et al.*, 2013). PPFP positive carcinomas were found to have elevated levels of phosphorylated AKT-protein kinase B (Dobson *et al.*, 2011). Although, PPFP was known to promote thyroid neoplasia, few reports suggested that additional molecular events are essential for the carcinogenesis (Cheung *et al.*, 2003; Diallo-Krou *et al.*, 2009). Additionally, expression of PPFP along with PAX8 had proved to exhibit opposite effects on the expressions of thyroid-specific genes as it decreased the levels of thyroid-stimulating hormone (thyrotropin) receptor (TSHR) and thyroglobulin (Tg) mRNA levels which may induce the malignant transformation (Espadinha *et al.*, 2007; Au *et al.*, 2006). Further, bioinformatic analysis for PPFP effector genes revealed that it regulates the expression of various genes like micro-RNA target genes, genes on chromosome 3p and genes involved in fatty acid, amino acid, and carbohydrate metabolism, etc. (Giordano *et al.*, 2006). Moreover, downregulation of NORE1A and upregulation of FGD3 were also found to be associated with the expression of PPFP (Foukakis *et al.*, 2006; Lacroix *et al.*, 2005). In contrast to its tumorigenic potential, PPFP was proved to inhibit angiogenesis which was confirmed by the decreased VEGF expression and increased TIMP-3 expression partially explaining the better prognosis associated with this fusion protein (Reddi *et al.*, 2010). Furthermore, in general, PPFP was hypothesized to exhibit both PPARγ-like activity and PPARγ antagonistic activity. Pioglitazone, a PPARγ agonist tested against PPFP expressing thyroid carcinoma mouse model reduced the tumor volume and prevented the metastatic transformation through increased adipogenic response (Dobson *et al.*, 2011). In this particular study, pioglitazone increased the PPARγ- like activity of PPFP thus transforming the thyroid carcinoma cells into adipocyte-like cells proving it to be a potent therapy for PPFP positive thyroid carcinoma suggesting the therapeutic potential of PPARγ agonists against PPFP positive FTCs (Dobson *et al.*, 2011; Placzkowski *et al.*, 2008).

PAX5 FUSIONS

As already mentioned, PAX5 transcription factor is a B-cell lineage-specific activator protein (BSAP) essential for the development and maintenance of B-lymphoid lineage. During B-cell development, PAX5 plays both transcription repressor and activator roles by suppressing the B-lineage inappropriate genes and inducing B-lineage-specific genes expression (Nebral *et al.*, 2009). Deregulation of this PAX5 gene through different chromosomal anomalies was frequently involved in the development of haematological malignancies. Extensive research on the chromosomal rearrangements of PAX5 has identified numerous fusion partners such as AUTS2, BRD1, C20orf112, DACH1, ELN, ESRRB, ETV6-TEL, FOXP1, HIPK1, IGH, JAK2, KIAA1549L, PML, POM121 and ZNF521, etc. (Figure 16.1) (Nebral *et al.*, 2007, 2009; Cazzaniga *et al.*, 2001; Strehl *et al.*, 2003; Bousquet *et al.*, 2007; Mullighan *et al.*, 2007; Denk *et al.*, 2014).

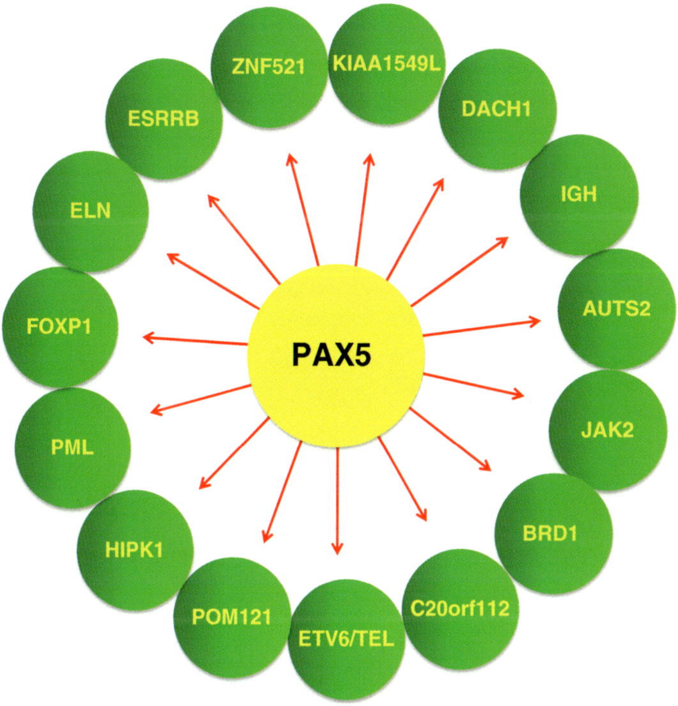

Figure 16.1: Different fusion partners of PAX5 gene.

PAX5-ELN

A novel chromosomal translocation involving chromosomes 7 and 9 was detected in two patients with B-ALL which was denoted as t(7;9)(q11;p13) and resulted in PAX5-ELN fusion transcript. In this translocation, the paired box domain of PAX5 is fused to the elastin (ELN) gene which inactivated the wild-type PAX5 and inhibited the CD19 transcription thus arresting the B-cell differentiation leading to increased population of pre-B-cells (Bousquet *et al.*, 2007; Denk *et al.*, 2014; Nebral *et al.*, 2007).

PAX5-PML

Nebral *et al.* (2007) first identified the translocation of chromosomes 9 and 15 i.e. t(9;15)(p13;q24) in childhood ALL resulting in the fusion of paired box domain, octapeptide and partial homeodomain of PAX5 to nearly the entire PML protein (Nebral *et al.*, 2007). The coiled-coil domain of PAX5 partner was found to be a key regulator of the oncogenic properties of PAX5-PML chimera (Qiu *et al.*, 2011). This fusion protein was shown to negatively regulate the activities of its wild-type partner genes; inhibit the PML SUMOylation and mediate the degradation of PML NBs contributing to apoptosis resistance which can be reverted by treating with arsenic trioxide (ATO). ATO was proved to inhibit the PAX5-PML mediated apoptosis resistance suggesting it to be a potential therapy for PAX5-PML positive ALL (Kurahashi *et al.*, 2011). However, further studies have reported that degradation of PML NBs was not essential for the induction of leukemogenesis. It was also reported that fusion-mediated deregulation of B-cell linker protein (BLNK) blocked the differentiation of pro-B-cells ultimately leading to ALL development (Imoto *et al.*, 2016).

CONCLUSION

In summary, PAX transcription factors were frequently reported to be deregulated by chromosomal rearrangements and involved in the development of both haematological and solid tumors. All the fusion proteins retained the DNA binding and transactivating domains of PAX proteins essential for the transcription factor activity. Further, it was confirmed that all the fusions were to be gain of function mutations resulting in the aberrant activation of PAX and their target genes. However, in addition to transactivation effect, the fusion proteins also exhibited transcriptional repressor activities. Further, the activation of PAX genes was governed by their partner genes. Therefore, targeting these fusion genes would have significant impact on the complications encountered during the treatment of PAX fusion positive cancers.

CONFLICT OF INTEREST

The authors express no conflict of interest.

REFERENCES

Ahn, E.H., Regulation of target genes of PAX3-FOXO1 in alveolar rhabdomyosarcoma, *Anticancer Res* **33**(5): 2029–2035 (2013).

Ahn, EH., G.E. Mercado, M. Laé, and M. Ladanyi, Identification of target genes of PAX3-FOXO1 in alveolar rhabdomyosarcoma, *Oncol Rep* **30**(2): 968–978 (2013).

Au, A.Y., C. McBride, Wilhelm K.G. Jr., R.J. Koenig, B. Speller, L. Cheung, M. Messina, J. Wentworth, V. Tasevski, D. Learoyd, B.G. Robinson, and R.J. Clifton-Bligh, PAX8-peroxisome proliferator-activated receptor gamma (PPARgamma) disrupts normal PAX8 or PPARgamma transcriptional function and stimulates follicular thyroid cell growth, *Endocrinology* **147**(1): 367–376 (2006).

Azuma, N., Y. Yamaguchi, H. Handa, K. Tadokoro, A. Asaka, E. Kawase, and M. Yamada, Mutations of the PAX6 gene detected in patients with a variety of optic-nerve malformations, *Am J Hum Genet* **72**(6): 1565–1570 (2003).

Barr, F.G., Chromosomal translocations involving paired box transcription factors in human cancer, *Int J Biochem Cell Biol* **29**(12): 1449–1461 (1997).

Barr, F.G., Gene fusions involving PAX and FOX family members in alveolar rhabdomyosarcoma, *Oncogene* **20**(40): 5736–5746 (2001).

Blake, J.A. and M.R. Ziman, Pax genes: regulators of lineage specification and progenitor cell maintenance, *Development* **141**(4): 737–751 (2014).

Bousquet, M., C. Broccardo, C. Quelen, F. Meggetto, E. Kuhlein, G. Delsol, N. Dastugue, and P. Brousset, A novel PAX5-ELN fusion protein identified in B-cell acute lymphoblastic leukemia acts as a dominant negative on wild-type PAX5, *Blood* **109**(8): 3417–3423 (2007).

Calhabeu, F., S. Hayashi, J.E. Morgan, F. Relaix, and P.S. Zammit, Alveolar rhabdomyosarcoma-associated proteins PAX3/FOXO1A and PAX7/FOXO1A suppress the transcriptional activity of MyoD-target genes in muscle stem cells, *Oncogene* **32**(5): 651–662 (2013).

Castro, P., L. Roque, J. Magalhães, and M. Sobrinho-Simões, A subset of the follicular variant of papillary thyroid carcinoma harbors the PAX8-PPARgamma translocation, *Int J Surg Pathol* **13**(3): 235–238 (2005).

Cazzaniga, G., M. Daniotti, S. Tosi, G. Giudici, A. Aloisi, E. Pogliani, L. Kearney, and A. Biondi, The paired box domain gene PAX5 is fused to ETV6/TEL in an acute lymphoblastic leukemia case, *Canc Res* **61**(12): 4666–4670 (2001).

Chang, B., L.J. Pang, Y. Qi, C.X. Liu, Y. Cao, H.A. Li, W.H. Hu, J.F. Jiang, W.J. Zhang, and F. Li, PAX — FKHR fusion genes and AChR-gamma in Chinese patients with rhabdomyosarcoma: diagnosis using formalin-fixed archival tissues, *Int J Surg Pathol* **17**(1): 6–15 (2009).

Charytonowicz, E., I. Matushansky, J.D. Doménech, M. Castillo-Martín, M. Ladanyi, C. Cordon-Cardo, and M. Ziman, PAX7-FKHR fusion gene inhibits myogenic differentiation via NF-kappaB upregulation, *Clin Transl Oncol* **14**(3): 197–206 (2012).

Cheung, L., M. Messina, A. Gill, A. Clarkson, D. Learoyd, L. Delbridge, J. Wentworth, J. Philips, R. Clifton-Bligh, and B.G. Robinson, Detection of the PAX8-PPAR gamma fusion oncogene in both follicular thyroid carcinomas and adenomas, *J Clin Endocrinol Metab* **88**(1): 354–357 (2003).

Crose, L.E., K.A. Galindo, J.G. Kephart, C. Chen, J. Fitamant, N. Bardeesy, R.C. Bentley, R.L. Galindo, J.T. Chi, and C.M. Linardic, Alveolar rhabdomyosarcoma-associated PAX3-FOXO1 promotes tumorigenesis via Hippo pathway suppression, *J Clin Invest* **124**(1): 285–286 (2014).

Dahl, E., H. Koseki, and R. Balling, Pax genes and organogenesis, *Bioessays* **19**(9): 755–765 (1997).

Denk, D., J. Bradtke, M. König, and S. Strehl, PAX5 fusion genes in t(7;9) (q11.2;p13) leukemia: a case report and review of the literature, *Mol Cytogenet* **7**(1): 13 (2014).

Diallo-Krou, E., J. Yu, L.A. Colby, K. Inoki, J.E. Wilkinson, D.G. Thomas, T.J. Giordano, and R.J. Koenig, Paired box gene 8-peroxisome proliferator-activated receptor-gamma fusion protein and loss of phosphatase and tensin homolog synergistically cause thyroid hyperplasia in transgenic mice, *Endocrinology* **150**(11): 5181–5190 (2009).

Dionyssiou, M.G., S. Ehyai, E. Avrutin, M.K. Connor, and J.C. McDermott, Glycogen synthase kinase 3β represses MYOGENIN function in alveolar rhabdomyosarcoma, *Cell Death Dis* **5**: e1094 (2014).

Dobson, M.E., E. Diallo-Krou, V. Grachtchouk, J. Yu, L.A. Colby, J.E. Wilkinson, T.J. Giordano, and R.J. Koenig, Pioglitazone induces a proadipogenic antitumor response in mice with PAX8-PPARgamma fusion protein thyroid carcinoma, *Endocrinology* **152**(11): 4455–4465 (2011).

Dwight, T., S.R. Thoppe, T. Foukakis, W.O. Lui, G. Wallin, A. Höög, T. Frisk, C. Larsson, and J. Zedenius, Involvement of the PAX8/peroxisome proliferator-activated receptor gamma rearrangement in follicular thyroid tumors, *J Clin Endocrinol Metab* **88**(9): 4440–4445 (2003).

Eberhardt, N.L., S.K. Grebe, B. McIver, and H.V. Reddi, The role of the PAX8/PPARgamma fusion oncogene in the pathogenesis of follicular thyroid cancer, *Mol Cell Endocrinol* **321**(1): 50–56 (2010).

Epstein, J., J. Cai, T. Glaser, L. Jepeal, and R. Maas, Identification of a Pax paired domain recognition sequence and evidence for DNA-dependent conformational changes, *J Biol Chem* **269**(11): 8355–8361 (1994).

Espadinha, C., B.M. Cavaco, and V. Leite, PAX8PPARgamma stimulates cell viability and modulates expression of thyroid-specific genes in a human thyroid cell line, *Thyroid* **17**(6): 497–509 (2007).

Foukakis, T., A.Y. Au, G. Wallin, J. Geli, L. Forsberg, R. Clifton-Bligh, B.G. Robinson, W.O. Lui, J. Zedenius, and C. Larsson, The Ras effector NORE1A is suppressed in follicular thyroid carcinomas with a PAX8-PPARgamma fusion, *J Clin Endocrinol Metab* **91**(3): 1143–1149 (2006).

Fredericks, W.J., N. Galili, S. Mukhopadhyay, G. Rovera, J. Bennicelli, F.G. Barr, F.J Rauscher 3rd, The PAX3-FKHR fusion protein created by the t(2;13) translocation in alveolar rhabdomyosarcomas is a more potent transcriptional activator than PAX3, *Mol Cell Biol* **15**(3): 1522–1535 (1995).

Gao, H., Y.L. Ou, K.R. Zhang, Z.B. Zhang, and W.L. Wang, Expression of fusion gene PAX3/PAX7-FKHR and chromosomal aberration in rhabdomyosarcoma, *Zhonghua Yi Xue Yi Chuan Xue Za Zhi* **24**(1): 42–47 (2007).

Giordano, T.J., A.Y. Au, R. Kuick, D.G. Thomas, D.R. Rhodes, Wilhelm K.G. Jr, M. Vinco, D.E. Misek, D. Sanders, Z. Zhu, R. Ciampi, S. Hanash, A. Chinnaiyan, R.J. Clifton-Bligh, B.G. Robinson, Y.E. Nikiforov, and R.J. Koenig, Delineation, functional validation, and bioinformatic evaluation of gene expression in thyroid follicular carcinomas with the PAX8-PPARG translocation, *Clin Cancer Res* **12**(7 Pt 1): 1983–1993 (2006).

Goulding, M.D., G. Chalepakis, U. Deutsch, J.R. Erselius, and P. Gruss, Pax-3, a novel murine DNA binding protein expressed during early neurogenesis, *EMBO J* **10**(5): 1135–1147 (1991).

Gregory Powell, J., X. Wang, B.L. Allard, M. Sahin, X.L. Wang, I.D. Hay, H.J. Hiddinga, S.S. Deshpande, T.G. Kroll, S.K. Grebe, N.L. Eberhardt, and B. McIver, The PAX8/PPARgamma fusion oncoprotein transforms immortalized human thyrocytes through a mechanism probably involving wild-type PPARgamma inhibition, *Oncogene* **23**(20): 3634–3641 (2004).

Hibi, Y., T. Nagaya, F. Kambe, T. Imai, H. Funahashi, A. Nakao, and H. Seo, Is thyroid follicular cancer in Japanese caused by a specific t(2; 3)(q13; p25) translocation generating Pax8-PPAR gamma fusion mRNA? *Endocr J* **51**(3): 361–366 (2004).

Hornby, S.J., S. Adolph, C.E. Gilbert, L. Dandona, and A. Foster, Visual acuity in children with coloboma: clinical features and a new phenotypic classification system, *Ophthalmology* **107**(3): 511–520 (2000).

Huang, S.C., R.A. Ghossein, J.A. Bishop, L. Zhang, T.C. Chen, H.Y. Huang, and C.R. Antonescu, Novel PAX3-NCOA1 Fusions in Biphenotypic Sinonasal

Sarcoma With Focal Rhabdomyoblastic Differentiation, *Am J Surg Pathol* **40**(1): 51–59 (2016).

Hwang, D.Y., G.C. Dworschak, S. Kohl, P. Saisawat, A. Vivante, A.C. Hilger, H.M. Reutter, N.A. Soliman, R. Bogdanovic, E.O. Kehinde, V. Tasic, and F. Hildebrandt, Mutations in 12 known dominant disease-causing genes clarify many congenital anomalies of the kidney and urinary tract, *Kidney Int* **85**(6): 1429–1433 (2014).

Imoto, N., F. Hayakawa, S. Kurahashi, T. Morishita, Y. Kojima, T. Yasuda, K. Sugimoto, S. Tsuzuki, T. Naoe, and H. Kiyoi, B Cell Linker Protein (BLNK) Is a Selective Target of Repression by PAX5-PML Protein in the Differentiation Block That Leads to the Development of Acute Lymphoblastic Leukemia, *J Biol Chem* **291**(9): 4723–4731 (2016).

Jonas, J.B., and K.A. Freisler, Bilateral congenital optic nerve head pits in monozygotic siblings, *Am J Ophthalmol* **124**(6): 844–846 (1997).

Klemke, M., N. Drieschner, G. Belge, K. Burchardt, K. Junker, and J. Bullerdiek, Detection of PAX8-PPARG fusion transcripts in archival thyroid carcinoma samples by conventional RT-PCR, *Genes Chromosomes Cancer* **51**(4): 402–408 (2012).

Klemke, M., N. Drieschner, A. Laabs, V. Rippe, G. Belge, J. Bullerdiek, and W. Sendt, On the prevalence of the PAX8-PPARG fusion resulting from the chromosomal translocation t(2;3)(q13;p25) in adenomas of the thyroid, *Cancer Genet* **204**(6): 334–339 (2011).

Kroll, T.G., P. Sarraf, L. Pecciarini, C.J. Chen, E. Mueller, B.M. Spiegelman, and J.A. Fletcher, PAX8-PPARgamma1 fusion oncogene in human thyroid carcinoma [corrected], *Science* **289**(5483): 1357–1360. Erratum in: *Science* **289**(5484): 1474 (2000).

Kubo, T., S. Shimose, J. Fujimori, T. Furuta, and M. Ochi, Prognostic value of PAX3/7-FOXO1 fusion status in alveolar rhabdomyosarcoma: Systematic review and meta-analysis, *Crit Rev Oncol Hematol* **96**(1): 46–53 (2015).

Kurahashi, S., F. Hayakawa, Y. Miyata, T. Yasuda, Y. Minami, S. Tsuzuki, A. Abe, and T. Naoe, PAX5-PML acts as a dual dominant-negative form of both PAX5 and PML, *Oncogene* **30**(15): 1822–1830 (2011).

Lacroix, L., V. Lazar, S. Michiels, H. Ripoche, P. Dessen, M. Talbot, B. Caillou, J.P. Levillain, M. Schlumberger, and J.M. Bidart, Follicular thyroid tumors with the PAX8-PPARgamma1 rearrangement display characteristic genetic alterations, *Am J Pathol* **167**(1): 223–231 (2005).

Lang, D., S.K. Powell, R.S. Plummer, K.P. Young, and B.A. Ruggeri, PAX genes: roles in development, pathophysiology, and cancer, *Biochem Pharmacol* **73**(1): 1–14 (2007).

Liu, L., J. Wu, S.S. Ong, and T. Chen, Cyclin-dependent kinase 4 phosphorylates and positively regulates PAX3-FOXO1 in human alveolar rhabdomyosarcoma cells, *PLoS One* **8**(2): e58193 (2013).

Lui, W.O., T. Foukakis, J. Lidén, S.R. Thoppe, T. Dwight, A. Höög, J. Zedenius, G. Wallin, M. Reimers, and C. Larsson, Expression profiling reveals a distinct transcription signature in follicular thyroid carcinomas with a PAX8-PPAR(gamma) fusion oncogene, *Oncogene* **24**(8): 1467–1476 (2005).

Mansouri, A., G. Goudreau, and P. Gruss, Pax genes and their role in organogenesis, *Cancer Res* **59**(7 Suppl): 1707s–1709s; discussion 1709s–1710s (1999).

Marshall, A.D., F. Picchione, R.I. Geltink, and G.C. Grosveld, PAX3-FOXO1 induces up-regulation of Noxa sensitizing alveolar rhabdomyosarcoma cells to apoptosis, *Neoplasia* **15**(7): 738–748 (2013).

Maulbecker, C.C. and P. Gruss, The oncogenic potential of Pax genes, *EMBO J* **12**(6): 2361–2367 (1993).

McIver, B., S.K. Grebe, and N.L. Eberhardt, The PAX8/PPAR gamma fusion oncogene as a potential therapeutic target in follicular thyroid carcinoma, *Curr Drug Targets Immune Endocr Metabol Disord* **4**(3): 221–234 (2004).

Mercado, G.E., and F.G. Barr, Fusions involving PAX and FOX genes in the molecular pathogenesis of alveolar rhabdomyosarcoma: recent advances, *Curr Mol Med* **7**(1): 47–61 (2007).

Mochizuki, K., T. Kondo, N. Oishi, I. Tahara, T. Inoue, K. Kasai, T. Nakazawa, T. Okamoto, N. Shibata, and R. Katoh, Low frequency of PAX8-PPARγ rearrangement in follicular thyroid carcinomas in Japanese patients, *Pathol Int* **65**(5): 250–253 (2015).

Mullighan, C.G., S. Goorha, I. Radtke, C.B. Miller, E. Coustan-Smith, J.D. Dalton, K. Girtman, S. Mathew, J. Ma, S.B. Pounds, X. Su, C.H. Pui, M.V. Relling, W.E. Evans, S.A. Shurtleff, and J.R. Downing, Genome-wide analysis of genetic alterations in acute lymphoblastic leukaemia, *Nature* **446**(7137): 758–764 (2007).

Nebral, K., D. Denk, A. Attarbaschi, M. König, G. Mann, O.A. Haas, and S. Strehl, Incidence and diversity of PAX5 fusion genes in childhood acute lymphoblastic leukemia, *Leukemia* **23**(1): 134–143 (2009).

Nebral, K., M. König, L. Harder, R. Siebert, O.A. Haas, and S. Strehl, Identification of PML as novel PAX5 fusion partner in childhood acute lymphoblastic leukaemia, *Br J Haematol* **139**(2): 269–274 (2007).

Pasca di Magliano, M., R. Di Lauro, and M. Zannini, Pax8 has a key role in thyroid cell differentiation, *Proc Natl Acad Sci USA*, **97**(24): 13144–13149 (2000).

Placzkowski, K.A., H.V. Reddi, S.K. Grebe, N.L. Eberhardt, and B. McIver, The Role of the PAX8/PPARgamma Fusion Oncogene in Thyroid Cancer, *PPAR Res* 2008: 672829 (2008).

Qiu, J.J., H. Chu, X. Lu, X. Jiang, and S. Dong, The reduced and altered activities of PAX5 are linked to the protein-protein interaction motif (coiled-coil domain) of the PAX5-PML fusion protein in t(9;15)-associated acute lymphocytic leukemia, *Oncogene* **30**(8): 967–977 (2011).

Raman, P., and R.J. Koenig, Pax-8-PPAR-γ fusion protein in thyroid carcinoma, *Nat Rev Endocrinol* **10**(10): 616–623 (2014).

Reddi, H.V., P. Madde, L.A. Marlow, J.A. Copland, B. McIver, S.K. Grebe, and N.L. Eberhardt, Expression of the PAX8/PPARγ Fusion Protein Is Associated with Decreased Neovascularization In Vivo: Impact on Tumorigenesis and Disease Prognosis, *Genes Cancer* **1**(5): 480–492 (2010).

Reddi, H.V., B. McIver, S.K. Grebe, and N.L. Eberhardt, The paired box-8/peroxisome proliferator-activated receptor-gamma oncogene in thyroid tumorigenesis, *Endocrinology* **148**(3): 932–935 (2007).

Relaix, F., M. Polimeni, D. Rocancourt, C. Ponzetto, B.W. Schäfer, and M. Buckingham, The transcriptional activator PAX3-FKHR rescues the defects of Pax3 mutant mice but induces a myogenic gain-of-function phenotype with ligand-independent activation of Met signaling in vivo, *Genes Dev* **17**(23): 2950–2965 (2003).

Ren, Y.X., F.G. Finckenstein, D.A. Abdueva, V. Shahbazian, B. Chung, K.I. Weinberg, T.J. Triche, H. Shimada, and M.J. Anderson, Mouse mesenchymal stem cells expressing PAX-FKHR form alveolar rhabdomyosarcomas by cooperating with secondary mutations, *Cancer Res* **68**(16): 6587–6597 (2008).

Rengaswamy, V., D. Zimmer, R. Süss, and J. Rössler, RGD liposome-protamine-siRNA (LPR) nanoparticles targeting PAX3-FOXO1 for alveolar rhabdomyosarcoma therapy, *J Control Release* **235**: 319–327 (2016).

Sanyanusin, P., L.A. Schimmenti, L.A. McNoe, T.A. Ward, M.E. Pierpont, M.J. Sullivan, W.B. Dobyns, and M.R. Eccles, Mutation of the PAX2 gene in a family with optic nerve colobomas, renal anomalies and vesicoureteral reflux, *Nat Genet* (1995); **9**(4): 358–364 *Erratum in: Nat Genet* **13**(1): 129 (1996).

Schmitt-Ney, M. and G. Camussi, The PAX3-FOXO1 fusion protein present in rhabdomyosarcoma interferes with normal FOXO activity and the TGF-β pathway, *PLoS One* **10**(3): e0121474 (2015).

Sharma, R., O. Sanchez-Ferras, and M. Bouchard, Pax genes in renal development, disease and regeneration, *Semin Cell Dev Biol* **44**: 97–106 (2015).

Skapek, S.X., J. Anderson, F.G. Barr, J.A. Bridge, J.M. Gastier-Foster, D.M. Parham, E.R. Rudzinski, T. Triche, and D.S. Hawkins, PAX-FOXO1 fusion status drives unfavorable outcome for children with rhabdomyosarcoma: a children's oncology group report, *Pediatr Blood Cancer* **60**(9): 1411–1417 (2013).

Sorensen, P.H., J.C. Lynch, S.J. Qualman, R. Tirabosco, J.F. Lim, H.M. Maurer, J.A. Bridge, W.M. Crist, T.J. Triche, and F.G. Barr, PAX3-FKHR and PAX7-FKHR gene fusions are prognostic indicators in alveolar rhabdomyosarcoma: a report from the children's oncology group, *J Clin Oncol* **20**(11): 2672–2679 (2002).

Strehl, S., M. König, M.N. Dworzak, K. Kalwak, and O.A. Haas, PAX5/ETV6 fusion defines cytogenetic entity dic(9;12)(p13;p13), *Leukemia* **17**(6): 1121–1123 (2003).

Stuart, E.T., and P. Gruss, PAX: developmental control genes in cell growth and differentiation, *Cell Growth Differ* **7**(3): 405–412 (1996).

Sublett, J.E., I.S. Jeon, and D.N. Shapiro, The alveolar rhabdomyosarcoma PAX3/FKHR fusion protein is a transcriptional activator, *Oncogene* **11**(3): 545–552 (1995).

Tekin, M., J.N. Bodurtha, W.E. Nance, and A. Pandya, Waardenburg syndrome type 3 (Klein-Waardenburg syndrome) segregating with a heterozygous deletion in the paired box domain of PAX3: a simple variant or a true syndrome? *Clin Genet* **60**(4): 301–304 (2001).

Thalhammer, V., L.A. Lopez-Garcia, D. Herrero-Martin, R. Hecker, D. Laubscher, M.E. Gierisch, M. Wachtel, P. Bode, P. Nanni, B. Blank, E. Koscielniak, and B.W. Schäfer, PLK1 phosphorylates PAX3-FOXO1, the inhibition of which triggers regression of alveolar Rhabdomyosarcoma, *Cancer Res* **75**(1): 98–110 (2015).

Underhill, D.A., PAX proteins and fables of their reconstruction, *Crit Rev Eukaryot Gene Expr* **22**(2): 161–177 (2012).

Vu-Phan, D., V. Grachtchouk, J. Yu, L.A. Colby, M.S. Wicha, and R.J. Koenig, The thyroid cancer PAX8-PPARG fusion protein activates Wnt/TCF-responsive cells that have a transformed phenotype, *Endocr Relat Cancer* **20**(5): 725–739 (2013).

Wang, Q., W.H. Fang, J. Krupinski, S. Kumar, M. Slevin, and P. Kumar, Pax genes in embryogenesis and oncogenesis, *J Cell Mol Med* **12**(6A): 2281–2294 (2008).

Wang, W., P. Kumar, W. Wang, J. Epstein, L. Helman, J.V. Moore, and S. Kumar, Insulin-like growth factor II and PAX3-FKHR cooperate in the oncogenesis of rhabdomyosarcoma, *Cancer Res* **58**(19): 4426–4433 (1998).

Wang, X., K.L. Bledsoe, R.P. Graham, Y.W. Asmann, D.S. Viswanatha, J.E. Lewis, J.T. Lewis, M.M. Chou, M.J. Yaszemski, J. Jen, J.J. Westendorf, and A.M. Oliveira, Recurrent PAX3-MAML3 fusion in biphenotypic sinonasal sarcoma, *Nat Genet* **46**(7): 666–668 (2014).

Wollnik, B., T. Tukel, O. Uyguner, A. Ghanbari, H. Kayserili, M. Emiroglu, and M. Yuksel-Apak, Homozygous and heterozygous inheritance of PAX3 mutations causes different types of Waardenburg syndrome, *Am J Med Genet A* **122A**(1): 42–45 (2003).

Wong, W.J., A. Lauria, J.L. Hornick, S. Xiao, J.A. Fletcher, and A. Marino-Enriquez, Alternate PAX3-FOXO1 oncogenic fusion in biphenotypic sinonasal sarcoma, *Genes Chromosomes Cancer* **55**(1): 25–29 (2016).

17

Retinoic Acid Receptor Alpha (RARα) Fusion Genes in Leukemia

*Ganesan Padmavathi, Javadi Monisha, Anand Anip, Krishan Kumar Thakur and Ajaikumar B. Kunnumakkara**

INTRODUCTION

RA produced by retinol and retinaldehyde dehydrogenase enzyme-mediated conversion of liposoluble vitamin A (retinol), which is a diet derived molecule essential for vision, has been reported to be involved in the regulation of differentiation and patterning of several progenitor cells (Rhinn and Dollé, 2012). Levels and distribution of RA in cells are tightly regulated through well programmed synthesis and degradation signaling cascades. It is well established to activate several transcription factors

*Author for correspondence: Ajaikumar B. Kunnumakkara, Cancer Biology Laboratory, Department of Biosciences and Bioengineering, Indian Institute of Technology Guwahati, Assam 781039, India. kunnumakkara@iitg.ernet.in

(that are otherwise transcriptional repressors) through interaction with nuclear receptor superfamily known as RA receptors (RARs) thereby inducing the expression of several downstream target genes involved in embryonic development, visual function and differentiation (Rhinn and Dollé, 2012). Moreover, external administration of RA to mouse embryonic stem cells was shown to trigger differentiation of ES into radial glial cells-type neural progenitors (Rhinn and Dollé, 2012; Bibel *et al.*, 2004). Aforementioned nuclear receptors, RAR and retinoid X receptors bind to all-trans-RA (ATRA) and 9-cis-RA, respectively, to induce retinoid signaling. However, due to lack of 9-cis-RA in embryos and adult tissues, the RXRs enable DNA binding activity of RAR–RXR heterodimer complex acting mainly as scaffold proteins (Mic *et al.*, 2003; Rhinn and Dollé, 2012). Both RARs and RXRs comprise three proteins each, namely, RARα, RARβ and RARγ and RXRα, RXRβ and RXRγ which are identified to be involved in retinoid signaling.

In the absence of ligand RA, the heterodimer RAR-RXR binds to RA-response elements (RAREs) of DNA and recruits different co-repressor complexes thus suppressing the expression of target genes. However, upon ligand binding, the heterodimer complex releases the co-repressor molecules through conformational changes and recruits co-activator complexes thus mediating chromatin remodeling and transcription pre-initiation complex assembly, finally leading to activation of gene expression (Rhinn and Dollé, 2012). Therefore, it is apparent that proper regulation of retinoid signaling is indispensable for the normal embryogenesis and other cellular processes. Aberrations in these receptor molecules have been found to result in severe developmental abnormalities and chronic diseases such as cancer. Especially, the chromosomal translocations involving the RAR genes have been frequently reported to be associated with APL characterized by accumulation of abnormal, heavily granulated promyelocytes. Notably, the first identified translocation of RARα-RARA involving PML gene, t(15;17) is regarded as the characteristic feature of APL (*De* Braekeleer *et al.*, 2014).

Apart from the most common t(15;17), several other rare translocations were also found in APL in which RARA gene was fused with different gene partners, namely, BCOR, FIP1L, NABP1, NPM, NuMA, PLZF,

PRKAR1A and STAT5B (Licht, 2006; De Braekeleer *et al.*, 2014). In addition to their dimerization effect, these partner genes also have essential inherent characteristics. For instance, NABP1 is a key factor of cellular response to DNA damage; NPM helps in maintaining the genomic stability; NuMA is a key component of the nuclear matrix; PLZF regulates the cell proliferation through the downregulation of *cyclin A2* and *c-myc*; PML helps to organize multiple proteins into large NBs and acts as a tumor suppressor; PRKAR1A involved in a cAMP-PKA signaling pathway; and STAT5B regulates cytokine signaling. Consequently, fusion of RARA with these genes interfered in their normal functioning and increased the tumorigenicity (Licht, 2006; De Braekeleer *et al.*, 2014). t(11;17)(q13;q21) resulted in the fusion of nuclear mitotic apparatus protein NuMA with RARA and interfered in retinoid signaling ultimately leading to the development of APL (Wells *et al.*, 1997). Similarly, STAT5B-RARA chimera delocalized from cytoplasm to nucleus and deregulated JAK-STAT5 signaling in addition to the retinoid signaling (Iwanaga *et al.*, 2009; Arnould *et al.*, 1999; Chen *et al.*, 2012). Interestingly, it has been found that fusion of STAT5B and RARA could be the result of small inversion at q21 of the chromosome 17 or a cryptic deletion, del(17)(q21.2q21.2) or a translocation, t(17;17)(q21.2;q21.2) (Kusakabe *et al.*, 2008; De Braekeleer *et al.*, 2014). t(5;17)(q35;q21) rearrangement resulting in the fusion of NPM gene with RARA was proved to block the myeloid differentiation inducing leukemogenesis (Pollock *et al.*, 2014; Redner *et al.*, 1996). t(X;17)(p11.2;q21) translocation resulted in the fusion of BCL6 corepressor (BCOR)-RARA which negatively regulates the RARA induced transcriptional activation (Yamamoto *et al.*, 2010). And, FIP1L gene is fused to RARA through t(4;17)(q12;q21) translocation (Buijs *et al.*, 2007). This chapter discusses the well characterized PML-RARA and PLZF-RARA fusion genes and their involvement in APL pathogenesis.

PML-RARA

Reciprocal translocation between the long arms q22 and q21 of chromosomes 15 and 17 written as t(15;17)(q22;q21) resulted in the fusion of promyelocytic leukemia (PML) and RAR alpha (RARA) genes (Figure 17.1) (Bennour *et al.*, 2013). The PML-RARA translocation remains a hallmark of APL, as around 98% of APL patients were found to be the carriers of t(15;17) translocation Sadrzadeh *et al.*, 2013; De Braekeleer *et al.*, 2014). The chimeric oncoprotein produced by this translocation comprised almost all of the RARA domains and was established as a major driving factor for APL (Ablain *et al.*, 2014; De Braekeleer *et al.*, 2014). Based on the BCR in PML gene, intron 6 (BCR1), exon 6 (BCR2) or intron 3 (BCR3), three variants of PML-RARA are produced, namely, long (L)-type, variant (V)-type, and short (S)-type, respectively (Figure 17.1) (Ruiz-Argüelles *et al.*, 2004). The shorter form lacks a NLS present in exon 6, therefore, delocalized to cytoplasm and associated with the poor response to ATRA and other chemotherapy ultimately resulting in poor prognosis (Vahdat *et al.*, 1994). Apart from the three M-BCR variants, based on alternative splicing, the long (L)-type PML-RARA exists in three isoforms: E5(+) E6(+), E5(−)E6(+), and E5(−)E6(−) which were found to be associated with time required for complete remission (Tan *et al.*, 2013). E5(−)E6(−) is characterized by the complete loss of NLS and localized to cytoplasm. Similar to (S)-type PML-RARA, the loss of NLS was found to be responsible for inhibiting differentiation and ATRA-dependent transcription which leads to poor sensitivity to ATRA treatment (Tan *et al.*, 2013).

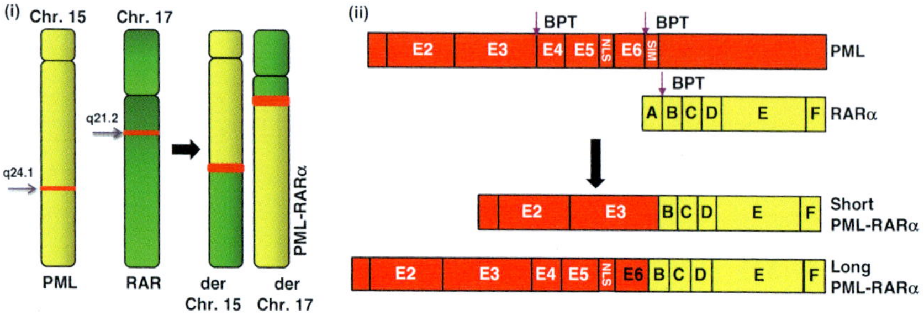

Figure 17.1: (i) Chromosomal translocation of PML-RARα; (ii) Splice variants of PML-RARα (A–F: exons).

Further, the PML-RARA was proved to be a transcriptional repressor of RARA and non-RARA target genes and to hamper PML nuclear body assembly thereby impeding several signaling pathways such as SUMOylation, senescence, etc. (Ablain *et al.*, 2014; Dos Santos *et al.*, 2013; Ivanschitz *et al.*, 2013). It was also known to induce the expression of the Notch ligand Jagged-1 (JAG1) thus stimulating Notch signaling pathway which is believed to be an important event of PML-RARA-mediated leukemogenesis (Figure 17.2) (Grieselhuber *et al.*, 2013). Moreover, PML-RARA and PU.1 bind to the RARA and PU.1 binding sites of DAPK2 promoter, respectively, and deregulate the expression of a proapoptotic protein DAPK2, thus interfering in neutrophil differentiation (Humbert *et al.*, 2014). The partner gene PML was proved to have tumor suppressor effects and found to play a major role in the RA-mediated terminal myeloid differentiation of precursor cells. It also regulated the expression of p21WAF1-CIP1 gene, which can control cell cycle progression and cellular differentiation. Therefore, t(15;17) translocation

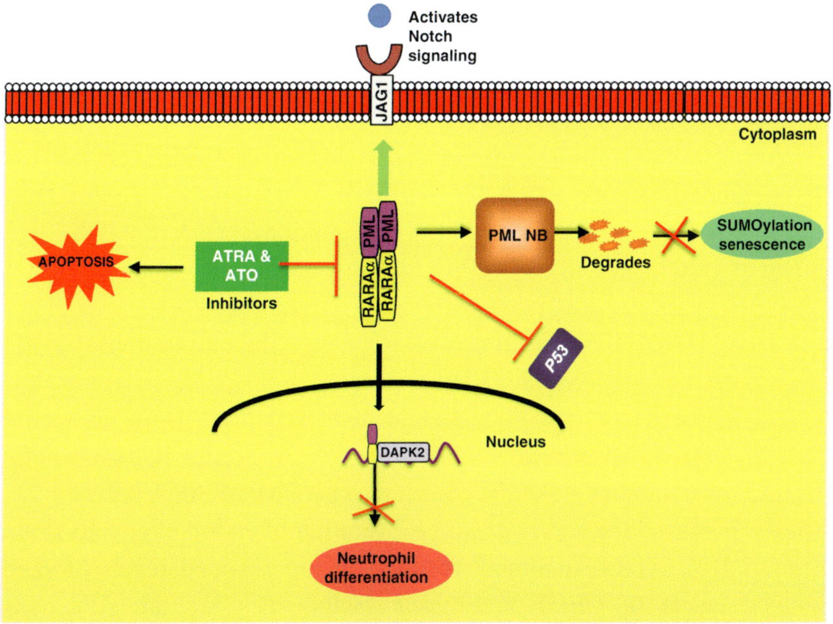

Figure 17.2: Mechanism of PML-RARAα induced APL.

inactivated PML and hampered its tumor suppressing effect and added to the complications of APL (Wang *et al.*, 1998). Initially, the only primary root of PML-RARA induced leukemogenesis was believed to be transcriptional repression of genes involved in myeloid differentiation resulting in increased self-renewal and strong anti-apoptotic effects in APL cells (Gaillard *et al.*, 2015; Vitaliano-Prunier *et al.*, 2014). However, later it has been proved to be associated with inhibition of P53 and activation of various cell cycle related genes as well ultimately resulting in increased proliferation of immature cells (Figure 17.2). It also altered the epigenetic profile of the promyeloid cells upon induction with additional secondary mutations (Gaillard *et al.*, 2015). It was also suggested that PML-RARA-mediated degradation of PML-nuclear bodies (PML-NBs) is a contributing factor for the APL pathogenesis (Figure 17.2). Recently, Liu *et al.* (2014) confounded this hypothesis showing that the DNA binding property of PML-RARA is necessary for leukemic transformation not the integrity of PML-NB (Liu *et al.*, 2014).

ATRA and arsenic trioxide (ATO) are successfully used in the treatment of APL as these compounds disparaged the chimeric oncoprotein by inducing proteasome-mediated degradation and PML moiety targeted degradation, respectively (Figure 17.2) (Ablain *et al.*, 2013). Deprivation of PML-RARA was associated with reformation of NBs which is specific for PML-RARA driven APL and increased myeloid cell differentiation (Ablain *et al.*, 2014; Vitaliano-Prunier *et al.*, 2014). In addition to the proteasome-mediated degradation, ATRA and ATO were shown to induce proteolysis of PML-RARA via the mammalian target of rapamycin pathway-mediated autophagy as well (Isakson *et al.*, 2010; Bøe *et al.*, 2010). It has been proved to change the emission profile and cargo of extracellular vesicles (EVs), heterogeneous membrane structures present in the secretome of leukemic cells and help in the molecular transfer and intercellular communication between hematopoietic, stromal, vascular and leukemic cells, etc. This PML-RARA induced EVs rapidly increased the survival and proliferation of endothelial cells (Fang *et al.*, 2016). ATRA treatment resulted in the elevated levels of IL-8, reduced levels of VEGF and tissue factor (TF) in both APL cells and their EVs which may contribute to ATRA induced cell remission in

APL (Fang *et al.*, 2016). ATRA treatment also resulted in the inhibition of isomerase Pin1 which leads to the degradation of PML-RARA (Wei *et al.*, 2015). The two effective therapeutic agents available for APL, ATRA and ATO, apart from degrading the fusion oncoprotein were also induced terminal differentiation through the removal of retinoid X receptor-α (RXRA) from PML-RARA thereby releasing it from DNA and inducing transcriptional activation which ultimately leads to APL maturation (Vitaliano-Prunier *et al.*, 2014). It has been proved that besides inducing differentiation of APL cells, RA reduced the growth of leukemia-initiating cells (LIC) as well and the (cAMP)-dependent phosphorylation site in PML-RARA is essential for this RA induced degradation and LIC clearance which helps in the long-term remission (Nasr *et al.*, 2008; Nasr and de Thè 2010). Another chromosomal rearrangement isochromosome 17q (iso(17q)) co-existing with PML-RARA translocation in APL was shown to respond well for ATRA/ATO therapy (Shepshelovich *et al.*, 2015). Above all, quantification of PML-RARA transcript after ATRA and ATO therapy was shown to be a better prognostic marker in childhood APL (Zhang *et al.*, 2012).

However, acquired mutations in either portion of PML-RARA were found to be associated with APL relapse and ATO resistance (Lou *et al.*, 2015; Goto *et al.*, 2011). For instance, regulation of PML-RARA by the overexpressed miRNA, miR125B1, inhibited the ATRA-induced proteolysis of PML-RARA and downregulation of SUMO E3-ligase PIAS1 inhibited the ATO induced SUMOylation degradation of PML-RARA thus developing resistance to ATRA/ATO therapy (Zeng *et al.*, 2014; Rabellino *et al.*, 2012). In addition, treatment of proteasome inhibitor, bortezomib stimulated the aberrant expression and intracellular accumulation of PML-RARA in APL cells inducing ER stress-related death and proved to have potential therapeutic effect against APL (Takenokuchi *et al.*, 2015). Remarkably, APL has been regarded as the first cancer successfully treated by differentiation therapy and it has been confirmed that successful inhibition of PML-RARA expression and induction of apoptosis can be achieved by treating APL cells (NB4 cells) with siRNA targeting the fusion oncogene (Chen *et al.*, 1993a; Luo *et al.*, 2014).

PLZF-RARA

Few APL patients (<1%) (Jovanovic *et al.*, 2011) were found to display resistance to RA treatment. Investigation of these retinoid resistance APL patients showed negative to PML-RARA aberration rather they harbor an alternative chromosomal rearrangement t(11;17)(q23;q21) where the retinoic acid receptor alpha (RARA) gene was fused with promyelocytic leukemia ZnF (PLZF) gene (Chen *et al.*, 1993b; Yang *et al.*, 2013; Rohr *et al.*, 2012). PLZF-RARA positive APL was found to be associated with unique clinical features like predominant blasts with regular nuclei, increased number of Pelger-like cells, expression of CD56 and resistance to conventional ATRA treatment (Sainty *et al.*, 2000; Brunel *et al.*, 1995). Unlike the wild-type RARA, the fused oncogenes tend to form homodimers and interfere with the normal retinoid signaling which blocks the cell differentiation and leads to the accumulation of promyelocytic cells (Hauksdóttir *et al.*, 2001). It contains the DNA- and RA-binding domains which are found responsible for the tumorigenic activity of the fusion gene (Grignani *et al.*, 1998). Moreover, it also prevented the ligand-dependent transactivation of wild-type RARs (Chen *et al.*, 1994). Deacetylation of histone protein by histone deacetylase enzymes is a key factor for transcriptional repression of various genes. In case of PML-RARA positive APL, RA treatment hampered this deacetylase activity, increased transcription of various downstream effectors and helped in disease remission. Interestingly, PLZF-RARA positive APL was found insensitive to RA treatment as it failed to inhibit the histone deacetylase activity due to the presence of a RA resistant N-CoR binding site in the N-terminal region of PLZF gene partner (Grignani *et al.*, 1998). However, treatment with combination of trichostatin A (TSA) and RA induced cell differentiation by inhibiting histone deacetylase activity (Grignani *et al.*, 1998; He *et al.*, 1998). Apart from TSA, granulocyte colony-stimulating factor (G-CSF), a hematopoietic growth factor, in combination with RA was also proved to induce terminal differentiation in APL cells (Jansen and Löwenberg, 2001).

PLZF-RARA was proved to act as an epigenetic regulator of around 413 genes including transcription factors that control haematopoiesis (Spicuglia *et al.*, 2011). Few *in vivo* assays evidenced that PLZF-RARA is involved in the up-regulation of tissue factor (TF) (Meng *et al.*, 2000). It was also determined that PLZF-RARA directly interplays with polycomb group (PcG) protein Bmi-1 and recruits the polycomb-repressive complex 1 (PRC1) PcG complex to RA response element. This complex remains active even after the degradation of PLZF-RARA by ATRA, resulting in poor prognosis (Boukarabila *et al.*, 2009). In an attempt to identify the regulators of PLZF-RARA expression, Yang and Shih (2013) found ubiquitin-specific peptidase 37 (USP37), a deubiquitinating enzyme, to be a potential regulator of PLZF-RARA levels as it interacts with the PLZF moiety and maintains the PLZF-RARA stability. Therefore, USP37 could be a key therapeutic target for the treatment of PLZF-RARA-associated APL (Yang and Shih, 2013).

CONCLUSION

Collectively, deregulation of retinoid signaling through translocation of RARA gene was found to be the major driving factor for the development of APL which can be successfully treated with ATRA and ATO. However, certain patients exert resistance to this conventional therapy warranting novel chemotherapeutics to target the RARA fusions and their upstream and downstream effectors; and to synergize the anti-tumor effect of ATRA and ATO. Moreover, the importance of newly identified RARA fusion genes also remains to be explored.

CONFLICT OF INTEREST

The authors express no conflict of interest.

REFERENCES

Ablain, J., M. Leiva, L. Peres, J. Fonsart, E. Anthony, and H. de Thé, Uncoupling RARA transcriptional activation and degradation clarifies the bases for APL response to therapies, *J Exp Med* **210**: 647–653 (2013).

Ablain, J., K. Rice, H. Soilihi, A. de Reynies, S. Minucci, and H. de Thé, Activation of a promyelocytic leukemia-tumor protein 53 axis underlies acute promyelocytic leukemia cure, *Nat Med* **20**: 167–174 (2014).

Arnould, C., C. Philippe, V. Bourdon, M.J. Gr goire, R. Berger, and P. Jonveaux, The signal transducer and activator of transcription STAT5b gene is a new partner of retinoic acid receptor alpha in acute promyelocytic-like leukaemia, *Hum Mol Genet* **8**: 1741–1749 (1999).

Bennour, A., I. Tabka, Y.B. Youssef, M. Zaier, S. Hizem, A. Khelif, A. Saad, and H. Sennana, A PML/RARA chimeric gene on chromosome 12 in a patient with acute promyelocytic leukemia (M4) associated with a new variant translocation: t(12;15;17)(q24;q24;q11), *Med Oncol* **30**: 409 (2013).

Bibel, M., J. Richter, K. Schrenk, K.L. Tucker, V. Staiger, M. Korte, M. Goetz, and Y.A Barde, Differentiation of mouse embryonic stem cells into a defined neuronal lineage, *Nat Neurosci* **7**(9): 1003–1009 (2004).

Bøe, S.O., and A. Simonsen, Autophagic degradation of an oncoprotein, *Autophagy* **6**: 964–965 (2010).

Boukarabila, H., A.J. Saurin, E. Batsché, N. Mossadegh, M. van Lohuizen, A.P. Otte, J. Pradel, C. Muchardt, M. Sieweke, and E. Duprez, The PRC1 Polycomb group complex interacts with PLZF/RARA to mediate leukemic transformation, *Genes Dev* **23**: 1195–1206 (2009).

Brunel, V., D. Sainty, N. Carbuccia, C. Arnoulet, R. Costello, MJ. Mozziconacci, J. Simonetti, L. Coignet, J. Gabert, and A.M. Stoppa, *et al.*, Unbalanced translocation t(5;17) in an typical acute promyelocytic leukemia, *Genes Chromosomes Canc* **14**: 307–312 (1995).

Buijs, A. and M. Bruin, Fusion of FIP1L1 and RARA as a result of a novel t(4;17)(q12;q21) in a case of juvenile myelomonocytic leukemia, *Leukemia* **21**(5): 1104–1108 (2007).

Chen, H., J. Pan, L. Yao, L. Wu, J. Zhu, W. Wang, C. Liu, Q. Han, G. Du, J. Cen, Y. Xue, D. Wu, M. Sun, and S. Chen, Acute promyelocytic leukemia with a STAT5b-RARα fusion transcript defined by array-CGH, FISH, and RT-PCR, *Canc Genet* **205**: 327–331 (2012).

Chen, S.J., A. Zelent, J.H. Tong, H.Q. Yu, Z.Y. Wang, J. Derré, R. Berger, S. Waxman, and Z. Chen, Rearrangements of the retinoic acid receptor alpha and promyelocytic leukemia zinc finger genes resulting from t(11;17)(q23;q21) in a patient with acute promyelocytic leukemia, *J Clin Invest* **91**: 2260–2267 (1993a).

Chen, Z., N.J. Brand, A. Chen, S.J. Chen, J.H. Tong, Z.Y. Wang, S. Waxman, and A. Zelent, Fusion between a novel Krüppel-like zinc finger gene and the retinoic acid receptor-alpha locus due to a variant t(11;17) translocation associated with acute promyelocytic leukaemia, *EMBO J* **12**: 1161–1167 (1993b).

Chen, Z., F. Guidez, P. Rousselot, A. Agadir, S.J. Chen, Z.Y. Wang, L. Degos, A. Zelent, S. Waxman, and C. Chomienne, PLZF-RAR alpha fusion proteins generated from the variant t(11;17)(q23;q21) translocation in acute promyelocytic leukemia inhibit ligand-dependent transactivation of wild-type retinoic acid receptors, *Proc Natl Acad Sci USA* **91**: 1178–1182 (1994).

De Braekeleer, E., N. Douet-Guilbert, and M. De Braekeleer, RARA fusion genes in acute promyelocytic leukemia: a review, *Expert Rev Hematol* **7**: 347–357 (2014).

Dos Santos, G.A., L. Kats, and P.P. Pandolfi, Synergy against PML-RARa: targeting transcription, proteolysis, differentiation, and self-renewal in acute promyelocytic leukemia, *J Exp Med* **210**: 2793–2802 (2013).

Fang, Y., D. Garnier, T.H. Lee, E. D'Asti, L. Montermini, B. Meehan, and J. Rak, PML-RARa modulates the vascular signature of extracellular vesicles released by acute promyelocytic leukemia cells, *Angiogenesis* **19**: 25–38 (2016).

Gaillard, C., T.A. Tokuyasu, G. Rosen, J. Sotzen, A. Vitaliano-Prunier, R. Roy, E. Passegué, H. de Thé, M.E. Figueroa, and S.C. Kogan, Transcription and methylation analyses of preleukemic promyelocytes indicate a dual role for PML/RARA in leukemia initiation, *Haematologica* **100**: 1064–1175 (2015).

Goto, E., A. Tomita, F. Hayakawa, A. Atsumi, H. Kiyoi, T. Naoe, Missense mutations in PML-RARA are critical for the lack of responsiveness to arsenic trioxide treatment, *Blood* **118**: 1600–1609 (2011).

Grieselhuber, N.R., J.M. Klco, A.M. Verdoni, T. Lamprecht, S.M. Sarkaria, L.D. Wartman, and T.J. Ley, Notch signaling in acute promyelocytic leukemia, *Leukemia* **27**: 1548–1557 (2013).

Grignani, F., S. De Matteis, C. Nervi, L. Tomassoni, V. Gelmetti, M. Cioce, M. Fanelli, M. Ruthardt, F.F. Ferrara, I. Zamir, C. Seiser, F. Grignani, M.A. Lazar, S. Minucci, and P.G. Pelicci, Fusion proteins of the retinoic acid receptor-alpha recruit histone deacetylase in promyelocytic leukaemia, *Nature* **391**: 815–818 (1998).

Hauksdóttir, H., and M.L. Privalsky, DNA recognition by the aberrant retinoic acid receptors implicated in human acute promyelocytic leukemia, *Cell Growth Differ* **12**: 85–98 (2001).

He, L.Z., F. Guidez, C. Tribioli, D. Peruzzi, M. Ruthardt, A. Zelent, and P.P. Pandolfi, Distinct interactions of PML-RARalpha and PLZF-RARalpha with co-repressors determine differential responses to RA in APL, *Nat Genet* **18**: 126–135 (1998).

Humbert, M., E.A. Federzoni, A. Britschgi, A.M. Schläfli, P.J. Valk, T. Kaufmann, T. Haferlach, G. Behre, H.U. Simon, B.E. Torbett, M.F. Fey, and M.P. Tschan, The tumor suppressor gene DAPK2 is induced by the myeloid transcription factors PU.1 and C/EBPα during granulocytic differentiation but repressed by PML-RARα in APL, *J Leukoc Biol* **95**: 83–93 (2014).

Isakson, P., M. Bjørås, S.O. Bøe, and A. Simonsen, Autophagy contributes to therapy-induced degradation of the PML/RARA oncoprotein, *Blood* **116**: 2324–2331 (2010).

Ivanschitz, L., H. De Thé, and M. Le Bras, PML, SUMOylation, and Senescence, *Front Oncol* **3**: 171 (2013).

Iwanaga, E., M. Nakamura, T. Nanri, T. Kawakita, K. Horikawa, H. Mitsuya, and N. Asou, Acute promyelocytic leukemia harboring a STAT5B-RARA fusion gene and a G596V missense mutation in the STAT5B SH2 domain of the STAT5B-RARA, *Eur J Haematol* **83**: 499–501 (2009).

Jansen, J.H. and B. Löwenberg, Acute promyelocytic leukemia with a PLZF-RARalpha fusion protein, *Semin Hematol* **38**: 37–41 (2001).

Jovanovic, J.V., K. Rennie, D. Culligan, A. Peniket, A. Lennard, J. Harrison, P. Vyas, and D. Grimwade, Development of real-time quantitative polymerase chain reaction assays to track treatment response in retinoid resistant acute promyelocytic leukemia, *Front Oncol* **1**: 35 (2011).

Kusakabe, M., K. Suzukawa, T. Nanmoku, N. Obara, Y. Okoshi, H.Y. Mukai, Y. Hasegawa, H. Kojima, Y. Kawakami, H. Ninomiya, and T. Nagasawa, Detection of the STAT5B-RARA fusion transcript in acute promyelocytic leukemia with the normal chromosome 17 on G-banding, *Eur J Haematol* **80**: 444–447 (2008).

Licht, J.D., Reconstructing a disease: What essential features of the retinoic acid receptor fusion oncoproteins generate acute promyelocytic leukemia? *Canc Cell* **9**: 73–74 (2006).

Liu, X., H. Yuan, L. Peres, S. Chen, Z. Chen, H. de The, J. Zhou, and J. Zhu, The DNA binding property of PML/RARA but not the integrity of PML nuclear bodies is indispensable for leukemic transformation, *PLoS One* **9**: e104906 (2014).

Lou, Y., Y. Ma, J. Sun, X. Ye, H. Pan, Y. Wang, W. Qian, H. Meng, W. Mai, J. He, H. Tong, and J. Jin, Evaluating frequency of PML-RARA mutations and conferring resistance to arsenic trioxide-based therapy in relapsed acute promyelocytic leukemia patients, *Ann Hematol* **94**: 1829–1837 (2015).

Luo, H., Y. Pan, X. Hao, and X. Cao, [Effect of siRNA targeting PML-RARa fusion gene on activity of the acute promyelocytic leukemia cell line NB4], *Sheng Wu Yi Xue Gong Cheng Xue Za Zhi* **31**: 850–854 (2014).

Meng, X., G. Cheng, and L. Wang, [hCG-PLZF-RARA transgenic mice develop leukemia resembling human chronic myeloid leukemia], *Zhonghua Zhong Liu Za Zhi* **22**: 22–25 (2000).

Mic, F.A., A. Molotkov, D.M. Benbrook, and G. Duester, Retinoid activation of retinoic acid receptor but not retinoid X receptor is sufficient to rescue lethal defect in retinoic acid synthesis, *Proc Natl Acad Sci USA* **100**(12): 7135–7140 (2003).

Nasr, R. and H. de Thé, Eradication of acute promyelocytic leukemia-initiating cells by PML/RARA-targeting, *Int J Hematol* **91**: 742–747 (2010).

Nasr, R., M.C. Guillemin, O. Ferhi, H. Soilihi, L. Peres, C. Berthier, P. Rousselot, M. Robledo-Sarmiento, V. Lallemand-Breitenbach, B. Gourmel, D. Vitoux, P.P. Pandolfi, C. Rochette-Egly, J. Zhu, and H. de Thé, Eradication of acute promyelocytic leukemia-initiating cells through PML-RARA degradation, *Nat Med* **14**: 1333–1342 (2008).

Pollock, S.L., EA. Rush, and R.L. Redner, NPM-RAR, not the RAR-NPM reciprocal t(5;17)(q35;q21) acute promyelocytic leukemia fusion protein, inhibits myeloid differentiation, *Leuk Lymphoma* **55**: 1383–1387 (2014).

Rabellino, A., B. Carter, G. Konstantinidou, S.Y. Wu, A. Rimessi, L.A. Byers, J.V. Heymach, L. Girard, C.M. Chiang, J. Teruya-Feldstein, and P.P. Scaglioni, The SUMO E3-ligase PIAS1 regulates the tumor suppressor PML and its oncogenic counterpart PML-RARA, *Canc Res* **72**: 2275–2284 (2012).

Redner, R.L., E.A. Rush, S. Faas, W.A. Rudert, and S.J. Corey, The t(5;17) variant of acute promyelocytic leukemia expresses a nucleophosmin-retinoic acid receptor fusion, *Blood* **87**: 882–886 (1996).

Rhinn, M. and P. Dollé, Retinoic acid signaling during development, *Development* **139**(5): 843–858 (2012).

Rohr, S.S., L.A. Pelloso, A. Borgo, De L.C. Nadai, M. Yamamoto, E.M. Rego, and M. de Lourdes L F Chauffaille, Acute promyelocytic leukemia associated with the PLZF-RARA fusion gene: two additional cases with clinical and laboratorial peculiar presentations, *Med Oncol* **29**: 2345–2347 (2012).

Ruiz-Argüelles, G.J., J. Garcés-Eisele, V. Reyes-Núñez, J.D. Gómez-Rangel, and G.J. Ruiz-Delgado, More on geographic hematology: the breakpoint cluster regions of the PML/RARalpha fusion gene in Mexican Mestizo patients with promyelocytic leukemia are different from those in Caucasians, *Leuk Lymphoma* **45**: 1365–1368 (2004).

Sadrzadeh, H., D.A. Kerr, P. Dal Cin, N.I. Lindeman, R.P. Hasserjian, K.K. Ballen, and A.T. Fathi, A unique PML-RARα rearrangement involving chromosomes 11, 15, and 17 in a patient with acute promyelocytic leukemia, *Exp Hematol* **41**: 769–771 (2013).

Sainty, D., V. Liso, A. Cantù-Rajnoldi, D. Head, M.J. Mozziconacci, C. Arnoulet, L. Benattar, S. Fenu, M. Mancini, E. Duchayne, F.X. Mahon, N. Gutierrez, F. Birg, A. Biondi, D. Grimwade, M. Lafage-Pochitaloff, A. Hagemeijer, and G. Flandrin, Groupe Français d'Hématologie Cellulaire; Groupe Français de Cytogénétique Hématologique; UK Cancer Cytogenetics Group; BIOMED 1 European Community-Concerted Action "Molecular Cytogenetic Diagnosis in Haematological Malignancies". A new morphologic classification system for acute promyelocytic leukemia distinguishes cases with underlying PLZF/RARA gene rearrangements, *Blood* **96**: 1287–1296 (2000).

Shepshelovich, D., N. Oniashvili, D. Parnes, A. Klein, E. Muchtar, J. Yeshaya, A. Aviram, E. Rabizadeh, and P. Raanani, Acute promyelocytic leukemia with isochromosome 17q and cryptic PML-RARA successfully treated with all-trans retinoic acid and arsenic trioxide, *Canc Genet* **208**: 575–579 (2015).

Spicuglia, S., C. Vincent-Fabert, T. Benoukraf, G. Tibéri, A.J. Saurin, J. Zacarias-Cabeza, D. Grimwade, K. Mills, B. Calmels, F. Bertucci, M. Sieweke, P. Ferrier, and E. Duprez, Characterisation of genome-wide PLZF/RARA target genes, *PLoS One* **6**: e24176 (2011).

Takenokuchi, M., K. Miyamoto, K. Saigo, and T. Taniguchi, Bortezomib Causes ER Stress-related Death of Acute Promyelocytic Leukemia Cells Through Excessive Accumulation of PML-RARA, *Anticancer Res* **35**: 3307–3316 (2015).

Tan, Y., S. Bian, Z. Xu, X. Chen, X. Qi, F. Ren, L. Li, H. Guo, A. Xu, L. Zhang, and H. Wang, The short isoform of the long-type PML-RARA fusion gene in acute promyelocytic leukaemia lacks sensitivity to all-trans-retinoic acid, *Br J Haematol* **162**: 93–97 (2013).

Vahdat, L., P. Maslak, Miller WH Jr, A. Eardley, G. Heller, D.A. Scheinberg, and Warrell R.P. Jr., Early mortality and the retinoic acid syndrome in acute promyelocytic leukemia: impact of leukocytosis, low-dose chemotherapy, PMN/RAR-alpha isoform, and CD13 expression in patients treated with all-trans retinoic acid, *Blood* **84**: 3843–3849 (1994).

Vitaliano-Prunier, A., J. Halftermeyer, J. Ablain, A. de Reynies, L. Peres, M. Le Bras, D. Metzger, and H. de Thé, Clearance of PML/RARA-bound promoters suffice to initiate APL differentiation, *Blood* **124**: 3772–3780 (2014).

Wang, Z.G., L. Delva, M. Gaboli, R. Rivi, M. Giorgio, C. Cordon-Cardo, F. Grosveld, and P.P. Pandolfi, Role of PML in cell growth and the retinoic acid pathway, *Science* **279**(5356): 1547–1551 (1998).

Wei, S., S. Kozono, L. Kats, M. Nechama, W. Li, J. Guarnerio, M. Luo, M.H. You, Y. Yao, A. Kondo, H. Hu, G. Bozkurt, N.J. Moerke, S. Cao, M. Reschke, C.H. Chen, E.M. Rego, F. Lo-Coco, LC. Cantley, T.H. Lee, H. Wu, Y. Zhang, P.P. Pandolfi, X.Z. Zhou, and K.P. Lu, Active Pin1 is a key target of all-trans retinoic acid in acute promyelocytic leukemia and breast cancer, *Nat Med* **21**: 457–466 (2015).

Wells, R.A., C. Catzavelos, and S. Kamel-Reid, Fusion of retinoic acid receptor alpha to NuMA, the nuclear mitotic apparatus protein, by a variant translocation in acute promyelocytic leukaemia, *Nat Genet* **17**: 109–113 (1997).

Yamamoto, Y., S. Tsuzuki, M. Tsuzuki, K. Handa, Y. Inaguma, and N. Emi, BCOR as a novel fusion partner of retinoic acid receptor alpha in a t(X;17)(p11;q12) variant of acute promyelocytic leukemia, *Blood* **116**(20): 4274–4283 (2010).

Yang, W.C. and H.M. Shih, The deubiquitinating enzyme USP37 regulates the oncogenic fusion protein PLZF/RARA stability, *Oncogene* **32**: 5167–5175 (2013).

Zeng, C.W., Z.H. Chen, X.J. Zhang, B.W. Han, K.Y. Lin, X.J. Li, P.P. Wei, H. Zhang, Y. Li, and Y.Q. Chen MIR125B1 represses the degradation of the PML-RARA oncoprotein by an autophagy-lysosomal pathway in acute promyelocytic leukemia, *Autophagy* **10**: 1726–1737 (2014).

Zhang, L., Z. Cao, Y. Zou, M. Ruan, Q. Li, J. Wang, and X. Zhu, Quantification of PML/RARa transcript after induction predicts outcome in children with acute promyelocytic leukemia, *Int J Hematol* **95**: 500–508 (2012).

18

RET-PTC Translocations and Thyroid Malignancies

*Ganesan Padmavathi, Devivasha Bordoloi, Anand Anip, Choudhary Harsha and Ajaikumar B. Kunnumakkara**

INTRODUCTION

Papillary thyroid carcinoma, abbreviated as PTC, is a common form of thyroid cancer with 80% occurrence (Prescott and Zeiger, 2015; Voskoboïnyk, 2009). In general, PTCs exhibited a remarkable prognosis with proper treatments including surgical removal and radiotherapy. However, a considerable number of cases poorly responded to therapy warranting a detailed analysis of the underlying molecular events of such PTCs (Prescott and Zeiger, 2015). Several decades of research further identified RET rearrangements to be one of the major tumor initiating events of PTCs with approximately 20% frequency and to be generated

*Author for correspondence: Ajaikumar B. Kunnumakkara, Cancer Biology Laboratory, Department of Biosciences and Bioengineering, Indian Institute of Technology Guwahati, Assam 781039, India. kunnumakkara@iitg.ernet.in

mainly by radiation (Voskoboĭnyk, 2009; Fusco and Santoro, 2007; Tallini and Asa, 2001). The rearranged forms of RET implicated in papillary thyroid carcinomas were generally denoted as PTC (Grieco *et al.*, 1990).

RET, or rearranged during transfection, is a transmembrane RTK protein often regarded as a proto-oncogene. Upon binding with the glial cell line-derived neurotrophic factor (GDNF) family of ligands, RET receptors were dimerized and autophosphorylated initiating signal transduction (Nikiforov, 2002; Tallini and Asa, 2001). Further, it was known to transduce intracellular signals through a multicompetent receptor complex that consists RET and GDNF family receptors (αGFRs) (Tallini and Asa, 2001). Apart from PTCs, RET gene was also implicated in follicular Hürthle cell carcinomas, Hirschsprung's disease, medullary thyroid carcinomas, multiple endocrine neoplasia type 2 (MEN2A, MEN2B), neuroblastoma and pheochromocytomas (de Vries *et al.*, 2012; Tahira *et al.*, 1990; Santoro *et al.*, 1990; Tallini and Asa, 2001; Romeo *et al.*, 1994; Eng, 1999).

RET-PTC REARRANGEMENTS

Large-scale chromosome folding was found to be responsible for the intrachromosomal rearrangements of RET-PTC by bringing the two partner genes in spatial proximity (Gandhi *et al.*, 2006). Prolonged exposure to IR was proved to generate these rearrangements leading to benign and malignant thyroid tumors (Sadetzki *et al.*, 2004; Romei and Elisei, 2012). Till date, more than 15 types of RET-PTCs have been identified all involving the fusion of tyrosine kinase domain of RET gene to various partner genes and exhibiting constitutive tyrosine kinase activity (Zhang *et al.*, 2015; Nikiforov, 2002; Tallini and Asa, 2001). The heterologous partner genes of rearranged RET were identified as CCDC6 (PTC1), ELKS, Htif1, Htifγ, KTN1, NCOA4 (PTC3/RFG/ELE1), PCM1, PRKAR1A, RFG5, RFG9 and RFP (Figure 18.1) (Tallini and Asa, 2001; Saenko *et al.*, 2003). Among them, RET-PTC1 and RET-PTC3 were the most commonly identified fusion transcripts in cancers (Nikiforov, 2002; Romei and Elisei, 2012; Tallini and Asa, 2001). Moreover, it was also believed that oncogenic features of PTCs may depend on the type of RET-PTC they possess (Nikiforov, 2002).

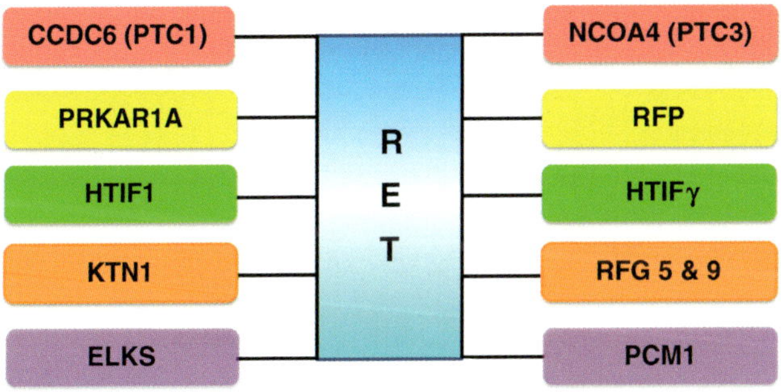

Figure 18.1: Fusion partners of RET gene.

Attributing to their constitutive tyrosine kinase activity, all these chimeras were shown to activate RAS, MAPK and PI3K signaling cascades (Figure 18.2) (Zhang *et al.*, 2015). Further, RET-PTC rearrangements were also known to activate phosphoinositide-dependent kinase 1 (PDK1), an important serine/threonine kinase involved in growth factor-signaling pathways, through PI3K independent phosphorylation which may be the underlying mechanism in RET-PTC-mediated thyroid carcinogenesis (Figure 18.2) (Kim *et al.*, 2003). However, additional genetic alterations are required to induce complete malignant transformation in RET-PTC expressing thyroid cells (Portella *et al.*, 1999). Furthermore, intrinsic tyrosine kinase activity of this protein induced the phosphorylation activation of STAT3 and its downstream targets like VEGF, cyclin D1 and ICAM-1 and enhanced the malignant transformation and proliferation *in vitro* (Figure 18.2) (Hwang *et al.*, 2003). This chapter deals with the role of the most common RET-PTCs (RET-PTC1 and RET-PTC3) in the development of thyroid cancer.

CCDC6-RET (RET-PTC1)

RET-PTC1 fusion had been originally found in about 20% of human PTC and produced by a chromosomal inversion denoted as inv(10)(q11.2q21) (Grieco *et al.*, 1990; Kondo *et al.*, 2006; Pierotti *et al.*, 1992; Sozzi *et al.*, 1994). The somatic RET-PTC1 fusion gene, mostly recognized as *CCDC6-RET* was known to be linked with sporadic and radiation-induced

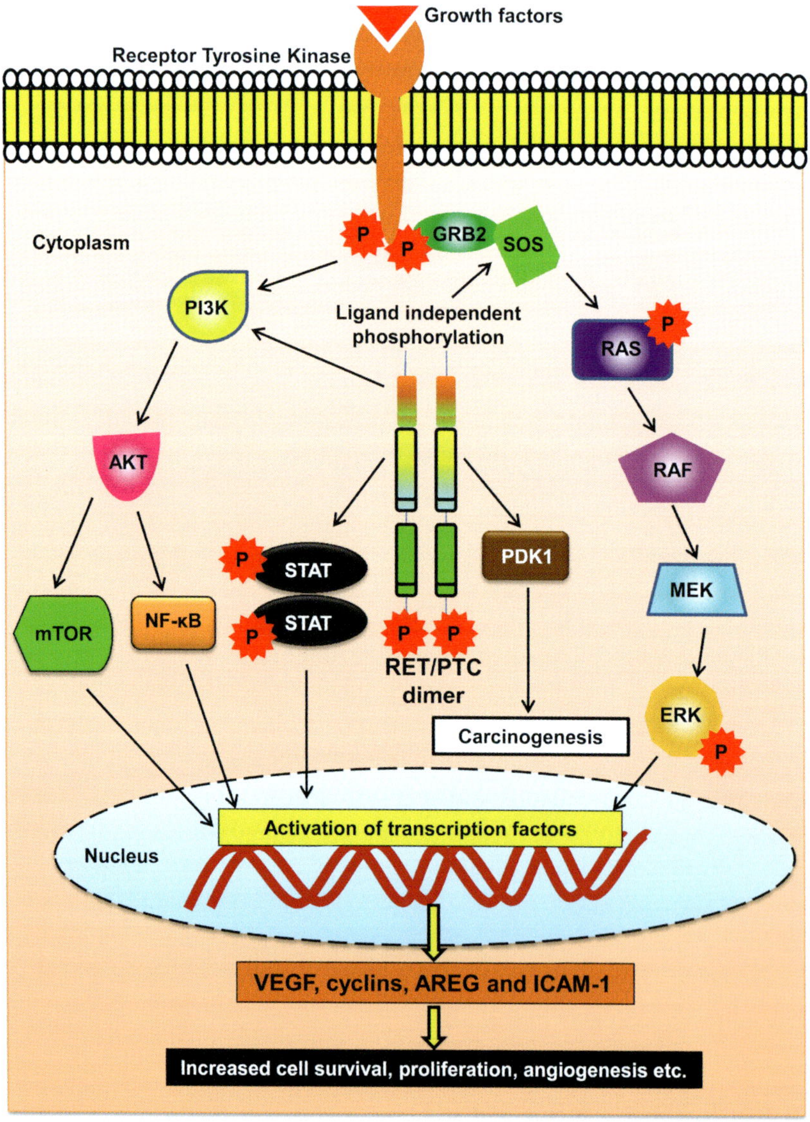

Figure 18.2: Schematic representation of RET-PTC induced tumorigenesis.

papillary thyroid cancers (Grieco *et al.*, 1990; Nikiforov and Nikiforova, 2011). It has been shown that hydrogen peroxide-mediated oxidative stress induced by the IR could cause this RET-PTC1 rearrangement (Ameziane-El-Hassani *et al.*, 2010). Further studies have claimed expression of

RET-PTC1 to deregulate the normal functions of the candidate genes involved in the fusion. For example, it has been shown to result in a sustained tyrosine kinase activity of RET gene and to negatively regulate the proapoptotic effect of the PTC1 gene thus driving tumorigenesis (Celetti *et al.*, 2004). In contrast to the normal PTC1, the fusion gene increased the phosphorylation and activity of CREB1 and its downstream targets AREG and cyclin A in thyroid papillary carcinomas (Leone *et al.*, 2010). In addition, expression of this chimeric protein was found to cooperate with TTF1 overexpression further adding to its tumorigenic potentials (Endo and Kobayashi, 2013). Moreover, RET-PTC1 fusion-induced actin reorganization and stress fiber formation which was found to be mediated by Rho, a small GTP-binding protein, and increased the survival signals in thyroid cells (Barone *et al.*, 2001). Interestingly, apart from PTCs, RET-PTC1 fusion has been detected in lung cancers as well. Treatment with vandetanib, a RET-inhibitor, restrained the AKT and ERK1/2 signaling pathways thus resulted in reduced cell viability of lung cancers both *in vitro* and *in vivo* suggesting AKT-ERK to be the underlying signaling pathways of the RET-PTC1 induced lung cancers (Suzuki *et al.*, 2013). All these reports insisted the use of protein kinase inhibitors to be the possible therapeutics for the treatment of RET-PTC1 overexpressing tumors. In line with this, RET kinase inhibitors like PP1 and ZD6474 were found to be effective against RET-PTC1 expressing thyroid cancers. These inhibitors were revealed to induce temporary cell cycle arrest at G1 phase by reducing the levels of G1 cyclins and increasing the levels of cdk inhibitor p27Kip1 and deregulated the fusion gene-induced MAPK pathway (Vitagliano *et al.*, 2004).

NCOA4-RET (RET-PTC3)

Aberrant chromosomal inversion of chromosome 10, known as inv(10)(q11.2q21) which linked the RET gene at q11.2 to the nuclear receptor coactivator 4 (NCOA4) (PTC3) gene at q21, was found in approximately 60–70% of papillary thyroid carcinomas signifying it to be a characteristic feature of this disease (Zheng, 2013; Gandhi *et al.*, 2010; Kitamura *et al.*, 1999). One of the fusion partners, RET, is a transmembrane RTK (Jhiang *et al.*, 2000; Okamoto *et al.*, 2013). This inversion relegated the tyrosine kinase domain of the RET gene to the

NCOA4 resulting in a constitutively active oncogenic tyrosine kinase and increased auto-phosphorylation (Okamoto *et al.*, 2013; Santoro *et al.*, 2006). The resulting fusion gene lacked the extracellular ligand-binding domain and the intracellular juxtamembrane domains of RET, thus relocating the fused product to cytoplasm and escaping it from the plasma membrane negative regulators such as PTPRJ leading to ligand-independent kinase activation through the coiled-coil dimerization domains of the fusion partner (Figure 18.2) (Santoro *et al.*, 2006). The auto-phosphorylated RTK was found to accelerate the BRAF-MAPK signaling by binding to growth factor receptor-bound protein 2 (GRB2)/son of sevenless (SOS) complexes and activating RAS proteins (Figure 18.2) (Santoro *et al.*, 2006). Lenvatinib (E7080), a tyrosine kinase inhibitor, was shown to exhibit anti-tumor effects against RET-PTC expressing cancer models through contained auto-phosphorylation of the oncogenic fusion product NCOA4-RET (Okamoto *et al.*, 2013). Besides thyroid carcinoma, this fusion gene has also been detected in very few cases of non-small cell lung cancers and lung adenocarcinomas (Wang *et al.*, 2012).

CONCLUSION

On the whole, it was proved that elevated levels of these RET-PTC chimeric proteins augment the tumorigenesis process to a greater extent through increased cell proliferation and malignant transformation henceforth, demanding extensive studies on these fused proteins and their management for the treatment concern.

CONFLICT OF INTEREST

The authors express no conflict of interest.

REFERENCES

Ameziane-El-Hassani, R., M. Boufraqech, O, Lagente-Chevallier U. Weyemi, M. Talbot, D. Métivier, F. Courtin, J.M. Bidart, M. El Mzibri, M. Schlumberger, and C. Dupuy, Role of H2O2 in RET-PTC1 chromosomal rearrangement produced by ionizing radiation in human thyroid cells, *Cancer Res* **70**(10): 4123–4132 (2010).

Barone, M.V., L. Sepe, R.M. Melillo, A. Mineo, G. Santelli, C. Monaco, M.D. Castellone, D. Tramontano, A. Fusco, and M. Santoro, RET-PTC1 oncogene signaling in PC Cl 3 thyroid cells requires the small GTP-binding protein Rho, *Oncogene* **20**(48): 6973–6982 (2001).

Celetti, A., A. Cerrato, F. Merolla, D. Vitagliano, G. Vecchio, and M. Grieco, H4(D10S170), a gene frequently rearranged with RET in papillary thyroid carcinomas: functional characterization, *Oncogene* **23**(1): 109–121 (2004).

de Vries, M.M., R. Celestino, P. Castro, C. Eloy, V. Máximo, J.E. van der Wal, J.T. Plukker, T.P. Links, R.M. Hofstra, M. Sobrinho-Simões, and P. Soares, RET-PTC rearrangement is prevalent in follicular Hürthle cell carcinomas, *Histopathology* **61**(5): 833–843 (2012).

Endo, T. and T. Kobayashi, Concurrent overexpression of RET-PTC1 and TTF1 confers tumorigenicity to thyrocytes, *EndocrRelat Cancer* **20**(6): 767–776 (2013).

Eng, C., RET proto-oncogene in the development of human cancer, *J ClinOncol* **17**(1): 380–393 (1999).

Fusco, A. and M. Santoro, 20 years of RET-PTC in thyroid cancer: clinico-pathological correlations, *Arq Bras EndocrinolMetabol* **51**(5): 731–735 (2007).

Gandhi, M., V. Evdokimova, and Y.E. Nikiforov, Mechanisms of chromosomal rearrangements in solid tumors: the model of papillary thyroid carcinoma, *Mol Cell Endocrinol* **321**(1): 36–43 (2010).

Gandhi, M., M. Medvedovic, J.R. Stringer, and Y.E. Nikiforov, Interphase chromosome folding determines spatial proximity of genes participating in carcinogenic RET-PTC rearrangements, *Oncogene* **25**(16): 2360–2366 (2006).

Grieco, M., M. Santoro, M.T. Berlingieri, R.M. Melillo, R. Donghi, I. Bongarzone, M.A. Pierotti, G. Della Porta, A. Fusco, and G. Vecchio, PTC is a novel rearranged form of the ret proto-oncogene and is frequently detected *in vivo* in human thyroid papillary carcinomas, *Cell* **60**(4): 557–563 (1990).

Hwang, J.H., D.W. Kim, J.M. Suh, H. Kim, J.H. Song, E.S. Hwang, K.C. Park, H.K. Chung, J.M. Kim, T.H. Lee, D.Y. Yu, and M. Shong, Activation of signal transducer and activator of transcription 3 by oncogenic RET-PTC (rearranged in transformation/papillary thyroid carcinoma) tyrosine kinase: roles in specific gene regulation and cellular transformation, *MolEndocrinol* **17**(6): 1155–1166 (2003).

Jhiang, S.M., The RET proto-oncogene in human cancers, *Oncogene* **19**(49): 5590–5597 (2000).

Kim, D.W., J.H. Hwang, J.M. Suh, H. Kim, J.H. Song, E.S. Hwang, I.Y. Hwang, K.C. Park, H.K. Chung, J.M. Kim, J. Park, B.A. Hemmings, and M. Shong, RET-PTC (rearranged in transformation/papillary thyroid carcinomas) tyrosine kinase phosphorylates and activates phosphoinositide-dependent kinase 1 (PDK1): an alternative phosphatidylinositol 3-kinase-independent pathway to activate PDK1, *MolEndocrinol* **17**(7): 1382–1394 (2003).

Kitamura, Y., K. Minobe, T. Nakata, K. Shimizu, S. Tanaka, M. Fujimori, S. Yokoyama, K. Ito, M. Onda, and M. Emi, RET-PTC3 is the most frequent form of gene rearrangement in papillary thyroid carcinomas in Japan, *J Hum Genet* **44**(2): 96–102 (1999).

Kondo, T., S. Ezzat, and S.L. Asa, Pathogenetic mechanisms in thyroid follicular-cell neoplasia, *Nat Rev Cancer* **6**(4): 292–306 (2006).

Leone, V., G. Mansueto, G.M. Pierantoni, M. Tornincasa, F. Merolla, A. Cerrato, M. Santoro, M. Grieco, A. Scaloni, A. Celetti, and A. Fusco, CCDC6 represses CREB1 activity by recruiting histone deacetylase 1 and protein phosphatase 1, *Oncogene* **29**(30): 4341–4351 (2010).

Nikiforov, Y.E. and M.N. Nikiforova, Molecular genetics and diagnosis of thyroid cancer, *Nat Rev Endocrinol* **7**(10): 569–580 (2011).

Nikiforov, Y.E. RET-PTC rearrangement in thyroid tumors, *EndocrPathol* **13**(1): 3–16 (2002).

Okamoto, K., K. Kodama, K. Takase, N.H. Sugi, Y. Yamamoto, M. Iwata, and A. Tsuruoka, Antitumor activities of the targeted multi-tyrosine kinase inhibitor lenvatinib (E7080) against RET gene fusion-driven tumor models, *Cancer Lett* **340**(1): 97–103 (2013).

Pierotti, M.A., M. Santoro, R.B. Jenkins, G. Sozzi, I. Bongarzone, M. Grieco, N. Monzini, M. Miozzo, M.A. Herrmann, A. Fusco, I.D. Hay, G.D. Porta, and G. Vecchio, Characterization of an inversion on the long arm of chromosome 10 juxtaposing D10S170 and RET and creating the oncogenic sequence RET-PTC, *Proc Natl AcadSci U S A* **89**(5): 1616–1620 (1992).

Portella, G., D. Vitagliano, C. Borselli, R.M. Melillo, D. Salvatore, J.L. Rothstein, G. Vecchio, A. Fusco, and M. Santoro, Human N-ras, TRK-T1, and RET-PTC3 oncogenes, driven by a thyroglobulin promoter, differently affect the expression of differentiation markers and the proliferation of thyroid epithelial cells, *Oncol Res* **11**(9): 421–427 (1999).

Prescott, J.D. and M.A. Zeiger, The RET oncogene in papillary thyroid carcinoma, *Cancer* **121**(13): 2137–2146 (2015).

Romei, C. and R. Elisei, RET-PTC translocations and clinico-pathological features in human papillary thyroid carcinoma, *Front Endocrinol* (Lausanne) **3**: 54 (2012).

Romeo, G., P. Ronchetto, Y. Luo, V. Barone, M. Seri, I. Ceccherini, B. Pasini, R. Bocciardi, M. Lerone, and H. Kääriäinen, *et al.*, Point mutations affecting the tyrosine kinase domain of the RET proto-oncogene in Hirschsprung's disease, *Nature* **367**(6461): 377–378 (1994).

Sadetzki, S., R. Calderon-Margalit, B. Modan, S. Srivastava, and R.M. Tuttle, RET-PTC activation in benign and malignant thyroid tumors arising in a population exposed to low-dose external-beam irradiation in childhood, *J ClinEndocrinolMetab* **89**(5): 2281–2289 (2004).

Saenko, V., T. Rogounovitch, Y. Shimizu-Yoshida, A. Abrosimov, E. Lushnikov, P. Roumiantsev, N. Matsumoto, M. Nakashima, S. Meirmanov, A. Ohtsuru, H. Namba, A. Tsyb, and S. Yamashita, Novel tumorigenic rearrangement, Delta rfp/ret, in a papillary thyroid carcinoma from externally irradiated patient, *Mutat Res* **527**(1–2): 81–90 (2003).

Santoro, M., R.M. Melillo, and A. Fusco, RET-PTC activation in papillary thyroid carcinoma: European Journal of Endocrinology Prize Lecture, *Eur J Endocrinol* **155**(5): 645–653 (2006).

Santoro, M., R. Rosati, M. Grieco, and M.T. Berlingieri, G.L. D'Amato, V. de Franciscis, and A. Fusco, The ret proto-oncogene is consistently expressed in human pheochromocytomas and thyroid medullary carcinomas, *Oncogene* **5**(10): 1595–1598 (1990).

Sozzi, G., I. Bongarzone, M. Miozzo, M.G. Borrello, M.G. Blutti, S. Pilotti, G. Della Porta, and M.A. Pierotti, A t(10;17) translocation creates the RET-PTC2 chimeric transforming sequence in papillary thyroid carcinoma, *Genes Chromosomes Cancer* **9**(4): 244–250 (1994).

Suzuki, M., H. Makinoshima, S. Matsumoto, A. Suzuki, S. Mimaki, K. Matsushima, K. Yoh, K. Goto, Y. Suzuki, G. Ishii, A. Ochiai, K. Tsuta, T. Shibata, T. Kohno, H. Esumi, and K. Tsuchihara, Identification of a lung adenocarcinoma cell line with CCDC6-RET fusion gene and the effect of RET inhibitors *in vitro* and *in vivo*, *Cancer Sci* **104**(7): 896–903 (2013).

Tahira, T., Y. Ishizaka, F. Itoh, T. Sugimura, and M. Nagao, Characterization of ret proto-oncogene mRNAs encoding two isoforms of the protein product in a human neuroblastoma cell line, *Oncogene* **5**(1): 97–102 (1990).

Tallini, G., and S.L. Asa, RET oncogene activation in papillary thyroid carcinoma, *AdvAnatPathol* **8**(6): 345–354 (2001).

Vitagliano, D., F. Carlomagno, M.L. Motti, G. Viglietto, Y.E. Nikiforov, M.N. Nikiforova, J.M. Hershman, A.J. Ryan, A. Fusco, R.M. Melillo, and M. Santoro, Regulation of p27Kip1 protein levels contributes to mitogenic effects of the RET-PTC kinase in thyroid carcinoma cells, *Cancer Res* **64**(11): 3823–3829 (2004).

Voskoboĭnyk, L.H., Oncogenes RET-PTC and mechanisms of their involvement in thyroid cancerogenesis, *UkrBiokhimZh* **81**(6): 17–25 (2009).

Wang, R., H. Hu, Y. Pan, Y. Li, T. Ye, C. Li, X. Luo, L. Wang, H. Li, Y. Zhang, F. Li, Y. Lu, Q. Lu, J. Xu, D. Garfield, L. Shen, H. Ji, W. Pao, Y. Sun, and H. Chen, RET fusions define a unique molecular and clinicopathologic subtype of non-small-cell lung cancer, *J ClinOncol* **30**(35): 4352–4359 (2012).

Zhang, T., Y. Lu, Q. Ye, M. Zhang, L. Zheng, X. Yin, P. Gavine, Z. Sun, Q. Ji, G. Zhu, and X. Su, An evaluation and recommendation of the optimal methodologies to detect RET gene rearrangements in papillary thyroid carcinoma, *Genes Chromosomes Cancer* **54**(3): 168–176 (2015).

Zheng, J. Oncogenic chromosomal translocations and human cancer (review), *Oncol Rep* **30**(5): 2011–2019 (2013).

19

RUNX1 or AML1 Fusion Genes in Leukemia and Other Cancers

*Ganesan Padmavathi, Javadi Monisha, Kishore Banik, Choudhary Harsha, Devivasha Bordoloi and Ajaikumar B. Kunnumakkara**

INTRODUCTION

Runt-related transcription factor family comprises three highly homologous transcription factors known as RUNX1, RUNX2 and RUNX3. RUNX genes together with CBFB-Pebpb2 were proved to play a vital role in deciding the fate of cell differentiation during embryogenesis and regarded as developmental regulators (Ito, 2004; De Braekeleer *et al.*, 2011; De Barkeeper *et al.*, 2009). RUNX1 was known to mediate definitive hematopoiesis and hematopoietic stem cell generation; RUNX2, osteogenesis; and RUNX3, neurogenesis and thymopoiesis (Okuda *et al.*,

*Author for correspondence: Ajaikumar B. Kunnumakkara, Cancer Biology Laboratory, Department of Biosciences and Bioengineering, Indian Institute of Technology Guwahati, Assam 781039, India. kunnumakkara@iitg.ernet.in

1998; North *et al.*, 2002; Levanon *et al.*, 2004; Ito, 2008; De Braekeleer *et al.*, 2009). Further, it has been discovered that they act as a heterodimeric transcription factor where the α- and β-subunits were produced by RUNX genes and CBFB-Pebpb2 (Ito, 2004). Subsequently, the Runt homology domain (RHD) of RUNX proteins was found to be responsible for heterodimer formation with CBFB-Pebpb2 and for effective DNA binding as well as transcription factor activities (De Braekeleer *et al.*, 2011; Ito, 2008). Besides RHD in the N-terminal, all the three proteins possess a transcription activation domain (TAD), a transcription inhibition domain and a VWRPY sequence in their C-terminal (De Braekeleer *et al.*, 2011).

Among the three proteins, RUNX1, also termed as AML1, CBFA2 or PEBP2aB, is our protein of interest as it is observed to be frequently involved in chromosomal translocation, tumor initiation and progression. Being a transcriptional regulator, RUNX1 can either induce or suppress the expression of target genes depending upon the interaction with other components of transcription factor complex. For example, it was shown to act as a transcriptional activator when binding with p300/CBP and histone acetyltransferase (HAT), whereas interaction with mSin3A, Groucho/TLE and histone deacetylase (HDAC) makes it a transcription repressor (De Braekeleer *et al.*, 2011).The common molecular targets regulated by RUNX1 are growth factors, transcription activators, surface receptors and signaling molecules such as BCL2, BLK, CDKN1A, FLT3, GM-CSF, IL-3, M-CSF receptor, MPO, MYB, STAT3, TCRA and TCRB, etc. (De Braekeleer *et al.*, 2009, 2011; Ito, 2004; Michaud *et al.*, 2003). Therefore, deregulation of this protein could aberrantly alter the expression profile of various important regulatory genes thus leading to the development of several diseases including hematological malignancies. The sustained deregulation of RUNX1 protein was attained through point mutation, gene amplification or through recurrent chromosomal translocations (De Braekeleer *et al.*, 2009). Further, this gene has been reported to be involved in translocation with more than 30 genes. However, only very few translocations were recurrently detected and identified to be associated with cancer development. Moreover, among the rearrangements identified, only 17 have been characterized at the molecular level. The frequent partner genes of RUNX1 are EAP, ETO, ETV6, EVI1, MDS1, MTG16 and PRDM16, etc. (Figure 19.1) (De Braekeleer *et al.*, 2009).

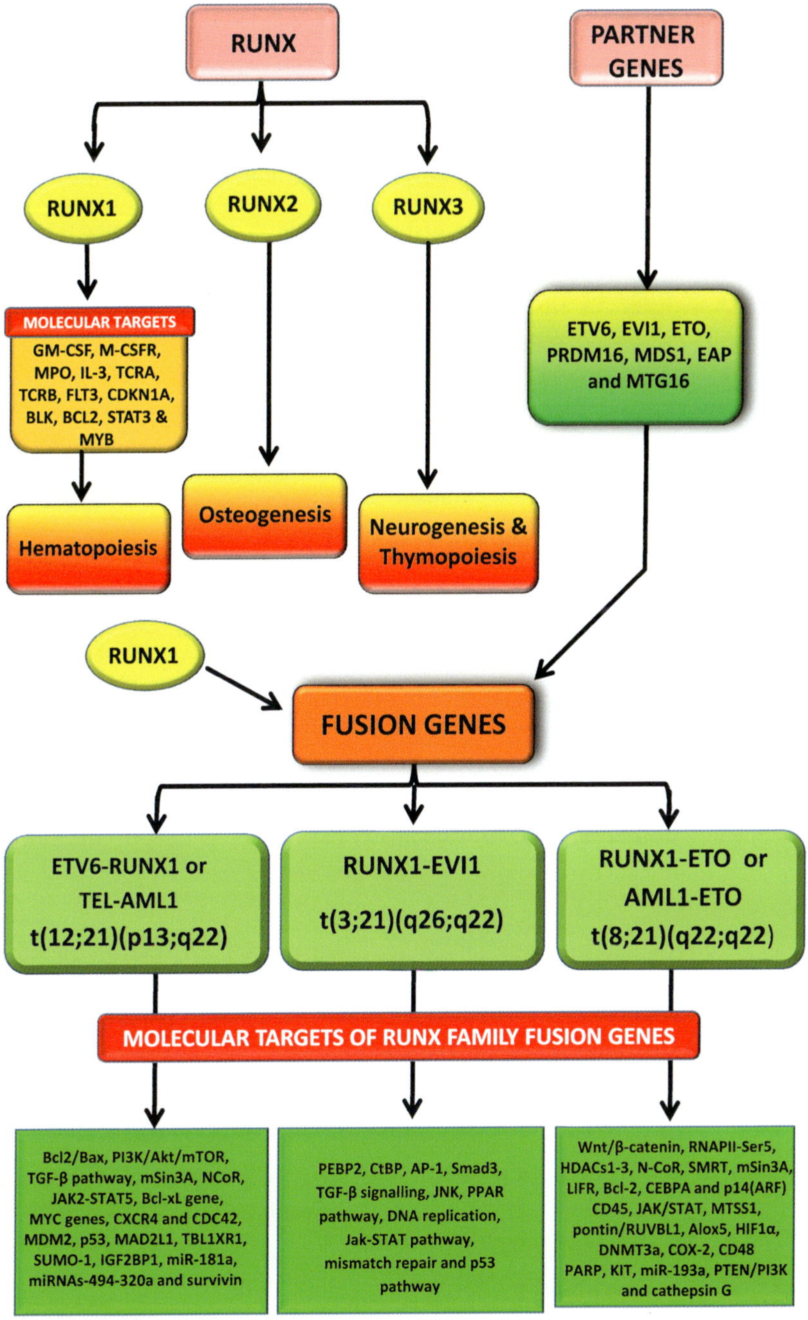

Figure 19.1: Fusion partner genes and molecular targets of RUNX family.

ETV6-RUNX1 (TEL-AML1)

The ETV6-RUNX1 fusion gene, also designated as TEL-AML1, is a chimeric transcription factor resulting from t(12;21)(p13;q22) chromosomal translocation. It was believed to be induced by DNA-damage-generated apoptogenic signals and the most common chromosomal aberration found in 25% of pediatric B cell precursor ALL (BCP-ALL) (Torrano *et al.*, 2011; Linka *et al.*, 2013; Eguchi-Ishimae *et al.*, 2001). However, similar to many other fusion genes, expression of ETV6-RUNX1 fusion was also detected in healthy individuals (Brassesco, 2008). RAG recombinase enzyme was found to play a major role in the ETV6-RUNX1 chromosomal rearrangement in ALL (Papaemmanuil *et al.*, 2014; Kuiper *et al.*, 2014). t(12;21) resulted in the fusion of dimerization domain of *ETV6* and DNA binding and activating regions of *RUNX1* (Romana *et al.*, 1995; Golub *et al.*, 1995; Zelent *et al.*, 2004; De Braekeleer *et al.*, 2009). Further, it was proved that ETV6/RUNX1 fusion is generally prenatal and produces clinically indolent preleukemic clone, which can develop into ALL at low frequency through further postnatal genetic alterations (Bateman *et al.*, 2010; Ford *et al.*, 1998; Wiemels *et al.*, 1999a, 1999b; Alpar *et al.*, 2015; Palmi *et al.*, 2014). Interestingly, only 1% of newborns with prenatal ETV6-RUNX1 developed leukemia later in their life supporting the hypothesis that t(12;21) alone is insufficient to develop leukemia. Further, it was discovered that in addition to t(12;21), deletion of normal TEL gene i.e. loss of heterozygosity at 12p through mitotic crossover and increased Bcl2/Bax ratio also contributed to leukemogenesis in these children (Ivanovski *et al.*, 2015; Sabaawy *et al.*, 2006).

Different mechanisms were proposed for the ETV6-RUNX1-induced leukemogenesis. Functional RUNX1 was found to be essential for normal fetal liver hematopoiesis as it is an important component of core binding complex (CBFα-RUNX1) and any mutation that causes functional deterioration of RUNX1 would result in development disorders. Consequently, fusion of RUNX1 with ETV6 produced a deregulated abnormal RUNX1 protein leading to acute leukemia (Okuda *et al.*, 1996; Wang *et al.*, 1996). Moreover, the DNA binding domain of RUNX1 and the dimerization and corepressor binding domains of ETV6 were found to be essential for the initiation and propagation of ALL (Morrow *et al.*, 2007). *In vivo* studies proved that ETV6-RUNX1 fusion induced the constitutive activation of PI3K-AKT-mTOR pathway which has been found to be essential for the maintenance of disease (Figure 19.1) (Fuka *et al.*, 2012). It was also shown to deregulate the TGF-β pathway giving growth advantage to the cells by developing resistance to TGF-β-mediated inhibition of proliferation (Ford *et al.*, 2009). Moreover, the fusion protein exerted transcriptional repressor activity for the RUNX1 target genes via interaction of both ETV6 and RUNX1 domains of chimera with corepressor molecules such as mSin3A and N-CoR, consequently blocking differentiation (Figure 19.1) (Fenrick *et al.*, 1999; Guidez *et al.*, 2000). In addition, by the virtue of helix loop helix (HLH) contributed by the ETV6 region, the ETV6-RUNX1 protein exhibited dominant negative effect on both wild-type ETV6 and RUNX1 activities which impaired the tumor suppressive ability of ETV6 in t(12;21) carrying leukemia (Gunji *et al.*, 2004). Further, the fusion protein has been reported to elevate erythropoietin receptor (*EPOR*) gene expression and to augment cell survival through the activation of JAK2-STAT5 pathway and up-regulation of anti-apoptotic *Bcl-xL* gene (Torrano *et al.*, 2011). Approximately 25% of ETV6-RUNX1 positive patients were also carriers of PAX5 mutations which were also known to activate STAT pathway and led to leukemogenesis (van der *et al.*, 2015). It also disrupted the transcriptional regulation of MYC genes and cytoskeletal regulatory genes as well as inhibited CXCR4 and CDC42 signaling (Figure 19.1) (Hajingabo *et al.*, 2014; Palmi *et al.*, 2014). In addition, it has been proposed that ETV6-RUNX1-induced reactive oxygen species may drive the accumulation of secondary mutations in B cells, thus facilitating the progression of preleukemic clones into fully transformed leukemic cells (Kantner *et al.*, 2013). Further, ETV6-RUNX1 fusion was also proved to upregulate MDM2, negative regulator of p53 levels by binding to RUNX1 motifs resulting in the inhibition of p53 which can be reverted using Nutlin-3, a small molecule inhibitor of MDM2-p53 interaction (Kaindl *et al.*, 2014). Above all, in a genome-wide screening method, more than 300 target genes were found to be deregulated by this fusion transcription factor (Linka *et al.*, 2013). It was also shown to impede the mitotic checkpoint through downregulation of its important component MAD2L1 (Krapf *et al.*, 2010). Moreover, additional molecular alterations like deletion of TBL1XR1 gene have been implicated in ETV6-RUNX1 positive ALL. Deletion of TBL1XR1 resulted in the disruption of SMRT-N-CoR functions leading to aberrant expression of various genes (Parker *et al.*, 2008). ETV6-RUNX1 chimeric protein was shown to be altered and localized into NBs by SUMO-1 which may contribute to malignant transformation (Chakrabarti *et al.*, 2000). mRNA levels of ETV6-RUNX1 was shown to be regulated by the oncofetal RNA-binding protein IGF2BP1 which is overexpressed in ETV6-RUNX1 positive ALL (Stoskus *et al.*, 2016). Moreover, miR-181a was also found to regulate ETV6-RUNX1 levels and vice versa. Increased levels of miR-181a caused reduction in ETV6-RUNX1 expression; induced cell differentiation, cell growth arrest and apoptosis (Yang *et al.*, 2015). Another two micro RNAs, miRNAs-494 and -320a essential for the regulation of survivin expression have been identified to be downregulated in ETV6-RUNX1 positive leukemia which was correlated with the anti-apoptotic effect of ETV6-RUNX1 which attributed to the increased expression of survivin (Figure 19.1) (Diakos *et al.*, 2010). Interestingly, unlike other fusion genes (e.g. BCR-ABL) involved in leukemia, expression of ETV6-RUNX1 was found to be correlated with better clinical behavior (Hakeem *et al.*, 2015). For instance, presence of this fusion increased the sensitivity to doxorubicin and etoposide treatment (Frost *et al.*, 2004). In few cases, ETV6-RUNX1 fusion acts as a tumor specific antigen and induces specific cytotoxic T-cell response leading to host anti-leukemia defense (Yotnda *et al.*, 1998).

RUNX1-ETO (AML1-ETO)

RUNX1-ETO oncoprotein is a repressive transcription factor resulting from the chromosomal rearrangement between chromosomes 8 and 21 i.e. t(8;21)(q22;q22) (LaFiura *et al.*, 2008; Esposito *et al.*, 2015). Approximately 12% of both adult and pediatric acute myeloid leukemia (AML) cases and 40% of the AML subclass FAB-M2 (French-American-British classification) were reported to harbor this fusion oncoprotein (Peterson and Zhang, 2004). Interestingly, recent studies proposed a novel mechanism where this translocation is induced by the activation of Wnt/β-catenin signaling cascade as Wnt3a activation increased the localization of β-catenin into RNA polymerase II transcription factories (RNAPII-Ser5), which brought the ETO and RUNX1 genes to close spatial proximity thereby assisting in the formation of RUNX1-ETO or AML1-ETO rearrangement (Ugarte *et al.*, 2015). The AML1-ETO protein comprises 177 N-terminal amino acid residues of AML1 which are necessary for hematopoiesis and almost the entire ETO protein which is known to act as a corepressor for variety of transcription factors (Erickson *et al.*, 1992). As already mentioned, RUNX1 is a well-known transcriptional activator which promotes granulocytic differentiation through the coordinated upregulation of lineage-specific target genes like MPO. But fusion with ETO causes it to act as a repressor rather than an activator and downregulates its target genes involved in differentiation. Similar to ETV6-RUNX1 gene, AML1-ETO also acts as a transcriptional repressor by interacting with nuclear corepressors such as HDACs1-3, N-CoR, SMRT and mSin3A (Figure 19.1) (Peterson and Zhang, 2004). In contrast to normal RUNX1 which was known to activate the promoters of leukemia inhibitory factor receptor (LIFR), the chimeric protein suppressed the LIFR promoter activity (Qadi *et al.*, 2016). It also reduced the expression of Bcl-2, CEBPA and p14 (ARF) in AML patients (Figure 19.1) (Zhuang *et al.*, 2013a, 2013b). Additionally, it suppressed CD45 levels which subsequently activated the JAK-STAT signaling pathway (Lo and Peterson, 2013). Though AML1-ETO was proved to be transcription repressor of various genes, it also acted as an activator of certain genes. For example, the chimeric fusion was shown to increase the expression of metastasis suppressor 1 (MTSS1) gene which was associated with better prognosis of AML patients (Schemionek *et al.*, 2015). It also elevated the expression of pontin-RUVBL1 thereby inducing cell cycle progression and increasing the disease aggressiveness (Breig *et al.*, 2014). Moreover, RUNX1-ETO9a, a splice isoform of RUNX1-ETO elevated the levels of Alox5 by the ZnF transcription factor KLF6 which in turn was activated by RUNX1-ETO itself contributing to the disease complexity (DeKelver *et al.*, 2013). In addition, it interacted with the hypoxia-inducible factor 1α (HIF1α) gene to transactivate DNMT3a resulting in DNA hypermethylation and poor prognosis (Figure 19.1) (Gao *et al.*, 2015). Further, it elevated the expression of cyclooxygenase (COX)-2 and β-catenin adding to the complications (Zhang *et al.*, 2013). AML1-ETO positive AML was induced at least in part by escape from host immune defense which was governed through CD48 downregulation-mediated decreased killing by NK cells (Elias *et al.*, 2014). Also, it has been reported that RUNX1-ETO enhanced the expansion of human hematopoietic stem cells (Mulloy *et al.*, 2002).

AML1-ETO expressing AML patients were found to be highly sensitive to PARP inhibition attributed to their impaired DNA-damage response (DDR) (Esposito *et al.*, 2015). However, activating mutations in c-KIT in addition to the signature t(8;21) translocation induced chemoresistance through increased DNA-repair efficiency (Wichmann *et al.*, 2015; Geng *et al.*, 2013). The nervy homology region 2 (NHR2) within ETO portion of the chimera was found to be responsible for its oligomerization-mediated oncogenic potential. Therefore, interference with this NHR2-mediated oligomerization by specific cell-penetrating peptides poses a great therapeutic potential (Bartel *et al.*, 2013). AML1-ETO was shown to function through an AML1-ETO-containing transcription factor complex (AETFC) with numerous hematopoietic transcription cofactors and DNA binding domains (Sun *et al.*, 2013). Increased IFN signaling reduced the effect of AML1-ETO fusion on the self-renewal and proliferation of leukemic cells (DeKelver *et al.*, 2014). AML1-ETO-fusion-associated overexpression of lymphoid enhancer-binding factor 1 (LEF1) gene resulted in the relapse-free survival (Fu *et al.*, 2014). Recently, Li *et al.* (2013) proved that AML1-ETO and miR-193a acted in a feedback circuitry where AML1-ETO-induced silencing of miR-193a expanded the oncogenicity of AML1-ETO and resulted in the activation of PTEN-PI3K pathway leading to leukemogenesis (Figure 19.1) (Li *et al.* 2013). AML1-ETO suppressed the expression of cathepsin G (CTSG), a serine protease, restoration of which could demodulate AML1-ETO, induce partial differentiation, growth inhibition and apoptosis suggesting it to be an effective target for the treatment of AML (Jin *et al.* 2013). Finally, as mentioned earlier, AML1-ETO has a splice isoform AML1-ETO9a. Expression of both the isoforms was detected in most of the AML patients. However, levels of AE9a were found to be lesser than that of AE itself. Similarly, response to standard treatment was also found to be poorer than that of AE (Li *et al.*, 2012).

RUNX1-EVI1

The N-terminal half of RUNX1 with runt homology domain is fused to the entire ZnF protein Evi-1 to produce a chimeric transcription factor through the t(3;21)(q26;q22) translocation and found to induce growth; inhibit differentiation and to play a key role in the progression of CML to an acute blast crisis (Mitani *et al.*, 1994). RUNX1-Evi1 blocked the wild-type RUNX1 induced transactivation of polyomavirus enhancer-binding protein 2 (PEBP2) by competitively binding to the PEBP2 sites (Tanaka *et al.*, 1995, 1998). Further reports proved that the inhibition of transactivation potential of wild-type RUNX1 was also mediated by the interaction of RUNX1-EVi1 with corepressor complex like CtBP (Izutsu *et al.*, 2002). In addition, the chimeric protein also enhanced the c-fos promoter transactivation and AP-1 activity similar to wild-type Evi-1 and was shown to interact with Smad3, mediator of TGF-β signaling through the Evi-1 portion and reduced its activity thereby interfering with TGF-β signaling ultimately leading to uncontrolled growth and leukemogenesis (Figure 19.1) (Tanaka *et al.*, 1995; Kurokawa *et al.*, 1998). The ZnF domain of the fusion protein was also shown to interact with JNK and deregulated its activity, thus preventing stress-induced apoptosis (Mitani *et al.*, 2004). Therefore, it was clearly proved that functions of both RUNX1 and Evi-1 portions of the fusion protein are essential for the leukemic transformation (Tanaka *et al.*, 1995). Recently, several additional molecular targets of RUNX1-EVi1 have been identified using microarray analysis which includes PPAR pathway, DNA replication, JAK-STAT pathway, MMR, nucleotide excision repair, p53 pathway, etc. (Shen *et al.*, 2015). However, extensive research is required to elucidate the actual downstream targets of this chimera.

CONCLUSION

Altogether, till date, more than 30 fusion partners of RUNX1 have been identified, all being the activators of RUNX1 thus producing constitutively active chimeric transcription factors. RUNX1 through these activating chromosomal rearrangements was consistently resulted in the deregulation of growth factors, transcription activators, surface receptors and signaling molecules involved in normal cellular functioning thus promoting cancer. However, the actual role of many of the RUNX fusion genes are not completely understood which requires extensive research for elucidating their function in respective cancers. Moreover, it is essential to identify novel therapeutic compounds to selectively inhibit the chimeric transcription factors which would result in better treatment outcomes.

CONFLICT OF INTEREST

The authors express no conflict of interest.

REFERENCES

Alpar, D., D. Wren, L. Ermini, M.B. Mansur, F.W. van Delft, C.M. Bateman, I. Titley, L. Kearney, T. Szczepanski, D. Gonzalez, A.M. Ford, N.E. Potter, and M. Greaves, Clonal origins of ETV6-RUNX1+ acute lymphoblastic leukemia: studies in monozygotic twins, *Leukemia* **29**(4): 839–846 (2015).

Bartel, Y., M. Grez, and C. Wichmann, Interference with RUNX1/ETO leukemogenic function by cell-penetrating peptides targeting the NHR2 oligomerization domain, *Biomed Res Int* **2013**: 297692 (2013).

Bateman, C.M., S.M. Colman, T. Chaplin, B.D. Young, T.O. Eden, M. Bhakta, E.J. Gratias, E.R. van Wering, G. Cazzaniga, C.J. Harrison, R. Hain, P. Ancliff, A.M. Ford, L. Kearney, and M. Greaves, Acquisition of genome-wide copy number alterations in monozygotic twins with acute lymphoblastic leukemia, *Blood* **115**(17): 3553–3558 (2010).

Brassesco, MS., Leukemia/lymphoma-associated gene fusions in normal individuals, *Genet Mol Res* **7**(3): 782–790 (2008).

Breig, O., S. Bras, N. Martinez, D. Soria, D. Osman, O. Heidenreich, and M. Haenlin, L. Waltzer, Pontin is a critical regulator for AML1-ETO-induced leukemia, *Leukemia* **28**(6): 1271–1279 (2014).

Burmeister, T., N. Gökbuget, S. Schwartz, L. Fischer, D. Hubert, A. Sindram, D. Hoelzer, and E. Thiel, Clinical features and prognostic implications of TCF3-PBX1 and ETV6-RUNX1 in adult acute lymphoblastic leukemia, *Haematologica* **95**(2): 241–246 (2010).

Chakrabarti, S.R., R. Sood, S. Nandi, and G. Nucifora, Posttranslational modification of TEL and TEL/AML1 by SUMO-1 and cell-cycle-dependent assembly into nuclear bodies, *Proc Natl Acad Sci USA* **97**(24): 13281–13285 (2000).

De Braekeleer, E., N. Douet-Guilbert, F. Morel, M.J. Le Bris, C. Férec, and M. De Braekeleer, RUNX1 translocations and fusion genes in malignant hemopathies, *Future Oncol* **7**(1): 77–91 (2011).

De Braekeleer, E., C. Férec, and M. De Braekeleer, RUNX1 translocations in malignant hemopathies, *Anticancer Res* **29**(4): 1031–1037 (2009).

DeKelver, R.C., B. Lewin, K. Lam, Y. Komeno, M. Yan, C. Rundle, M.C. Lo, and D.E. Zhang, Cooperation between RUNX1-ETO9a and novel transcriptional partner KLF6 in upregulation of Alox5 in acute myeloid leukemia, *PLoS Genet* **9**(10): e1003765 (2013).

DeKelver, R.C., B. Lewin, S. Weng, M. Yan, J. Biggs, and D.E. Zhang, RUNX1-ETO induces a type I interferon response which negatively effects t(8;21)-induced increased self-renewal and leukemia development, *Leuk Lymphoma* **55**(4): 884–891 (2014).

Diakos. C., S. Zhong, Y. Xiao, M. Zhou, G.M. Vasconcelos, G. Krapf, R.F. Yeh, S. Zheng, M. Kang, J.K. Wiencke, M.S. Pombo-de-Oliveira, R. Panzer-Grümayer, and J.L. Wiemels, TEL-AML1 regulation of survivin and apoptosis via miRNA-494 and miRNA-320a, *Blood* **116**(23): 4885–4893 (2010).

Eguchi-Ishimae, M., M. Eguchi, E. Ishii, S. Miyazaki, K. Ueda, N. Kamada, and S. Mizutani, Breakage and fusion of the TEL (ETV6) gene in immature B lymphocytes induced by apoptogenic signals, *Blood* **97**(3): 737–743 (2001).

Elias, S., R. Yamin, L. Golomb, P. Tsukerman, N. Stanietsky-Kaynan, D. Ben-Yehuda, and O. Mandelboim, Immune evasion by oncogenic proteins of acute myeloid leukemia, *Blood* **123**(10): 1535–1543 (2014).

Erickson, P., J. Gao, K.S. Chang, T. Look, E. Whisenant, S. Raimondi, R. Lasher, J. Trujillo, J. Rowley, and H. Drabkin, Identification of breakpoints in t(8;21) acute myelogenous leukemia and isolation of a fusion transcript, AML1/ETO, with similarity to Drosophila segmentation gene, runt, *Blood* **80**(7): 1825–1831 (1992).

Esposito, M.T., L. Zhao, T.K. Fung, J.K. Rane, A. Wilson, N. Martin, J. Gil, A.Y. Leung, A. Ashworth, and C.W. So, Synthetic lethal targeting of oncogenic transcription factors in acute leukemia by PARP inhibitors, *Nat Med* **21**(12): 1481–1490 (2015).

Fenrick, R., J.M. Amann, B. Lutterbach, L. Wang, J.J. Westendorf, J.R. Downing, and S.W. Hiebert, Both TEL and AML-1 contribute repression domains to the t(12;21) fusion protein, *Mol Cell Biol* **19**(10): 6566–6574 (1999).

Ford, A.M., C.A. Bennett, C.M. Price, M.C. Bruin, E.R. Van Wering, and M. Greaves, Fetal origins of the TEL-AML1 fusion gene in identical twins with leukemia, *Proc Natl Acad Sci USA* **95**(8): 4584–4588 (1998).

Ford, A.M., C. Palmi, C. Bueno, D. Hong, P. Cardus, D. Knight, G. Cazzaniga, T. Enver, and M. Greaves, The TEL-AML1 leukemia fusion gene dysregulates the TGF-beta pathway in early B lineage progenitor cells, *J Clin Invest* **119**(4): 826–836 (2009).

Frost, B.M., E. Forestier, G. Gustafsson, P. Nygren, M. Hellebostad, O.G. Jonsson, J. Kanerva, K. Schmiegelow, R. Larsson, and G. Lönnerholm, Translocation t(12;21) is related to *in vitro* cellular drug sensitivity to doxorubicin and etoposide in childhood acute lymphoblastic leukemia, *Blood* **104**(8): 2452–2457 (2004).

Fu, Y., H. Zhu, W. Wu, J. Xu, T. Chen, B. Xu, S. Qian, J. Li, and P. Liu, Clinical significance of lymphoid enhancer-binding factor 1 expression in acute myeloid leukemia, *Leuk Lymphoma* **55**(2): 371–377 (2014).

Fuka, G., H.P. Kantner, R. Grausenburger, A. Inthal, E. Bauer, G. Krapf, U. Kaindl, M. Kauer, M.N. Dworzak, D. Stoiber, O.A. Haas, and R. Panzer-Grümayer, Silencing of ETV6/RUNX1 abrogates PI3K/AKT/mTOR signaling and impairs reconstitution of leukemia in xenografts, *Leukemia* **26**(5): 927–933 (2012).

Gao, X.N., F. Yan, J. Lin, L. Gao, X.L. Lu, S.C. Wei, N. Shen, J.X. Pang, Q.Y. Ning, Y. Komeno, A.L. Deng, Y.H. Xu, J.L. Shi, Y.H. Li, D.E. Zhang, C. Nervi, S.J. Liu, and L. Yu, AML1/ETO cooperates with HIF1α to promote leukemogenesis through DNMT3a transactivation, *Leukemia* **29**(8): 1730–1740 (2015).

Geng, S.X., X. Du, J.Y. Weng, X. Huang, Z.S. Lu, L.Y. Zhong, R. Guo, S.J. Wu, and P. Wu, [C-kit mutation in acute myeloid leukemia patients with AML1-ETO fusion gene and its clinical significance], *Zhongguo Shi Yan Xue Ye Xue Za Zhi* **21**(4): 839–842 (2013).

Golub, T.R., G.F. Barker, S.K. Bohlander, S.W. Hiebert, D.C. Ward, P. Bray-Ward, E. Morgan, S.C. Raimondi, J.D. Rowley, and D.G. Gilliland, Fusion of the TEL gene on 12p13 to the AML1 gene on 21q22 in acute lymphoblastic leukemia, *Proc Natl Acad Sci USA* **92**(11): 4917–4921 (1995).

Guidez, F., K. Petrie, A.M. Ford, H. Lu, C.A. Bennett, A. MacGregor, J. Hannemann, Y. Ito, J. Ghysdael, M. Greaves, L.M. Wiedemann, and A. Zelent, Recruitment of the nuclear receptor corepressor N-CoR by the TEL moiety of the childhood leukemia-associated TEL-AML1 oncoprotein, *Blood* **96**(7): 2557–2561 (2000).

Gunji, H., K. Waga, F. Nakamura, K. Maki, K. Sasaki, Y. Nakamura, and K. Mitani, TEL/AML1 shows dominant-negative effects over TEL as well as AML1, *Biochem Biophys Res Commun* **322**(2): 623–630 (2004).

Hajingabo, L.J., S. Daakour, M. Martin, R. Grausenburger, R. Panzer-Grümayer, F. Dequiedt, N. Simonis, and J.C. Twizere, Predicting interactome network perturbations in human cancer: application to gene fusions in acute lymphoblastic leukemia, *Mol Biol Cell* **25**(24): 3973–3985 (2014).

Hakeem, A., A.A. Shiekh, G.M. Bhat, and A.R. Lone, Prognostification of ALL by Cytogenetics, *Indian J Hematol Blood Transfus* **31**(3): 322–331 (2015).

Ito, Y., Oncogenic potential of the RUNX gene family: 'overview', *Oncogene* **23**(24): 4198–4208 (2004).

Ito, Y., RUNX genes in development and cancer: regulation of viral gene expression and the discovery of RUNX family genes, *Adv Cancer Res* **99**: 33–76 (2008).

Ivanovski, I., L. Garavelli, O. Djurić, A. Ćirović, D. Škorić, and P.I. Ivanovski, Mitotic crossover promotes leukemogenesis in children born with TEL-AML1 via the generation of loss of heterozygosity at 12p, *Pediatr Med Chir* **37**(2): pmc.2015.112 (2015).

Izutsu, K., M. Kurokawa, Y. Imai, M. Ichikawa, T. Asai, K. Maki, K. Mitani, and H. Hirai The t(3;21) fusion product, AML1/Evi-1 blocks AML1-induced transactivation by recruiting CtBP, *Oncogene* **21**(17): 2695–2703 (2002).

Jin, W., K. Wu, Y.Z. Li, W.T. Yang, B. Zou, F. Zhang, J. Zhang, and K.K. Wang, AML1-ETO targets and suppresses cathepsin G, a serine protease, which is able to degrade AML1-ETO in t(8;21) acute myeloid leukemia, *Oncogene* **32**(15): 1978–1987 (2013).

Kaindl, U., M. Morak, C. Portsmouth, A. Mecklenbräuker, M. Kauer, M. Zeginigg, A. Attarbaschi, O.A. Haas, and R. Panzer-Grümayer, Blocking ETV6/RUNX1-induced MDM2 overexpression by Nutlin-3 reactivates p53 signaling in childhood leukemia, *Leukemia* **28**(3): 600–608 (2014).

Kantner, H.P., W. Warsch, A. Delogu, E. Bauer, H. Esterbauer, E. Casanova, V. Sexl, and D. Stoiber, ETV6/RUNX1 induces reactive oxygen species and drives the accumulation of DNA damage in B cells, *Neoplasia* **15**(11): 1292–1300 (2013).

Krapf, G., U. Kaindl, A. Kilbey, G. Fuka, A. Inthal, R. Joas, G. Mann, J.C. Neil, O.A. Haas, and E.R. Panzer-Grümayer, ETV6/RUNX1 abrogates mitotic checkpoint function and targets its key player MAD2L1, *Oncogene* **29**(22): 3307–3312 (2010).

Kuiper, R.P., and E. Waanders, A RAG driver on the road to pediatric ALL, *Nat Genet* **46**(2): 96–98 (2014).

Kurokawa, M., K. Mitani, Y. Imai, S. Ogawa, Y. Yazaki, and H. Hirai, The t(3;21) fusion product, AML1/Evi-1, interacts with Smad3 and blocks transforming growth factor-beta-mediated growth inhibition of myeloid cells, *Blood* **92**(11): 4003–4012 (1998).

LaFiura, K.M., H. Edwards, J.W. Taub, L.H. Matherly, J.A. Fontana, A.N. Mohamed, Y. Ravindranath, and Y. Ge, Children's Oncology Group, Identification and characterization of novel AML1-ETO fusion transcripts in pediatric t(8;21) acute myeloid leukemia: a report from the Children's Oncology Group, *Oncogene* **27**(36): 4933–4942 (2008).

Levanon, D., and Y. Groner, Structure and regulated expression of mammalian RUNX genes, *Oncogene* **23**(24): 4211–4219 (2004).

Li, L.M., Z.X. Chen, J.N. Cen, H.J. Shen, L. Yao, Y.Y. Wang, and X.F. Qi, Monitoring the expression ratio of AML1-ETO9a isoform in t(8;21) acute myeloid leukemia and its significance, *Zhonghua Xue Ye Xue Za Zhi* **33**(1): 1–5 (2012).

Li. Y., L. Gao, X. Luo, L. Wang, X. Gao, W. Wang, J. Sun, L. Dou, J. Li, C. Xu, L. Wang, M. Zhou, M. Jiang, J. Zhou, M.A. Caligiuri, C. Nervi, C.D. Bloomfield, G. Marcucci, and L. Yu, Epigenetic silencing of microRNA-193a contributes to leukemogenesis in t(8;21) acute myeloid leukemia by activating the PTEN/PI3K signal pathway, *Blood* **121**(3): 499–509 (2013).

Linka, Y., S. Ginzel, M. Krüger, A. Novosel, M. Gombert, E. Kremmer, J. Harbott, R. Thiele, A. Borkhardt, and P. Landgraf, The impact of TEL-AML1 (ETV6-RUNX1) expression in precursor B cells and implications for leukaemia using three different genome-wide screening methods, *Blood Cancer J* **3**: e151 (2013).

Lo, M.C., and L.F. Peterson, Combined gene expression and DNA occupancy profiling as a strategy to identify therapeutic target(s) in t(8;21) acute myeloid leukemia, *Crit Rev Eukaryot Gene Expr* **23**(2): 103–113 (2013).

Michaud, J., H.S. Scott, and R. Escher, AML1 interconnected pathways of leukemogenesis, *Cancer Invest* **21**(1): 105–136 (2003).

Mitani, K., S. Ogawa, T. Tanaka, H. Miyoshi, M. Kurokawa, H. Mano, Y. Yazaki, M. Ohki, and H. Hirai, Generation of the AML1-EVI-1 fusion gene in the t(3;21)(q26;q22) causes blastic crisis in chronic myelocytic leukemia, *EMBO J* **13**(3): 504–510 (1994).

Mitani, K., Molecular mechanisms of leukemogenesis by AML1/EVI-1, *Oncogene* **23**(24): 4263–4269 (2004).

Morrow, M., A. Samanta, D. Kioussis, H.J. Brady, and O. Williams, TEL-AML1 preleukemic activity requires the DNA binding domain of AML1 and the dimerization and corepressor binding domains of TEL, *Oncogene* **26**(30): 4404–4414 (2007).

Mulloy, J.C., J. Cammenga, K.L. MacKenzie, F.J. Berguido, M.A. Moore, and S.D. Nimer, The AML1-ETO fusion protein promotes the expansion of human hematopoietic stem cells, *Blood* **99**(1): 15–23 (2002).

North, T.E., M.F. de Bruijn, T. Stacy, L. Talebian, E. Lind, C. Robin, M. Binder, E. Dzierzak, and N.A. Speck, Runx1 expression marks long-term repopulating hematopoietic stem cells in the midgestation mouse embryo, *Immunity* **16**(5): 661–672 (2002).

Okuda, T., Z. Cai, S. Yang, N. Lenny, C.J. Lyu, J.M. van Deursen, H. Harada, and J.R. Downing, Expression of a knocked-in AML1-ETO leukemia gene inhibits the establishment of normal definitive hematopoiesis and directly generates dysplastic hematopoietic progenitors, *Blood* **91**(9): 3134–3143 (1998).

Okuda, T., J. van Deursen, S.W. Hiebert, G. Grosveld, and J.R. Downing, AML1, the target of multiple chromosomal translocations in human leukemia, is essential for normal fetal liver hematopoiesis, *Cell* **84**(2): 321–330 (1996).

Palmi, C., G. Fazio, A.M. Savino, J. Procter, L. Howell, V. Cazzaniga, M. Vieri, G. Longinotti, I. Brunati, V. Andrè, P. Della Mina, A. Villa, M. Greaves, A. Biondi, G. D'Amico, A. Ford, and G. Cazzaniga, Cytoskeletal regulatory gene expression and migratory properties of B-cell progenitors are affected by the ETV6-RUNX1 rearrangement, *Mol Cancer Res* **12**(12): 1796–1806 (2014).

Papaemmanuil, E., I. Rapado, Y. Li, N.E. Potter, D.C. Wedge, J. Tubio, L.B. Alexandrov, Van P. Loo, SL. Cooke, J. Marshall, I. Martincorena, J. Hinton, G. Gundem, F.W. van Delft, S. Nik-Zainal, D.R. Jones, M. Ramakrishna, I. Titley, L. Stebbings, C. Leroy, A. Menzies, J. Gamble, B. Robinson, L. Mudie, K. Raine, S. O'Meara, J.W. Teague, A.P. Butler, G. Cazzaniga, A. Biondi, J. Zuna, H. Kempski, M. Muschen, A.M. Ford, M.R. Stratton, M. Greaves, and P.J. Campbell, RAG-mediated recombination is the predominant driver of oncogenic rearrangement in ETV6-RUNX1 acute lymphoblastic leukemia, *Nat Genet* **46**(2): 116–125 (2014).

Parker, H., Q. An, K. Barber, M. Case, T. Davies, Z. Konn, A. Stewart, S. Wright, M. Griffiths, F.M. Ross, A.V. Moorman, A.G. Hall, J.A. Irving, C.J. Harrison, and J.C. Strefford, The complex genomic profile of ETV6-RUNX1 positive acute lymphoblastic leukemia highlights a recurrent deletion of TBL1XR1, *Genes Chromosomes Cancer* **47**(12): 1118–1125 (2008).

Peterson, L.F., and D.E. Zhang, The 8;21 translocation in leukemogenesis, *Oncogene* **23**(24): 4255–4262, Review. PubMed PMID: 15156181 (2004).

Qadi, AA., PC. Taberlay, JL. Phillips, A. Young, AC. West, KH. Brettingham-Moore, JL. Dickinson, AF. Holloway, The leukemia inhibitory factor receptor gene is a direct target of RUNX1, *J Cell Biochem* **117**(1): 49–58 (2016).

Romana, S.P., M. Mauchauffé, M. Le Coniat, I. Chumakov, D. Le Paslier, R. Berger, and O.A. Bernard, The t(12;21) of acute lymphoblastic leukemia results in a tel-AML1 gene fusion, *Blood* **85**(12): 3662–3670 (1995).

Sabaawy, H.E., M. Azuma, L.J. Embree, H.J. Tsai, M.F. Starost, and D.D. Hickstein, TEL-AML1 transgenic zebrafish model of precursor B cell acute lymphoblastic leukemia, *Proc Natl Acad Sci USA* **103**(41): 15166–15171 (2006).

Schemionek, M., Kharabi B. Masouleh, Y. Klaile, U. Krug, K. Hebestreit, C. Schubert, M. Dugas, T. Büchner, B. Wörmann, W. Hiddemann, W.E. Berdel, T.H. Brümmendorf, C. Müller-Tidow, and S. Koschmieder, Identification of the Adapter Molecule MTSS1 as a Potential Oncogene-Specific Tumor Suppressor in Acute Myeloid Leukemia, *PLoS One* **10**(5): e0125783 (2015).

Shen, L., J. Zhu, F. Chen, W. Lin, J. Cai, J. Zhong, and H. Zhong, RUNX1-Evi-1 fusion gene inhibited differentiation and apoptosis in myelopoiesis: an in vivo study, *BMC Cancer* **15**: 970 (2015).

Stoskus, M., G. Vaitkeviciene, A. Eidukaite, and L. Griskevicius, ETV6/RUNX1 transcript is a target of RNA-binding protein IGF2BP1 in t(12;21)(p13;q22)-positive acute lymphoblastic leukemia, *Blood Cells Mol Dis* **57**: 30–34 (2016).

Sun, X.J., Z. Wang, L. Wang, Y. Jiang, N. Kost, T.D. Soong, W.Y. Chen, Z. Tang, T. Nakadai, O. Elemento, W. Fischle, A. Melnick, D.J. Patel, S.D. Nimer, and R.G. Roeder, A stable transcription factor complex nucleated by oligomeric AML1-ETO controls leukaemogenesis, *Nature* **500**(7460): 93–97 (2013).

Tanaka, K., T. Tanaka, M. Kurokawa, Y. Imai, S. Ogawa, K. Mitani, Y. Yazaki, and H. Hirai, The AML1/ETO(MTG8) and AML1/Evi-1 leukemia-associated chimeric oncoproteins accumulate PEBP2beta(CBFbeta) in the nucleus more efficiently than wild-type AML1, *Blood* **91**(5): 1688–1699 (1998).

Tanaka, T., K. Mitani, M. Kurokawa, S. Ogawa, K. Tanaka, J. Nishida, Y. Yazaki, Y. Shibata, and H. Hirai, Dual functions of the AML1/Evi-1 chimeric protein in the mechanism of leukemogenesis in t(3;21) leukemias, *Mol Cell Biol* **15**(5): 2383–2392 (1995).

Torrano, V., J. Procter, P. Cardus, M. Greaves, and A.M. Ford, ETV6-RUNX1 promotes survival of early B lineage progenitor cells via a dysregulated erythropoietin receptor, *Blood* **118**(18): 4910–4918 (2011).

Ugarte, G.D., M.F. Vargas, M.A. Medina, P. León, D. Necuñir, A.A. Elorza, S.E. Gutiérrez, R.T. Moon, A. Loyola, and G.V. De Ferrari, Wnt signaling induces transcription, spatial proximity, and translocation of fusion gene partners in human hematopoietic cells, *Blood* **126**(15): 1785–1789 (2015).

van der Weyden, L., G. Giotopoulos, K. Wong, A.G. Rust, C.D. Robles-Espinoza, H. Osaki, B.J. Huntly, and D.J. Adams, Somatic drivers of B-ALL in a model of ETV6-RUNX1; Pax5(+/-) leukemia, *BMC Cancer* **15**: 585 (2015).

Wang, Q., T. Stacy, M. Binder, M. Marin-Padilla, A.H. Sharpe, and N.A. Speck Disruption of the Cbfa2 gene causes necrosis and hemorrhaging in the central nervous system and blocks definitive hematopoiesis, *Proc Natl Acad Sci U S A* **93**(8): 3444–3449 (1996).

Wichmann, C., Quagliano-Lo I. Coco, Ö. Yildiz, L. Chen-Wichmann, H. Weber, T. Syzonenko, C. Döring, C. Brendel, K. Ponnusamy, A. Kinner, C. Brandts,

R. Henschler, and M. Grez, Activating c-KIT mutations confer oncogenic cooperativity and rescue RUNX1/ETO-induced DNA damage and apoptosis in human primary CD34+ hematopoietic progenitors, *Leukemia* **29**(2): 279–289 (2015).

Wiemels, J.L., G. Cazzaniga, M. Daniotti, O.B. Eden, G.M. Addison, G. Masera, V. Saha, A. Biondi, and M.F. Greaves, Prenatal origin of acute lymphoblastic leukaemia in children, *Lancet* **354**(9189): 1499–1503 (1999a).

Wiemels, J.L., A.M. Ford, E.R. Van Wering, A. Postma, and M. Greaves, Protracted and variable latency of acute lymphoblastic leukemia after TEL-AML1 gene fusion in utero, *Blood* **94**(3): 1057–1062 (1999b).

Yang, Y.L., C.T. Yen, C.H. Pai, H.Y. Chen, S.L. Yu, C.Y. Lin, C.Y. Hu, S.T. Jou, D.T. Lin, S.R. Lin, and S.W. Lin, A Double Negative Loop Comprising ETV6/RUNX1 and MIR181A1 Contributes to Differentiation Block in t(12;21)-Positive Acute Lymphoblastic Leukemia, *PLoS One* **10**(11): e0142863 (2015).

Yotnda, P., F. Garcia, M. Peuchmaur, B. Grandchamp, M. Duval, F. Lemonnier, E. Vilmer, and P. Langlade-Demoyen, Cytotoxic T cell response against the chimeric ETV6-AML1 protein in childhood acute lymphoblastic leukemia, *J Clin Invest* **102**(2): 455–462 (1998).

Zelent, A., M. Greaves, and T. Enver, Role of the TEL-AML1 fusion gene in the molecular pathogenesis of childhood acute lymphoblastic leukaemia, *Oncogene* **23**(24): 4275–4283 (2004).

Zhang, Y., J. Wang, J. Wheat, X. Chen, S. Jin, H. Sadrzadeh, A.T. Fathi, R.T. Peterson, A.L. Kung, D.A. Sweetser, and J.R. Yeh, AML1-ETO mediates hematopoietic self-renewal and leukemogenesis through a COX/β-catenin signaling pathway, *Blood* **121**(24): 4906–4916 (2013).

Zhuang, W.Y., J.N. Cen, Y. Zhao, and Z.X. Chen, Epigenetic silencing of Bcl-2, CEBPA and p14(ARF) by the AML1-ETO oncoprotein contributing to growth arrest and differentiation block in the U937 cell line, *Oncol Rep* **30**(1): 185–192 (2013a).

Zhuang, W.Y., Z.Y. Li, Y. Zhao, J.N. Cen, W.Z. Zhuang, and Z.X. Chen, Effect of AML1-ETO fusion protein on the expression of BCL-2, *Zhongguo Shi Yan Xue Ye Xue Za Zhi* **21**(6): 1394–1398 (2013b).

20

Recently Discovered Fusion Genes and Their Implications in Cancer

*Ganesan Padmavathi, Devivasha Bordoloi, Javadi Monisha, Nand K. Roy, Choudhary Harsha and Ajaikumar B. Kunnumakkara**

INTRODUCTION

Discovery of Philadelphia chromosome further encouraged the identification of plenty of novel chromosomal translocations and associated fusion transcripts, most of them being abnormally activated fusion tyrosine kinases and transcription factors (Chinnaiyan and Palanisamy, 2010). Moreover, detection of these fusion proteins and their deregulation in cancer served as diagnostic and prognostic biomarkers, treatment targets and also used

*Author for correspondence: Ajaikumar B. Kunnumakkara, Cancer Biology Laboratory, Department of Biosciences and Bioengineering, Indian Institute of Technology Guwahati, Assam 781039, India. kunnumakkara@iitg.ernet.in

to classify the complex neoplasms as certain fusion genes were exclusively associated with particular cancers (Chinnaiyan and Palanisamy, 2010; Aman, 1999). For example, BCR-ABL, RET-PTC, TMPRSS2-ERG, BRD4-NUT, MYB-NFIB fusion genes were specifically involved in the tumorigenesis of leukemia, thyroid cancers, prostate cancers, NUT midline carcinoma and ACC, respectively, therefore regarded as hallmark of respective malignancies. In the previous chapters, we have discussed the implication of commonly occurring and frequently studied fusion genes and their oncogenic potential in the development and maintenance of several neoplasms including both haematological and solid tumors. However, several other fusion transcripts have been discovered in small population of tumors and are not fully characterized for their exact function and downstream targets. Therefore, the scope of this chapter is to discuss such fusion genes and their associated cancers in detail.

SOLID TUMORS AND ASSOCIATED FUSION GENES

Tumors of non-liquid and non-cystic origin such as bone, muscle and organs were regarded as solid tumors which can be either benign or malignant. Depending on the tissue of origin, the solid tumors were categorized into carcinomas, sarcomas and adenomas. Plenty of fusion transcripts and their impact on tumorigenesis of these cancers have been unfolded by several decades of research. However, a number of novel fusion genes are also being identified every day. These newly identified translocations and their involvement in cancer development are not yet completely explored and less cited in literature. In the following section, we tried to expose such translocations associated with different solid tumors.

CD74-NRG1

CD74-NRG1 fusion identified in lung adenocarcinoma was known to induce the disease via activation of PI3K-AKT pathway (Fernandez-Cuesta *et al.*,

2014; Duruisseaux and Wislez, 2014). It has also been shown to induce cancer stem cell-like properties through the phosphorylation activation of ErbB2/3 and PI3K/Akt/NF-κB and IGF2/IGF1R signaling pathways (Murayama *et al.*, 2016).

CD74-ROS

CD74-ROS is a chimeric tyrosine kinase detected in non-small cell lung cancers, overexpression of which enhanced the phosphorylation of extended synaptotagmin-like protein 1 (E-Syt1) contributing to the invasiveness of the disease (Jun *et al.*, 2012).

CIC-DUX4

This fusion has been identified in primitive small round cell sarcomas (SRCSs), distinct variant of Ewing-like sarcoma, and generated by t(4;19)(q35;q13.1) translocation (Choi *et al.*, 2013; Italiano *et al.*, 2012; Tardío *et al.*, 2015). Fusion of double homeobox 4 (DUX4) gene increased the transactivation potential of the CIC gene and induced activation of various downstream targets thus resulting in malignant transformation *in vitro* (Kawamura-Saito *et al.*, 2006). Similarly, another fusion gene involving the CIC gene has also been detected in SRCs, CIC-FOXO4 with t(X;19)(q13;q13.3) translocation (Sugita *et al.*, 2014). Other than CIC-DUX4 and CIC-FOXO4, three fusions: BCOR-CCNB3, BCOR-MAML3 and ZC3H7B-BCOR have also been detected in small blue round cell tumors (SBRCTs) (Specht *et al.*, 2016).

EIF3E-RSPO2

Seshagiri *et al.* (2012) reported a novel fusion protein EIF3E-RSPO2 in colon cancer involving R-spondin, a secreted protein that can alter canonical Wnt signaling pathway (Yoon and Lee, 2012; Seshagiri *et al.*, 2012; Shinmura *et al.*, 2014). This protein is the product of fusion of exon 1 of EIF3E with exon 2 of RSPO2 gene. WGS analysis revealed that the genomic deletion placed the exon1 of EIF3E in close proximity to the 5′ end of RSPO2 supporting their fusion. It has been reported to deregulate the Wnt signaling target genes (Seshagiri *et al.*, 2012). However, extensive research is needed in deciphering the actual role of this fusion protein in the development of colon cancer.

ESRRA-C11orf20

Estrogen-related receptor alpha (ESRRA) gene encoding a nuclear receptor similar to that of estrogen receptor is fused with C11orf20, an open reading frame sequence, to form ESRRA–C11orf20 translocation. The breakpoint was found to occur in the long arm of chromosome 11 at q13.1 region (Micci *et al.*, 2014a). In 2011, it was first detected in serous ovarian carcinomas by deep paired-end mRNA and respective genomic region sequencing and shown to have high frequency of occurrence, as in a total of 67 tumor samples analyzed, 15% expressed this fusion protein (Salzman *et al.*, 2011). In contrast to the previous study, recently Micci *et al.* (2014a) showed that the frequency of ESRRA–C11orf20 fusion in serous ovarian carcinomas is very low (Micci *et al.*, 2014a). It is doubtful that this fusion has any decisive role in tumorigenesis and may be the consequence of other functionally important genetic events or a "passenger" to other structural rearrangements as the distance between these two partner genes was found very less as 11 kb (Micci *et al.*, 2014a). Only two studies were reported on this fusion gene to date and both are showing conflicting results. Therefore, more extensive studies need to be performed to reveal the actual role of this fusion transcript.

FIG-ROS1

FIG-ROS1 fusion gene produced by a microdeletion on 6q21 i.e. del(6)(q21q21) occurred in glioblastoma and intrahepatic cholangiocarcinoma (ICC) (Charest *et al.*, 2003a, 2003b; Saborowski *et al.*, 2013). This deletion-induced fusion protein resulted in the constitutive activation of the RTK through subcellular localization to the Golgi apparatus. The oncogenic transforming potential of the chimera is also attributed to the interaction and localization of FIG-ROS1 to the Golgi apparatus (Charest *et al.*, 2003a). This chimeric tyrosine kinase was shown to induce the activation of SH2 domain-containing phosphatase-2 (SHP-2)/PI3K/

mTOR signaling axis (Charest *et al.*, 2006). Subsequently, in the development of ICC, deregulation of AKT signaling by the chimeric protein was found to be the key mechanism, inhibition of which suppressed cell proliferation, colony-formation, cell cycle progression, migration and invasion, and induced apoptosis (Deng *et al.*, 2014). CD74-ROS1, SLC34A2-ROS1 and TPM3-ROS1 are the other fusion proteins involving the RTK ROS and were associated with non-small cell lung cancer (Rimkunas *et al.*, 2012; Hong *et al.*, 2016; Jun *et al.*, 2012; Wiesner *et al.*, 2014).

HMGA2-LPP

The high mobility group (HMG) protein gene HMGA2, also known as HMGIC from chromosome 12, was linked with the LIM protein family gene LPP from chromosome 3 by t(3;12)(q27-28;q14-15) translocation in a subset of lipomas and pulmonary chondroid hamartomas (Petit *et al.*, 1996; Rogalla *et al.*, 2000). The resultant fusion protein retained the active LIM domains of LPP thus acting as a potent transcription factor. This transactivation function of the HMGA2-LPP protein was further enhanced when co-expressed with the wild-type HMGA2 which may be a key factor in lipomagenesis (Crombez *et al.*, 2005). Besides adipogenesis, the over-expression of HMGA2-LPP chimera also induced chondrogenesis through the upregulation of alpha 2 type XI collagen gene (COL11A2) (Kubo *et al.*, 2006).

MTAP-ANRIL

Very recently, Xie *et al.* (2016) identified this fusion in melanoma cell lines, derived from metastasized tumors which remains to be further characterized (Xie *et al.*, 2016).

NAB2-STAT6

The early growth response (EGR)-binding domain of NGFI-A binding protein 2 (NAB2), also known as EGR1 binding protein 2, was fused to the activation domain of STAT6 to form the NAB2-STAT6, recurrently observed in meningeal hemangiopericytoma and solitary fibrous tumors (SFT). Further, it has been found to be the driving factor of SFTs and to increase the expression of EGR-responsive genes (Robinson *et al.*, 2013; Nakada *et al.*, 2015; Barthelmeß *et al.*, 2014; Fritchie *et al.*, 2016).

PLAG1 Fusions

In certain cases of lipoblastomas, chromosomal rearrangement involving 8q12 was observed where the entire coding sequence of pleiomorphic adenoma gene 1 (PLAG1) was fused to the promotor regions of either hyaluronic acid synthase 2 (HAS2) or collagen 1 alpha 2 (COL1A2) or RAD51L1 genes (Hibbard *et al.*, 2000; Yoshida *et al.*, 2014). The PLAG1-HAS2 fusion was produced by a peculiar intrachromosomal rearrangement between 8q12.1 and 8q24.1 but the PLAG1-COL1A2 and PLAG1-RAD51L1 were produced by the translocation of 8q12 with 7q22 or 14q24, respectively (Morerio *et al.*, 2005; Yoshida *et al.*, 2014). Recently, two more fusion partners of PLAG1 have been detected in lipoblastoma, namely, COL3A1 and RAB2A (Yoshida *et al.*, 2014). Further, CHCHD7, CTNNB1, LIFR and TCEA1genes were also found to be rearranged with PLAG1 in pleomorphic salivary gland adenomas (Asp *et al.*, 2006; Aström *et al.*, 1999; Voz *et al.*, 1998). All these fusions were shown to induce the overexpression of PLAG1 gene (Yoshida *et al.*, 2014). PLAG1 is a well-known oncogene, expression of which was highly upregulated by the fusion-mediated promotor swapping thus initiating the development of lipoblastoma (Hibbard *et al.*, 2000; Yoshida *et al.*, 2014). Moreover, PLAG1 rearrangements and its overexpression remain as potential biomarkers of lipoblastoma (Yoshida *et al.*, 2014).

PTPRK-RSPO3

The PTPRK-RSPO3 fusion gene resulting from the fusion of either exon1 or exon 7 of PTPRK with exon2 of R-spondin (RSPO3) gene was reported to be associated with colon cancer (Seshagiri *et al.*, 2012). This rearrangement was generated by chromosomal inversions that placed RSPO3 close to PTPRK on chromosome 6. In the PTPRK(e1)–RSPO3(e2) in frame fusion, only the secretion signal sequence was replaced with that of PTPRK keeping the whole coding sequence of RSPO3 intact. Whereas, in PTPRK(e7)–RSPO3(e2) fusion, a 70 kDa protein consisting of first 387 amino acids of PTPRK along with its secretion signal sequence is fused with 34-327 amino acids of RSPO3 lacking its native signal sequence. It was also reported that RSPO-gene fusions in colon cancer upregulated Wnt signaling target genes in a similar fashion to tumors with adenomatous polyposis coli (APC) mutations (Seshagiri *et al.*, 2012). Therefore, targeting the RSPO3 portion of the fusion transcript would promote differentiation providing a better prognosis (Storm *et al.*, 2016).

SDK1-AMACR

It was identified in Chinese prostate cancer samples and found to exhibit as a transcription-mediated chimeric RNA and correlated with the increased expression of AMACR (alpha-methylacyl-CoA racemase) which is believed to mediate prostate carcinogenesis (Zhang *et al.*, 2015).

SYT-SSX

A team of scientists working on cancer genetics in the Institute of Cancer Research, London, for the first time observed a consistent chromosomal translocation occurring in patients with synovial sarcoma (SS) in 1987 (Smith *et al.*, 1987). The finding led to extensive research aimed at elucidating the cytogenetic basis of this disease. Other groups also confirmed the evidence of chromosomal translocation in synovial sarcoma and categorically described that the translocation involved chromosome Xp11.2 and chromosome 18q11.2. Further, t(X;18)(p11;q11) chromosomal translocation was also subsequently reported in synovial sarcoma of orofacial, submandibular, thoracic and cardiac region but absent in other cases of soft tissue tumor proving its specificity to synovial sarcoma and potential as a genetic marker of the disease (Bridge *et al.*, 1988; Udayakumar *et al.*, 2002; Iyengar *et al.*, 1995; Yano *et al.*, 2004; Ladanyi, 2001). Further studies by the same UK-based group who first reported the chromosomal translocation, identified the candidate genes involved as SYT and SSX genes located in chromosome 18 and chromosome X, respectively, which are the principal mediators in causing synovial sarcoma. More specifically, the fusion was found to occur between SYT4 and any one of the SSX genes from SSX1 to SSX9 (Turc-Carel *et al.*, 1987; Clark *et al.*, 1994; Dimitriadis *et al.*, 2009). Among them, SYT-SSX1 and SYT-SSX2 were most commonly associated with SS and the other fusion transcripts were found in very rare cases (Dimitriadis *et al.*, 2009). In line with this, clinical data also suggested that more than 95% of synovial sarcoma cases were found to be positive for the t(X;18)(p11.2;q11.2) translocation with SYT-SSX1 transcript present in 55% patients and SYT-SSX2 in 42.5% patients. This implicated the use of SYT-SSX proteins as potential diagnostic markers for SS (Przybyl *et al.*, 2012; Yoneda *et al.*, 2013). The wild-type SYT protein localized in NBs plays a central role in SS acting as a transcriptional activator. Hence, it was also referred as SS18 protein. Fusion of the C-terminal domain of SSX with SYT resulted in a potent transcriptional co-activator and mediated the transactivation of different target genes. Additionally, as almost entire sequence of SYT was fused to SSX, the resultant chimera possessed both transcriptional activating and repressing domains (Brett *et al.*, 1997; Ladanyi, 2001). Further, it was proved to play a critical role in regulating the Wnt/β-catenin pathway (Barham *et al.*, 2013; Trautmann *et al.*, 2014). The other molecular targets of this chimeric protein were found to be E-cadherin, AXIN2, p300, miR-17, COM1, IGF2, CD44, p21WAF1/CIP1, NCOA3, hBRM/hSNF2α chromatin remodeling complex and polycomb subunit Bmil or Bmi1, etc. (Saito, 2013; Saito *et al.*, 2006; Thaete *et al.*, 1999; Nagai *et al.*, 2001; Ladanyi, 2001; Dimitriadis *et al.*, 2009; Eid *et al.*, 2000; Cironi *et al.*, 2016; Minami *et al.*, 2014; Sun *et al.*, 2011; Barco *et al.*, 2009; Ishida *et al.*, 2007; de Bruijn *et al.*, 2006). Moreover, recent reports claimed that the SS18-SSX fusion protein can also be used as a therapeutic target for synovial sarcoma as knockdown of SS18-SSX1 splice variant in synovial carcinoma related cell lines led to decreased cell viability and increased apoptosis (Carmody *et al.*, 2014). Further supporting this claim, truncated SSX domain of this fusion protein was reported to inhibit the localization of the protein and suppress the proliferation of synovial carcinoma cells (Yoneda *et al.*, 2013).

TBL1XR1-HMGA1

TBL1XR1-HMGA1 fusion gene was formed by the translocation of chromosomes 3 and 6 denoted as t(3;6)(q26;p21) and first identified in splenic hemangioma (Panagopoulos *et al.*, 2016).

TFE3 Translocations

Chromosomal translocations linking the transcription factor TFE3 gene at Xp11.2 to six different genes, namely, ASPSCR1 at 17q25, SFPQ at 1p34 and PRCC at 1q21, PSF at 1q34, CLTC at 17q23, PARP14 at 3q23 and NONO at Xq12 are frequently seen in alveolar soft part sarcoma (ASPS) and renal cell carcinomas (RCCs) (Kobos *et al.*, 2013; Pérot *et al.*, 2003; Huang *et al.*, 2015). The functional domains of TFE3 remained intact in these translocations resulting in a transcriptional activator protein with greater potency than the normal TFE3 (Medendorp *et al.*, 2009). Further, all these fusions in addition to MALAT1-TFEB fusion were found to regulate various cellular processes involved in tumorigenesis such as E-cadherin, TGFβ, cyclin D1 and D3, p21 and ETS transcription factors activation; mTORC1 signaling; folliculin signaling; CD40L-mediated lymphocyte activation and Rb-dependent cell cycle arrest (Kauffman *et al.*, 2014; Müller-Höcker *et al.*, 2008). Interestingly, the oncogenic effect of these translocations in pediatric and young adult carcinomas was found to be indolent unlike the aggressive effect found in case of older patients (Kuroda *et al.*, 2012).

ASPSCR1-TFE3 resulting from t(X;17)(p11.2;q25) was detected in both alveolar soft part sarcoma and renal cell carcinomas, whereas the other two fusions are unique to RCCs (Kobos *et al.*, 2013; Martignoni *et al.*, 2011). Fusion of ASPSCR1 to TFE3 significantly increased the transactivation potential of the latter and upregulated various target genes including CYP17A1 and UPP1 by direct binding of the fusion product (Kobos *et al.*, 2013). Moreover, increased expression of a protease enzyme cathepsin K was observed in ASPSCR1-TFE3-mediated alveolar soft part sarcoma and not in carcinoma thus distinguishing from sarcoma giving it a diagnostic advantage (Martignoni *et al.*, 2011).

The t(X;1)(p11.2;q21) translocation in which the entire TFE3 is juxtaposed to the N-terminal proline-rich domain of PRCC, the most common fusion partner of TFE3 was surprisingly associated with the complete loss of wild-type TFE3 gene in RCC (Pérot *et al.*, 2003; Argani *et al.*, 2002; Meloni *et al.*, 1993; Onder *et al.*, 2006; Sidhar *et al.*, 1996; Skalsky *et al.*, 2001; Weterman *et al.*, 1996). Further, this fusion protein was determined to cooperate with the pre-mRNA splicing factors; to disrupt the interaction with MAD2B; and to deregulate mitotic checkpoint in RCCs (Skalsky *et al.*, 2001; Weterman *et al.*, 2001). Despite the cell proliferating effect of PRCC-TFE3, a recent study demonstrated that it can delay the cell cycle progression by binding to the promotor of cyclin-dependent kinase inhibitor p21(WAF1/CIP1), and inducing its expression thus driving the pRb-dependent cell cycle arrest. The PRCC-TFE3 induced cell cycle arrest was proposed to be inhibited by additional mutations during the initial phases of RCC development (Medendorp *et al.*, 2009). Like ASPSCR1-TFE3 alveolar soft part sarcoma, expression of cathepsin K was detected in PRCC-TFE3 carcinoma as well (Martignoni *et al.*, 2011).

PSF-TFE3 fusion protein resulting from t(X;1)(p11.2;q34) translocation was observed to induce anchorage-independent growth and dedifferentiation and to sequester TFE3 and p53 proteins leading to their inactivation in RCC cells (Mathur *et al.*, 2003, 2007). Two more translocations involving the TFE3 gene viz. t(X;10)(p11;q23), and t(X;19)(p11;q13) were identified. However, the exact description of the partner genes remains elusive (Huang *et al.*, 2015).

HAEMATOLOGICAL MALIGNANCIES AND ASSOCIATED FUSION GENES

Tumors of body fluids including blood and lymph are categorized as haematological malignancies which include all type of leukemias and lymphomas. After the discovery of Philadelphia chromosome in leukemia, thousands of studies have been carried out on deciphering the role of the resultant BCR-ABL chimera in the development of leukemia. Likewise, several other fusion genes are also being consistently discovered in different types of haematological malignancies in which some are well characterized whereas some remain elusive. In this section of the chapter, we will discuss the identification and role of uncharacterized fusion genes of haematological cancers.

CTLA4-CD28

Fusion of the extracellular domain of CTLA4 and the cytoplasmic domain of CD28 was identified in T-cell lymphoma. The partner genes were having contrary functions in T-cell signaling, whereas the fusion gene resulted in the increased phosphorylation of Akt and ERK (Yoo *et al.*, 2016).

NUP98-NSD1

NUP98 fusions with various partner genes have been detected in AML however, with very less frequency (Nebral *et al.*, 2005). NSD1 was one of the partner genes fused to NUP98 by the t(5;11)(q35;p15.5) translocation, which was found to be associated with 5q deletion as well (Jaju *et al.*, 2001). However, NUP98-NSD1 without 5q deletion was also reported in AML (Panarello *et al.*, 2002). In addition to AML, NUP98-NSD1 had been detected in myelodysplastic syndrome (MDS) as well, yet, the fusion was found to be resulted from cryptic insertion of NUP98 to the NSD1/5q35 locus and not from the t(5;11) translocation (La *et al.*, 2004). Further, NUP98-NSD1 chimera induced leukemogenesis through the upregulation of proto-oncogenes like HoxA7, HoxA9, HoxA10 and Meis1 by preventing their EZH2-mediated transcriptional repression which was attributed to the fusion-mediated deregulation of H3K36 methylation and histone acetylation (Wang *et al.*, 2007). Interestingly, it has been found to cooperate with another activating mutation FLT3-ITD in 70% of the cases (Thanasopoulou *et al.*, 2014). Moreover, it was seen to be associated with poor prognosis thereby indicating the requirement of novel treatment strategies (Hollink *et al.*, 2011; Shiba *et al.*, 2013; Akiki *et al.*, 2013). Various other fusion partners of NUP98 include NSD3, HOXA9, HOXA11, HOXA13, HOXC13, HOXD11, HOXD13, DDX10, RAP1GDS1, LEDGF, PMX1, TOP1, JARID1A and ANKRD28. All these fusion genes were associated with different haematological malignancies. Moreover, fusion of NUP98 with the homeobox genes was found to be the most common rearrangement (Panagopoulos *et al.*, 2003; de Rooij *et al.*, 2013; Ishikawa *et al.*, 2007).

PCM1-JAK2

t(8;9)(p22;p24) translocation was known to ligate the coiled-coil domain of PCM1 to the kinase domain of non-RTK JAK2 and reported to be associated with both acute and chronic leukemia and with T-cell lymphoma (Reiter *et al.*, 2005; Bousquet *et al.*, 2005; Adélaïde *et al.*, 2006). The t(8;9) translocation induced the oligomerization and activation of the JAK2 kinase which in turn phosphorylated and activated STAT5 ultimately resulting in the activation of suppressors of cytokine signaling 2 and 3 (SOCS2 & SOCS3) (Hoeller *et al.*, 2011; Ehrentraut *et al.*, 2013).

TCF3-PBX1

t(1;19)(q23;p13) translocation produced the fusion of N-terminal transactivation domain of transcription factor 3 (TCF3), also known as E2A gene and C-terminal DNA-binding homeodomain of pre-B-cell leukemia homeobox 1 (PBX1) gene, which is most commonly observed in precursor-B-cell ALL (pre B-ALL) and deregulated the Wnt, apoptosis, cell cycle regulation and JunD transcriptional pathways (Scheele *et al.*, 2009; Hajingabo *et al.*, 2014; Tirado *et al.*, 2015; Diakos *et al.*, 2014). In addition to this, overexpression of the proto-oncogene BCL6 has also been observed in t(1;19) positive B-lymphoblastic leukemia suggesting a correlation between TCF3-PBX1 translocation and BCL6 expression (Deucher *et al.*, 2015). Interestingly, the C-terminal homeodomain of PBX1 portion was empirically proved to have very less or no effect on the fusion-induced transactivation of growth related genes supporting the possible interaction of E2A elements with unidentified coactivator complexes which may have a decisive role in this context (Bayly *et al.*, 2000). Moreover, this TCF3-PBX1 translocation as sole abnormality presented an intermediate prognosis, whereas additional cytogenetic changes especially hyperdiploidy increased the complications (Tirado *et al.*, 2015). Though TCF3-PBX1 was thought to be associated with better clinical behavior, CNS relapse was commonly observed in these cases which proved the requirement of altered CNS-directed chemotherapy regimen for the fusion positive ALL (ElGendi *et al.*, 2014).

ZMYND11-MBTD1

t(10;17)(p15;q21) chromosomal rearrangement associated with minimally differentiated AML was recently identified to fuse the otherwise tumor suppressor gene ZMYND11 to the chromatin protein MBTD1. It was found to deregulate the HOXA expression contributing to leukemogenesis (de Rooij *et al.*, 2016).

Apart from the above mentioned genes, several other fusion genes have been identified in various cancers (*http://cancer.sanger.ac.uk/cosmic/fusion*). However, their molecular bases have not been completely understood. Such chimeric genes are listed below: ACBD6/RRP15 (Stephens *et al.*, 2009), ACSL3/ETV1 (Attard *et al.*, 2008), ACTB/GLI1 (Bridge *et al.*, 2012), AGTRAP/BRAF (Palanisamy *et al.*, 2010), ARID1A/MAST2 (Robinson *et al.*, 2011), BCR/JAK2 (Lane *et al.*, 2008), CANT1/ETV4 (Han *et al.*, 2008), CDH11/USP6 (Oliveira *et al.*, 2004), CDKN2D/WDFY2 (Kannan *et al.*, 2014), CEP89/BRAF (Wiesner *et al.*, 2014), CIC/DUX4 (Graham *et al.*, 2012), CIC/FOXO4 (Sugita *et al.*, 2014), CLCN6/BRAF (Jones *et al.*, 2013), CLIP1/ROS1 (Wiesner *et al.*, 2014), COL1A1/PDGFB (Navarro *et al.*, 1998), COL1A1/USP6 (Panagopoulos *et al.*, 2008), DNAJB1/PRKACA (Graham *et al.*, 2015), EPC1/PHF1 (Micci *et al.*, 2006), ERC1/ROS1 (Wiesner *et al.*, 2014), ERO1L/FERMT2 (Stephens *et al.*, 2009), ETV6/ITPR2 (Stephens *et al.*, 2009), EWSR1/NFATC1 (Arbajian *et al.*, 2013), EWSR1/NFATC2 (Szuhai *et al.*, 2009), EWSR1/SMARCA5 (Sumegi *et al.*, 2011), EWSR1/SP3 (Wang *et al.*, 2007), EWSR1/YY1 (Panagopoulos *et al.*, 2013), EWSR1/ZNF384 (Martini *et al.*, 2002), EWSR1/ZNF444 (Brandal *et al.*, 2009), EZR/ROS1 (Lee *et al.*, 2013), FCHSD1/BRAF (Dessars *et al.*, 2007), GNAI1/BRAF (Jones *et al.*, 2013), GPBP1L1/MAST2 (Robinson *et al.*, 2011), HEY1/NCOA2 (Wang *et al.*, 2012), HLA-A/ROS1 (Wiesner *et al.*, 2014), HMGA2/ALDH2 (Kazmierczak *et al.*, 1995), HMGA2/CCNB1IP1 (Mine *et al.*, 2001), HMGA2/COX6C (Kurose *et al.*, 2000), HMGA2/EBF1 (Nilsson *et al.*, 2006), HMGA2/FHIT (Geurts *et al.*, 1997), HMGA2/LHFP (Petit *et al.*, 1999), HMGA2/NFIB (Geurts *et al.*, 1998), HMGA2/RAD51B (Takahashi *et al.*, 2001), HMGA2/WIF1 (Queimado *et al.*, 2007), HN1/USH1G (Stephens *et al.*, 2009), HNRNPA2B1/ETV1 (Han *et al.*, 2008), HOOK3/RET (Ciampi *et al.*, 2007), INTS4/GAB2 (Stephens *et al.*, 2009), IRF2BP2-CDX1 (Nyquist *et al.*, 2012), JAZF1/PHF1 (Micci *et al.*, 2006), JAZF1/SUZ12 (Koontz *et al.*, 2001), KIAA1598/ROS1 (Wiesner *et al.*, 2014), KIF5B/RET (Kohno *et al.*, 2012), KLK2/ETV1 (Pflueger *et al.*, 2011), KLK2/ETV4 (Hermans *et al.*, 2008), KMT2A/ACTN4 (Yang *et al.*, 2014), KMT2A/BTBD18 (Alonso *et al.*, 2010), KMT2A/CASP8AP2 (Park *et al.*, 2009), KMT2A/CT45A2 (Cerveira *et al.*, 2010), KMT2A/FRYL (Robinson *et al.*, 2008), KMT2A/KIAA0284 (Burmeister *et al.*, 2008), KMT2A/KIAA1524 (Coenen *et al.*, 2011), KMT2A/MAPRE1 (Fu *et al.*, 2005), KMT2A/MYO1F (Taki *et al.*, 2005), KMT2A/NRIP3 (Balgobind *et al.*, 2009), KMT2A/PDS5A (Put *et al.*, 2012), KMT2A/PRRC1 (Douet-Guilbert *et al.*, 2014), KMT2A/SARNP (Hashii *et al.*, 2004), KMT2A/SORBS2 (Pession *et al.*, 2006), KMT2A/TOP3A (Herbaux *et al.*, 2012), LMNA/NTRK1 (Wiesner *et al.*, 2014), LSM14A/BRAF (Wiesner *et al.*, 2014), MBOAT2/PRKCE (Stephens *et al.*, 2009), MBTD1-CXorf67 (Dewaele *et al.*, 2014), MEAF6/PHF1 (Micci *et al.*, 2014b), MKRN1/BRAF (Jones *et al.*, 2013), MYO5A/ROS1 (Wiesner *et al.*, 2014), NACC2/NTRK2 (Jones *et al.*, 2013), NFIA/EHF (Stephens *et al.*, 2009), NFIX/MAST1 (Robinson *et al.*, 2011), NUP107/LGR5 (Wang *et al.*, 2012), OMD/USP6 (Oliveira *et al.*, 2005), PLA2R1/RBMS1 (Stephens *et al.*, 2009), PLXND1/TMCC1 (Stephens *et al.*, 2009), PPFIBP1/ROS1 (Wiesner *et al.*, 2014), PWWP2A/ROS1 (Wiesner *et al.*, 2014), QKI/NTRK2 (Jones *et al.*, 2013), RAF1/DAZL (Stephens *et al.*, 2009), RGS22/SYCP1 (Stephens *et al.*, 2009), RNF130/BRAF (Jones *et al.*, 2013), SDC4/ROS1 (Gainor *et al.*, 2013), SEC16A/NOTCH1 (Robinson *et al.*, 2011), SEC31A/JAK2 (Van *et al.*, 2011), SEPT8/AFF4 (Stephens *et al.*, 2009), SLC26A6/PRKAR2A (Stephens *et al.*, 2009), SS18L1/SSX1 (Storlazzi *et al.*, 2003), SSBP2/JAK2 (Poitras *et al.*, 2008), TADA2A/MAST1 (Robinson *et al.*, 2011), TCF12/NR4A3 (Sjögren *et al.*, 2001), TFG/NR4A3 (Hisaoka *et al.*, 2004), TFG/NTRK1 (Greco *et al.*, 1995), THRAP3/USP6 (Oliveira *et al.*, 2005), TP53/NTRK1 (Wiesner *et al.*, 2014), TPM3/NTRK1 (Butti *et al.*, 1995), VTI1A/TCF7L2 (Bass *et al.*, 2011), YWHAE/FAM22 (O'Meara *et al.*, 2012), ZCCHC8/ROS1 (Wiesner *et al.*, 2014) and ZNF700/MAST1 (Robinson *et al.*, 2011).

CONCLUSION

Overall in this chapter, we have discussed the discovery and role of various uncommon and recently identified fusion proteins in the tumorigenesis of solid and haematological malignancies. Besides their impact in tumorigenesis process, the possible diagnostic and treatment values were also described. However, detailed reports are required to completely unfold the function of these chimeric proteins.

CONFLICT OF INTEREST

The authors express no conflict of interest.

REFERENCES

Adélaïde, J., C. Pérot, V. Gelsi-Boyer, C. Pautas, A. Murati, C. Copie-Bergman, M. Imbert, M. Chaffanet, D. Birnbaum, and M.J. Mozziconacci, A t(8;9) translocation with PCM1-JAK2 fusion in a patient with T-cell lymphoma, *Leukemia* **20**: 536–537 (2006).

Akiki, S., S.A. Dyer, D. Grimwade, A. Ivey, N. Abou-Zeid, J. Borrow, S. Jeffries, J. Caddick, H. Newell, S. Begum, K. Tawana, J. Mason, M. Velangi, and M. Griffiths, NUP98-NSD1 fusion in association with FLT3-ITD mutation identifies a prognostically relevant subgroup of pediatric acute myeloid leukemia patients suitable for monitoring by real time quantitative PCR, *Genes Chromosomes Cancer* **52**: 1053–1064 (2013).

Alonso, C.N., C. Meyer, M.S. Gallego, J.G. Rossi, A.P. Mansini, P.L. Rubio, A. Medina, R. Marschalek, and M.S. Felice, BTBD18: A novel MLL partner gene in an infant with acute lymphoblastic leukemia and inv(11)(q13;q23), *Leuk Res* **34**: e294–e296 (2010).

Aman, P., Fusion genes in solid tumors, *Semin Cancer Biol* **9**: 303–318 (1999).

Arbajian, E., L. Magnusson, O. Brosjö, J. Wejde, A.L. Folpe, K.H. Nord, and F. Mertens, A benign vascular tumor with a new fusion gene: EWSR1-NFATC1 in hemangioma of the bone, *Am J Surg Pathol* **37**: 613–616 (2013).

Argani, P., C.R. Antonescu, J. Couturier, J.C. Fournet, R. Sciot, M. Debiec-Rychter, B. Hutchinson, V.E. Reuter, L. Boccon-Gibod, C. Timmons, N. Hafez, and M. Ladanyi, PRCC-TFE3 renal carcinomas: morphologic, immunohistochemical, ultrastructural, and molecular analysis of an entity associated with the t(X;1)(p11.2;q21), *Am J Surg Pathol* **26**: 1553–1566 (2002).

Asp, J., F. Persson, M. Kost-Alimova, and G. Stenman, CHCHD7-PLAG1 and TCEA1-PLAG1 gene fusions resulting from cryptic, intrachromosomal 8q rearrangements in pleomorphic salivary gland adenomas, *Genes Chromosomes Cancer* **45**: 820–828 (2006).

Aström, A.K., M.L. Voz, K. Kas, E. Röijer, B. Wedell, N. Mandahl, W. Van de Ven, J. Mark, and G. Stenman, Conserved mechanism of PLAG1 activation in salivary gland tumors with and without chromosome 8q12 abnormalities: identification of SII as a new fusion partner gene, *Cancer Res* **59**: 918–923 (1999).

Attard, G., J. Clark, L. Ambroisine, I.G. Mills, G. Fisher, P. Flohr, A. Reid, S. Edwards, G. Kovacs, D. Berney, C. Foster, C.E. Massie, A. Fletcher, J.S. De Bono, P. Scardino, J. Cuzick, and C.S. Cooper, Transatlantic Prostate Group. Heterogeneity and clinical significance of ETV1 translocations in human prostate cancer, *Br J Cancer* **99**: 314–320 (2008).

Balgobind, B.V., C.M. Zwaan, C. Meyer, R. Marschalek, R. Pieters, H.B. Beverloo, and M.M. Van den Heuvel-Eibrink, NRIP3: a novel translocation partner of MLL detected in a pediatric acute myeloid leukemia with complex chromosome 11 rearrangements, *Haematologica* **94**: 1033 (2009).

Barco, R., C.B. Garcia, and J.E. Eid, The synovial sarcoma-associated SYT-SSX2 oncogene antagonizes the polycomb complex protein Bmi1. *PLoS One* **4**: e5060 (2009).

Barham, W., A.L. Frump, T.P. Sherrill, C.B. Garcia, K. Saito-Diaz, M.N. VanSaun, B. Fingleton, L. Gleaves, D. Orton, M.R. Capecchi, T.S. Blackwell, E. Lee, F. Yull, and J.E. Eid, Targeting the Wnt pathway in synovial sarcoma models, *Cancer Discov* **3**: 1286–1301 (2013).

Barthelmeß, S., H. Geddert, C. Boltze, E.A. Moskalev, M. Bieg, H. Sirbu, B. Brors, S. Wiemann, A. Hartmann, A. Agaimy, and F. Haller, Solitary fibrous tumors/hemangiopericytomas with different variants of the NAB2-STAT6 gene fusion are characterized by specific histomorphology and distinct clinicopathological features, *Am J Pathol* **184**: 1209–1218 (2014).

Bass, A.J., M.S. Lawrence, L.E. Brace, A.H. Ramos, Y. Drier, K. Cibulskis, C. Sougnez, D. Voet, G. Saksena, A. Sivachenko, R. Jing, M. Parkin, T. Pugh, R.G. Verhaak, N. Stransky, A.T. Boutin, J. Barretina, D.B. Solit, E. Vakiani, W. Shao, Y. Mishina, M. Warmuth, J. Jimenez, D.Y. Chiang, S. Signoretti,

W.G. Kaelin, N. Spardy, W.C. Hahn, Y. Hoshida, S. Ogino, R.A. Depinho, L. Chin, L.A. Garraway, C.S. Fuchs, J. Baselga, J. Tabernero, S. Gabriel, E.S. Lander, G. Getz, and M. Meyerson, Genomic sequencing of colorectal adenocarcinomas identifies a recurrent VTI1A-TCF7L2 fusion, *Nat Genet* **43**: 964–968 (2011).

Bayly, R. and D.P. LeBrun, Role for homodimerization in growth deregulation by E2a fusion proteins, *Mol Cell Biol* **20**: 5789–5796 (2000).

Bousquet, M., C. Quelen, V. De Mas, E. Duchayne, B. Roquefeuil, G. Delsol, G. Laurent, N. Dastugue, and P. Brousset, The t(8;9)(p22;p24) translocation in atypical chronic myeloid leukaemia yields a new PCM1-JAK2 fusion gene, *Oncogene* **24**: 7248–7252 (2005).

Brandal, P., I. Panagopoulos, B. Bjerkehagen, and S. Heim, t(19;22)(q13;q12) Translocation leading to the novel fusion gene EWSR1-ZNF444 in soft tissue myoepithelial carcinoma, *Genes Chromosomes Cancer* **48**: 1051–1056 (2009).

Brett, D., S. Whitehouse, P. Antonson, J. Shipley, C. Cooper, and G. Goodwin, The SYT protein involved in the t(X;18) synovial sarcoma translocation is a transcriptional activator localized in nuclear bodies, *Hum Mol Genet* **6**: 1559–1564 (1997).

Bridge, J.A., R.S. Bridge, D.A. Borek, B. Shaffer, and C.W. Norris, Translocation t(X;18) inorofacial synovial sarcoma, *Cancer* **62**: 935–937 (1988).

Bridge, J.A., K. Sanders, D. Huang, M. Nelson, J.R. Neff, D. Muirhead, C. Walker, T.A. Seemayer, and J. Sumegi, Pericytoma with t(7;12) and ACTB-GLI1 fusion arising in bone, *Hum Pathol* **43**: 1524–1529 (2012).

Burmeister, T., C. Meyer, G. Thiel, R. Reinhardt, E. Thiel, and R. Marschalek, A MLL-KIAA0284 fusion gene in a patient with secondary acute myeloid leukemia and t(11;14)(q23;q32), *Blood Cells Mol Dis* **41**: 210–214 (2008).

Butti, M.G., I. Bongarzone, G. Ferraresi, P. Mondellini, M.G. Borrello, and M.A. Pierotti, A sequence analysis of the genomic regions involved in the rearrangements between TPM3 and NTRK1 genes producing TRK oncogenes in papillary thyroid carcinomas, *Genomics* **28**: 15–24 (1995).

Carmody Soni, E.E., S. Schlottman, H.V. Erkizan, A. Uren, and J.A. Toretsky, Loss of SS18-SSX1 inhibits viability and induces apoptosis in synovial sarcoma, *Clin Orthop Relat Res* **472**: 874–882 (2014).

Catalogue of somatic mutations in cancer: http://cancer.sanger.ac.uk/cosmic/fusion.

Cerveira, N., C. Meyer, J. Santos, L. Torres, S. Lisboa, M. Pinheiro, S. Bizarro, C. Correia, L. Norton, R. Marschalek, and M.R. Teixeira, A novel spliced fusion of MLL with CT45A2 in a pediatric biphenotypic acute leukemia, *BMC Cancer* **10**: 518 (2010).

Charest, A., V. Kheifets, J. Park, K. Lane, K. McMahon, C.L. Nutt, and D. Housman, Oncogenic targeting of an activated tyrosine kinase to the Golgi apparatus in a glioblastoma, *Proc Natl Acad Sci USA* **100**: 916–921 (2003a).

Charest, A., K. Lane, K. McMahon, J. Park, E. Preisinger, H. Conroy, and D. Housman, Fusion of FIG to the receptor tyrosine kinase ROS in a glioblastoma with an interstitial del(6)(q21q21), *Genes Chromosomes Cancer* **37**: 58–71 (2003b).

Charest, A., E.W. Wilker, M.E. McLaughlin, K. Lane, R. Gowda, S. Coven, K. McMahon, S. Kovach, Y. Feng, M.B. Yaffe, T. Jacks, and D. Housman, ROS fusion tyrosine kinase activates a SH2 domain-containing phosphatase-2/phosphatidylinositol 3-kinase/mammalian target of rapamycin signaling axis to form glioblastoma in mice. *Cancer Res* **66**: 7473–7481 (2006).

Chinnaiyan, A.M. and N. Palanisamy, Chromosomal aberrations in solid tumors, *Prog Mol Biol Transl Sci* **95**: 55–94 (2010).

Choi, E.Y., D.G. Thomas, J.B. McHugh, R.M. Patel, D. Roulston, S.M. Schuetze, R. Chugh, J.S. Biermann, and D.R. Lucas, Undifferentiated small round cell sarcoma with t(4;19)(q35;q13.1) CIC-DUX4 fusion: a novel highly aggressive soft tissue tumor with distinctive histopathology, *Am J Surg Pathol* **37**: 1379–1386 (2013).

Ciampi, R., T.J. Giordano, K. Wikenheiser-Brokamp, R.J. Koenig, and Y.E. Nikiforov, HOOK3-RET: a novel type of RET-PTC rearrangement in papillary thyroid carcinoma, *Endocr Relat Cancer* **14**: 445–452 (2007).

Cironi, L., T. Petricevic, V. Fernandes Vieira, P. Provero, C. Fusco, S. Cornaz, G. Fregni, I. Letovanec, M. Aguet, and I. Stamenkovic, The fusion protein SS18-SSX1 employs core Wnt pathway transcription factors to induce a partial Wnt signature in synovial sarcoma, *Sci Rep* **6**: 22113 (2016).

Clark, J., P.J. Rocques, A.J. Crew, S. Gill, J. Shipley, A.M. Chan, B.A. Gusterson, and C.S. Cooper, Identification of novel genes, SYT SSX. and, involved in the t(X;18)(p11.2;q11.2) translocation found in human synovial sarcoma, *Nat Genet* **7**: 502–508 (1994).

Coenen, E.A., C.M. Zwaan, C. Meyer, R. Marschalek, R. Pieters, L.T. van der Veken, H.B. Beverloo, and M.M. van den Heuvel-Eibrink, KIAA1524: A novel MLL translocation partner in acute myeloid leukemia, *Leuk Res* **35**: 133–135 (2011).

Crombez, K.R., E.M. Vanoirbeek, W.J. Van de Ven, and M.M. Petit, Transactivation functions of the tumor-specific HMGA2/LPP fusion protein are augmented by wild-type HMGA2, *Mol Cancer Res* **3**: 63–70 (2005).

de Bruijn, D.R., S.V. Allander, A.H. van Dijk, M.P. Willemse, J. Thijssen, J.J. van Groningen, P.S. Meltzer, and A.G. van Kessel, The synovial-sarcoma-associated SS18-SSX2 fusion protein induces epigenetic gene (de)regulation, *Cancer Res* **66**: 9474–9482 (2006).

de Rooij, J.D., I.H. Hollink, S.T. Arentsen-Peters, J.F. van Galen, H. Berna Beverloo, A. Baruchel, J. Trka, D. Reinhardt, E. Sonneveld, M. Zimmermann, T.A. Alonzo, R. Pieters, S. Meshinchi, M.M. van den Heuvel-Eibrink, and C.M. Zwaan, NUP98/JARID1A is a novel recurrent abnormality in pediatric acute megakaryoblastic leukemia with a distinct HOX gene expression pattern, *Leukemia* **27**: 2280–2288 (2013).

de Rooij, J.D., M.M. van den Heuvel-Eibrink, W.J. Kollen, E. Sonneveld, G.J. Kaspers, H.B. Beverloo, M. Fornerod, R. Pieters, and C.M. Zwaan, Recurrent translocation t(10;17)(p15;q21) in minimally differentiated acute myeloid leukemia results in ZMYND11/MBTD1 fusion, *Genes Chromosomes Cancer* **55**: 237–241 (2016).

Deng, G., C. Hu, L. Zhu, F. Huang, W. Huang, H. Xu, and W. Nie, Downregulation of ROS-FIG inhibits cell proliferation, colony-formation, cell cycle progression, migration and invasion, while inducing apoptosis in intrahepatic cholangiocarcinoma cells, *Int J Mol Med* **34**: 661–668 (2014).

Dessars, B., L.E. De Raeve, H. El Housni, C.J. Debouck, P.J. Sidon, R. Morandini, D. Roseeuw, G.E. Ghanem, G. Vassart, and P. Heimann, Chromosomal translocations as a mechanism of BRAF activation in two cases of large congenital melanocytic nevi, *J Invest Dermatol* **127**: 1468–1470 (2007).

Deucher, A.M., Z. Qi, J. Yu, T.I. George, and J.E. Etzell, BCL6 expression correlates with the t(1;19) translocation in B-lymphoblastic leukemia, *Am J Clin Pathol* **143**: 547–557 (2015).

Dewaele, B., J. Przybyl, A. Quattrone, J. Finalet Ferreiro, V. Vanspauwen, E. Geerdens, V. Gianfelici, Z. Kalender, A. Wozniak, P. Moerman, R. Sciot, S. Croce, F. Amant, P. Vandenberghe, J. Cools, and M. Debiec-Rychter, Identification of a novel, recurrent MBTD1-CXorf67 fusion in low-grade endometrial stromal sarcoma, *Int J Cancer* **134**: 1112–1122 (2014).

Diakos, C., Y. Xiao, S. Zheng, L. Kager, M. Dworzak, and J.L. Wiemels, Direct and indirect targets of the E2A-PBX1 leukemia-specific fusion protein, *PLoS One* **9**: e87602 (2014).

Dimitriadis, E., D. Rontogianni, A. Kyriazoglou, A. Takou, K. Frangia, N. Pandis, and T. Trangas, Novel SYT-SSX fusion transcript variants in synovial sarcoma, *Cancer Genet Cytogenet* **195**: 54–58 (2009).

Douet-Guilbert, N., J.R. Eveillard, C. Meyer, V. Ugo, M.J. Le Bris, A. Basinko, F. Morel, R. Marschalek, and M. De Braekeleer. MLL partner genes in secondary acute lymphoblastic leukemia: report of a new partner PRRC1 and review of the literature, *Leuk Res* **38**: 1316–1319 (2014).

Duruisseaux, M. and M. Wislez, CD74-NRG1: a new fusion gene in lung adenocarcinomas characterizing mucinous adenocarcinomas, *Bull Cancer* **101**: 529–530 (2014).

Ehrentraut, S., S. Nagel, M.E. Scherr, B. Schneider, H. Quentmeier, R. Geffers, M. Kaufmann, C. Meyer, M. Prochorec-Sobieszek, R.P. Ketterling, R.A. Knudson, A.L. Feldman, M.E. Kadin, H.G. Drexler, and R.A. MacLeod, t(8;9)(p22;p24)/PCM1-JAK2 activates SOCS2 and SOCS3 via STAT5, *PLoS One* **8**: e53767 (2013).

Eid, J.E., A.L. Kung, R. Scully, and D.M. Livingston, p300 interacts with the nuclear proto-oncoprotein SYT as part of the active control of cell adhesion, *Cell* **102**: 839–848 (2000).

ElGendi, H.M., A.A. Abdelmaksoud, D.G. Eissa, and S.A. Abusikkien, Impact of TCF3 rearrangement on CNS relapse in egyptian pediatric acute lymphoblastic leukemia, *Pediatr Hematol Oncol* **31**: 638–646 (2014).

Fernandez-Cuesta, L., D. Plenker, H. Osada, R. Sun, R. Menon, F. Leenders, S. Ortiz-Cuaran, M. Peifer, M. Bos, J. Daßler, F. Malchers, J. Schöttle, W. Vogel, I. Dahmen, M. Koker, R.T. Ullrich, G.M. Wright, P.A. Russell, Z. Wainer, B. Solomon, E. Brambilla, H. Nagy-Mignotte, D. Moro-Sibilot, C.G. Brambilla, S. Lantuejoul, J. Altmüller, C. Becker, P. Nürnberg, J.M. Heuckmann, E. Stoelben, I. Petersen, J.H. Clement, J. Sänger, L.A. Muscarella, A. la Torre, V.M. Fazio, I. Lahortiga, T. Perera, S. Ogata, M. Parade, D. Brehmer, M. Vingron, L.C. Heukamp, R. Buettner, T. Zander, J. Wolf, S. Perner, S. Ansén, S.A. Haas, Y. Yatabe, and R.K. Thomas, CD74-NRG1 fusions in lung adenocarcinoma, *Cancer Discov* **4**: 415–422 (2014).

Yuzawa, S., H. Nishihara, L. Wang, M. Tsuda, T. Kimura, M. Tanino, and S. Tanaka, Analysis of NAB2-STAT6 Gene Fusion in 17 Cases of Meningeal Solitary Fibrous Tumor/Hemangiopericytoma: Review of the Literature, *Am J Surg Pathol* **40**: 1031–1040 (2016).

Fu, J.F., H.C. Hsu, and L.Y. Shih, MLL is fused to EB1 (MAPRE1), which encodes a microtubule-associated protein, in a patient with acute lymphoblastic leukemia, *Genes Chromosomes Cancer* **43**: 206–210 (2005).

Gainor, J.F. and A.T. Shaw, Novel targets in non-small cell lung cancer: ROS1 and RET fusions, *Oncologist* **18**: 865–875 (2013). doi: 10.1634/theoncologist.2013-0095.

Geurts, J.M., E.F. Schoenmakers, E. Röijer, A.K. Aström, G. Stenman, and W.J. van de Ven, Identification of NFIB as recurrent translocation partner gene of HMGIC inpleomorphic adenomas, *Oncogene* **16**: 865–872 (1998).

Geurts, J.M., E.F. Schoenmakers, E. Röijer, G. Stenman, and W.J. Van de Ven, Expression of reciprocal hybrid transcripts of HMGIC and FHIT in a pleomorphic adenoma of theparotid gland, *Cancer Res* **57**: 13–17 (1997).

Graham, C., S. Chilton-MacNeill, M. Zielenska, and G.R. Somers, The CIC-DUX4 fusion transcript is present in a subgroup of pediatric primitive round cell sarcomas, *Hum Pathol* **43**: 180–189 (2012).

Graham, R.P., L. Jin, D.L. Knutson, S.M. Kloft-Nelson, P.T. Greipp, N. Waldburger, S. Roessler, T. Longerich, L.R. Roberts, A.M. Oliveira, K.C. Halling, P. Schirmacher, and M.S. Torbenson, DNAJB1-PRKACA is specific for fibrolamellar carcinoma, *Mod Pathol* **28**: 822–829 (2015).

Greco, A., C. Mariani, C. Miranda, A. Lupas, S. Pagliardini, M. Pomati, and M.A. Pierotti, The DNA rearrangement that generates the TRK-T3 oncogene involves a novel gene on chromosome 3 whose product has a potential coiled-coil domain, *Mol Cell Biol* **15**: 6118–6127 (1995).

Hajingabo, L.J., S. Daakour, M. Martin, R. Grausenburger, R. Panzer-Grümayer, F. Dequiedt, N. Simonis, and J.C. Twizere, Predicting interactome network perturbations in human cancer: application to gene fusions in acute lymphoblastic leukemia, *Mol Biol Cell* **25**: 3973–3985 (2014).

Han, B., R. Mehra, S.M. Dhanasekaran, J. Yu, A. Menon, R.J. Lonigro, X. Wang, Y. Gong, L. Wang, S. Shankar, B. Laxman, R.B. Shah, S. Varambally, N. Palanisamy, S.A. Tomlins, C. Kumar-Sinha, and A.M. Chinnaiyan, A fluorescence *in situ* hybridization screen for E26 transformation-specific aberrations: identification of DDX5-ETV4 fusion protein in prostate cancer, *Cancer Res* **68**: 7629–7637 (2008).

Hashii, Y., J.Y. Kim, A. Sawada, S. Tokimasa, F. Hiroyuki, H. Ohta, K. Makiko, Y. Takihara, K. Ozono, and J. Hara, A novel partner gene CIP29 containing a SAP domain with MLL identified in infantile myelomonocytic leukemia, *Leukemia* **18**: 1546–1548 (2004).

Herbaux, C., S. Poulain, C. Meyer, R. Marschalek, A. Renneville, J. Fernandes, O. Theisen, S. Tricot, M. Simon, P. Duthilleul, and A. Daudignon, TOP3A, a new partner gene fused to MLL in an adult patient with de novo acute myeloid leukaemia, *Br J Haematol* **157**: 128–131 (2012).

Hermans, K.G., A.A. Bressers, H.A. van der Korput, N.F. Dits, G. Jenster, and J. Trapman, Two unique novel prostate-specific and androgen-regulated fusion partners of ETV4 in prostate cancer, *Cancer Res* **68**: 3094–3098 (2008).

Hibbard, M.K., H.P. Kozakewich, P. Dal Cin, R. Sciot, X. Tan, S. Xiao, and J.A. Fletcher, PLAG1 fusion oncogenes in lipoblastoma, *Cancer Res* **60**: 4869–4872 (2000).

Hisaoka, M., T. Ishida, T. Imamura, and H. Hashimoto, TFG is a novel fusion partner of NOR1 in extraskeletal myxoid chondrosarcoma, *Genes Chromosomes Cancer* **40**: 325–328 (2004).

Hoeller, S., C. Walz, A. Reiter, S. Dirnhofer, and A. Tzankov, PCM1-JAK2-fusion: a potential treatment target in myelodysplastic-myeloproliferative and other hemato-lymphoid neoplasms, *Expert Opin Ther Targets* **15**: 53–62 (2011).

Hollink, I.H., M.M. van den Heuvel-Eibrink, S.T. Arentsen-Peters, M. Pratcorona, S. Abbas, J.E. Kuipers, J.F. van Galen, H.B. Beverloo, E. Sonneveld, G.J. Kaspers, J. Trka, A. Baruchel, M. Zimmermann, U. Creutzig, D. Reinhardt, R. Pieters, P.J. Valk, and C.M. Zwaan, NUP98/NSD1 characterizes a novel poor prognostic group in acute myeloid leukemia with a distinct HOX gene expression pattern, *Blood* **118**: 3645–3656 (2011).

Hong, Y., W.J. Kim, C.Y. Bang, J.C. Lee, and Y.M. Oh, Identification of Alternative Splicing and Fusion Transcripts in Non-Small Cell Lung Cancer by RNA Sequencing, *Tuberc Respir Dis* (*Seoul*) **79**: 85–90 (2016).

Huang, W., M. Goldfischer, S. Babyeva, Y. Mao, K. Volyanskyy, N. Dimitrova, J.T. Fallon, and M. Zhong, Identification of a novel PARP14-TFE3 gene fusion from 10-year-old FFPE tissue by RNA-seq, *Genes Chromosomes Cancer* [Epub ahead of print] (2015).

Ishida, M., M. Miyamoto, S. Naitoh, D. Tatsuda, T. Hasegawa, T. Nemoto, H. Yokozeki, K. Nishioka, A. Matsukage, M. Ohki, and T. Ohta, The SYT-SSX fusion protein down-regulates the cell proliferation regulator COM1 in t(x;18) synovial sarcoma, *Mol Cell Biol* **27**: 1348–1355 (2007).

Ishikawa, M., F. Yagasaki, D. Okamura, T. Maeda, Y. Sugahara, I. Jinnai, and M. Bessho, A novel gene, ANKRD28 on 3p25, is fused with NUP98 on 11p15 in a cryptic 3-way translocation of t(3;5;11)(p25;q35;p15) in an adult patient with myelodysplastic syndrome/acute myelogenous leukemia, *Int J Hematol* **86**: 238–245 (2007).

Italiano, A., Y.S. Sung, L. Zhang, S. Singer, R.G. Maki, J.M. Coindre, and C.R. Antonescu, High prevalence of CIC fusion with double-homeobox (DUX4) transcription factors in EWSR1-negative undifferentiated small blue round cell sarcomas, *Genes Chromosomes Cancer* **51**: 207–218 (2012).

Iyengar, V., A.S. Lineberger, S. Kerman, and N.A. Burton, Synovial sarcoma of the heart. Correlation with cytogenetic findings, *Arch Pathol Lab Med* **119**: 1080–1082 (1995).

Jaju, R.J., C. Fidler, O.A. Haas, A.J. Strickson, F. Watkins, K. Clark, N.C. Cross, J.F. Cheng, P.D. Aplan, L. Kearney, J. Boultwood, and J.S. Wainscoat, A novel gene, NSD1, is fused to NUP98 in the t(5;11)(q35;p15.5) in de novo childhood acute myeloid leukemia, *Blood* **98**: 1264–1267 (2001).

Jones, D.T., B. Hutter, N. Jäger, A. Korshunov, M. Kool, H.J. Warnatz, T. Zichner, S.R. Lambert, M. Ryzhova, D.A. Quang, A.M. Fontebasso, A.M. Stütz, S. Hutter, M. Zuckermann, D. Sturm, J. Gronych, B. Lasitschka, S. Schmidt, H. Seker-Cin, H. Witt, M. Sultan, M. Ralser, P.A. Northcott, V. Hovestadt, S. Bender, E. Pfaff, S. Stark, D. Faury, J. Schwartzentruber, J. Majewski, U.D. Weber, M. Zapatka, B. Raeder, M. Schlesner, C.L. Worth, C.C. Bartholomae, C. von Kalle, C.D. Imbusch, S. Radomski, C. Lawerenz, P. van Sluis, J. Koster, R. Volckmann, R. Versteeg, H. Lehrach, C. Monoranu, B. Winkler, A. Unterberg, C. Herold-Mende, T. Milde, A.E. Kulozik, M. Ebinger, M.U. Schuhmann, Y.J. Cho, S.L. Pomeroy, A. von Deimling, O. Witt, M.D. Taylor, S. Wolf, M.A. Karajannis, C.G. Eberhart, W. Scheurlen, M. Hasselblatt, K.L. Ligon, M.W. Kieran, J.O. Korbel, M.L. Yaspo, B. Brors, J. Felsberg, G. Reifenberger, V.P. Collins, N. Jabado, R. Eils, P. Lichter, and S.M. Pfister, International Cancer Genome Consortium PedBrain Tumor Project. Recurrent somatic alterations of FGFR1 and NTRK2 in pilocytic astrocytoma, *Nat Genet* **45**: 927–932 (2013).

Jun, H.J., H. Johnson, R.T. Bronson, S. de Feraudy, F. White, and A. Charest, The oncogenic lung cancer fusion kinase CD74-ROS activates a novel invasiveness pathway through E-Syt1 phosphorylation, *Cancer Res* **72**: 3764–3774 (2012).

Kannan, K., C. Coarfa, K. Rajapakshe, S.M. Hawkins, M.M. Matzuk, A. Milosavljevic, and L. Yen, CDKN2D-WDFY2 is a cancer-specific fusion gene recurrent in high-grade serous ovarian carcinoma, *PLoS Genet* **10**: e1004216 (2014).

Kauffman, E.C., C.J. Ricketts, S. Rais-Bahrami, Y. Yang, M.J. Merino, D.P. Bottaro, R. Srinivasan, and W.M. Linehan, Molecular genetics and cellular features of TFE3 and TFEB fusion kidney cancers, *Nat Rev Urol* **11**: 465–475 (2014).

Kawamura-Saito, M., Y. Yamazaki, K. Kaneko, N. Kawaguchi, H. Kanda, H. Mukai, T. Gotoh, T. Motoi, M. Fukayama, H. Aburatani, T. Takizawa, and T. Nakamura, Fusion between CIC and DUX4 up-regulates PEA3 family genes in Ewing-like sarcomas with t(4;19)(q35;q13) translocation, *Hum Mol Genet* **15**: 2125–2137 (2006).

Kazmierczak, B., Y. Hennig, S. Wanschura, P. Rogalla, S. Bartnitzke, W. Van de Ven, and J. Bullerdiek, Description of a novel fusion transcript between HMGI-C, a gene encoding for a member of the high mobility group proteins, and the mitochondrial aldehyde dehydrogenase gene, *Cancer Res* **55**: 6038–6039 (1995).

Kobos, R., M. Nagai, M. Tsuda, M.Y. Merl, T. Saito, M. Laé, Q. Mo, A. Olshen, S. Lianoglou, C. Leslie, I. Ostrovnaya, C. Antczak, H. Djaballah, and

M. Ladanyi, Combining integrated genomics and functional genomics to dissect the biology of a cancer-associated, aberrant transcription factor, the ASPSCR1-TFE3 fusion oncoprotein, *J Pathol* **229**: 743–754 (2013).

Kohno, T., H. Ichikawa, Y. Totoki, K. Yasuda, M. Hiramoto, T. Nammo, H. Sakamoto, K. Tsuta, K. Furuta, Y. Shimada, R. Iwakawa, H. Ogiwara, T. Oike, M. Enari, A.J. Schetter, H. Okayama, A. Haugen, V. Skaug, S. Chiku, I. Yamanaka, Y. Arai, S. Watanabe, I. Sekine, S. Ogawa, C.C. Harris, H. Tsuda, T. Yoshida, J. Yokota, and T. Shibata, KIF5B-RET fusions in lung adenocarcinoma, *Nat Med* **18**: 375–377 (2012).

Koontz, J.I., A.L. Soreng, M. Nucci, F.C. Kuo, P. Pauwels, H. van Den Berghe, P. Dal Cin, J.A. Fletcher, and J. Sklar, Frequent fusion of the JAZF1 and JJAZ1 genes in endometrial stromal tumors, *Proc Natl Acad Sci USA* **98**: 6348–6353 (2001).

Kubo, T., Y. Matsui, T. Goto, K. Yukata, and N. Yasui, Overexpression of HMGA2-LPP fusion transcripts promotes expression of the alpha 2 type XI collagen gene, *Biochem Biophys Res Commun* **340**: 476–481 (2006).

Kuroda, N., S. Mikami, C.C. Pan, R.J. Cohen, O. Hes, M. Michal, Y. Nagashima, Y. Tanaka, K. Inoue, T. Shuin, and G.H. Lee, Review of renal carcinoma associated with Xp11.2 translocations/TFE3 gene fusions with focus on pathobiological aspect, *Histol Histopathol* **27**: 133–140 (2012).

Kurose, K., N. Mine, D. Doi, Y. Ota, K. Yoneyama, H. Konishi, T. Araki, and M. Emi, Novel gene fusion of COX6C at 8q22-23 to HMGIC at 12q15 in a uterine leiomyoma, *Genes Chromosomes Cancer* **27**: 303–307 (2000).

La Starza, R., P. Gorello, R. Rosati, A. Riezzo, A. Veronese, E. Ferrazzi, M.F. Martelli, M. Negrini, and C. Mecucci, Cryptic insertion producing two NUP98/NSD1 chimeric transcripts in adult refractory anemia with an excess of blasts, *Genes Chromosomes Cancer* **41**: 395–399 (2004).

Ladanyi, M., Fusions of the SYT and SSX genes in synovial sarcoma, *Oncogene* **20**: 5755–5762 (2001).

Lane, S.W., D.J. Fairbairn, C. McCarthy, A. Nandini, J. Perry-Keene, and G.A. Kennedy, Leukaemia cutis in atypical chronic myeloid leukaemia with a t(9;22) (p24;q11.2) leading to BCR-JAK2 fusion, *Br J Haematol* **142**: 503 (2008).

Lee, J., S.E. Lee, S.Y. Kang, I.G. Do, S. Lee, S.Y. Ha, J. Cho, W.K. Kang, J. Jang, S.H. Ou, and K.M. Kim, Identification of ROS1 rearrangement in gastric adenocarcinoma, *Cancer* **119**: 1627–1635 (2013).

Martignoni, G., S. Gobbo, P. Camparo, M. Brunelli, E. Munari, D. Segala, M. Pea, F. Bonetti, P.B. Illei, G.J. Netto, M. Ladanyi, M. Chilosi, and

P. Argani, Differential expression of cathepsin K in neoplasms harboring TFE3 gene fusions, *Mod Pathol* **24**: 1313–1319 (2011).

Martini, A., R. La Starza, H. Janssen, C. Bilhou-Nabera, A. Corveleyn, R. Somers, A. Aventin, R. Foà, A. Hagemeijer, C. Mecucci, and P. Marynen, Recurrent rearrangement of the Ewing's sarcoma gene, EWSR1, or its homologue, TAF15, with the transcription factor CIZ/NMP4 in acute leukemia, *Cancer Res* **62**: 5408–5412 (2002).

Mathur, M., S. Das, and H.H. Samuels, PSF-TFE3 oncoprotein in papillary renal cell carcinoma inactivates TFE3 and p53 through cytoplasmic sequestration, *Oncogene* **22**: 5031–5044 (2003).

Mathur, M. and H.H. Samuels, Role of PSF-TFE3 oncoprotein in the development of papillary renal cell carcinomas, *Oncogene* **26**: 277–283 (2007).

Medendorp, K., J.J. van Groningen, L. Vreede, L. Hetterschijt, L. Brugmans, W.H. van den Hurk, and A.G. van Kessel, The renal cell carcinoma-associated oncogenic fusion protein PRCCTFE3 provokes p21 WAF1/CIP1-mediated cell cycle delay, *Exp Cell Res* **315**: 2399–2409 (2009).

Meloni, A.M., R.M. Dobbs, J.E. Pontes, and A.A. Sandberg, Translocation (X;1) in papillary renal cell carcinoma. A new cytogenetic subtype, *Cancer Genet Cytogenet* **65**: 1–6 (1993).

Micci, F., L. Gorunova, S. Gatius, X. Matias-Guiu, B. Davidson, S. Heim, and I. Panagopoulos, MEAF6/PHF1 is a recurrent gene fusion in endometrial stromal sarcoma, *Cancer Lett* **347**: 75–78 (2014a).

Micci, F., I. Panagopoulos, B. Bjerkehagen, and S. Heim, Consistent rearrangement of chromosomal band 6p21 with generation of fusion genes JAZF1/PHF1 and EPC1/PHF1 in endometrial stromal sarcoma, *Cancer Res* **66**: 107–112 (2006).

Micci, F., I. Panagopoulos, J. Thorsen, B. Davidson, C.G. Tropé, and S. Heim, Low frequency of ESRRA-C11orf20 fusion gene in ovarian carcinomas, *PLoS Biol* **12**: e1001784 (2014b).

Minami, Y., S. Kohsaka, M. Tsuda, K. Yachi, N. Hatori, M. Tanino, T. Kimura, H. Nishihara, A. Minami, N. Iwasaki, and S. Tanaka, SS18-SSX-regulated miR-17 promotes tumor growth of synovial sarcoma by inhibiting p21WAF1/CIP1, *Cancer Sci* **105**: 1152–1159 (2014).

Mine, N., K. Kurose, H. Konishi, T. Araki, H. Nagai, and M. Emi, Fusion of a sequence from HEI10 (14q11) to the HMGIC gene at 12q15 in a uterine leiomyoma, *Jpn J Cancer Res* **92**: 135–139 (2001).

Morerio, C., A. Rapella, C. Rosanda, E. Tassano, C. Gambini, G. Romagnoli, and C. Panarello, PLAG1-HAS2 fusion in lipoblastoma with masked 8q intrachromosomal rearrangement, *Cancer Genet Cytogenet* **156**: 183–184 (2005).

Müller-Höcker, J., G. Babaryka, I. Schmid, and A. Jung, Overexpression of cyclin D1, D3, and p21 in an infantile renal carcinoma with Xp11.2 TFE3-gene fusion, *Pathol Res Pract* **204**: 589–597 (2008).

Murayama, T., T. Nakaoku, M. Enari, T. Nishimura, K. Tominaga, A. Nakata, A. Tojo, S. Sugano, T. Kohno, and N. Gotoh, Oncogenic Fusion Gene CD74-NRG1 Confers Cancer Stem Cell-like Properties in Lung Cancer through a IGF2 Autocrine/Paracrine Circuit, *Cancer Res* **76**: 974–983 (2016).

Nagai, M., S. Tanaka, M. Tsuda, S. Endo, H. Kato, H. Sonobe, A. Minami, H. Hiraga, H. Nishihara, H. Sawa, and K. Nagashima, Analysis of transforming activity of human synovial sarcoma-associated chimeric protein SYT-SSX1 bound to chromatin remodeling factor hBRM/hSNF2 alpha, *Proc Natl Acad Sci USA* **98**: 3843–3848 (2001).

Nakada, S., H. Minato, T. Takegami, N. Kurose, H. Ikeda, M. Kobayashi, Y. Sasagawa, T. Akai, T. Kato, N. Yamamoto, and T. Nojima, NAB2-STAT6 fusion gene analysis in two cases of meningeal solitary fibrous tumor/hemangiopericytoma with late distant metastases, *Brain Tumor Pathol* **32**: 268–274 (2015).

Navarro, M., M.P. Simon, C. Migeon, C. Turc-Carel, and F. Pedeutour, COL1A1-PDGFB fusion in a ring chromosome 4 found in a dermatofibrosarcoma protuberans, *Genes Chromosomes Cancer* **23**: 263–266 (1998).

Nebral, K., M. König, H.H. Schmidt, D. Lutz, W.R. Sperr, K. Kalwak, S. Brugger, M.N. Dworzak, O.A. Haas, and S. Strehl, Screening for NUP98 rearrangements in hematopoietic malignancies by fluorescence *in situ* hybridization, *Haematologica* **90**: 746–752 (2005).

Nilsson, M., F. Mertens, M. Höglund, N. Mandahl, and I. Panagopoulos, Truncation and fusion of HMGA2 in lipomas with rearrangements of 5q32-->q33 and 12q14-->q15, *Cytogenet Genome Res* **112**: 60–66 (2006).

Nyquist, K.B., I. Panagopoulos, J. Thorsen, L. Haugom, L. Gorunova, B. Bjerkehagen, A. Fosså, M. Guriby, T. Nome, R.A. Lothe, R.I. Skotheim, S. Heim, and F. Micci, Whole-transcriptome sequencing identifies novel IRF2BP2-CDX1 fusion gene brought about by translocation t(1;5)(q42;q32) in mesenchymal chondrosarcoma, *PLoS One* **7**: e49705 (2012).

Oliveira, A.M., B.L. Hsi, S. Weremowicz, A.E. Rosenberg, P. Dal Cin, N. Joseph, J.A. Bridge, A.R. Perez-Atayde, and J.A. Fletcher, USP6 (Tre2) fusion oncogenes in aneurysmal bone cyst, *Cancer Res* **64**: 1920–1923 (2004).

Oliveira, A.M., A.R. Perez-Atayde, P. Dal Cin, M.C. Gebhardt, C.J. Chen, J.R. Neff, G.D. Demetri, A.E. Rosenberg, J.A. Bridge, and J.A. Fletcher,

Aneurysmal bone cyst variant translocations upregulate USP6 transcription by promoter swapping with the ZNF9, COL1A1, TRAP150, and OMD genes, *Oncogene* **24**: 3419–3426 (2005).

O'Meara, E., D. Stack, C.H. Lee, A.J. Garvin, T. Morris, P. Argani, J.S. Han, J. Karlsson, D. Gisselson, I. Leuschner, M. Gessler, N. Graf, J.A. Fletcher, and M.J. O'Sullivan, Characterization of the chromosomal translocation t(10;17)(q22;p13) in clear cell sarcoma of kidney, *J Pathol* **227**: 72–80 (2012).

Onder, A.M., U. Teomete, P. Argani, S. Toledano, G. Zilleruelo, and M.M. Rodriguez, PRCC-TFE3 renal cell carcinoma in a boy with a history of contralateral mesoblastic nephroma, *Pediatr Nephrol* **21**: 1471–1475 (2006).

Palanisamy, N., B. Ateeq, S. Kalyana-Sundaram, D. Pflueger, K. Ramnarayanan, S. Shankar, B. Han, Q. Cao, X. Cao, K. Suleman, C. Kumar-Sinha, S.M. Dhanasekaran, Y.B. Chen, R. Esgueva, S. Banerjee, C.J. LaFargue, J. Siddiqui, F. Demichelis, P. Moeller, T.A. Bismar, R. Kuefer, D.R. Fullen, T.M. Johnson, J.K. Greenson, T.J. Giordano, P. Tan, S.A. Tomlins, S. Varambally, M.A. Rubin, C.A. Maher, and A.M. Chinnaiyan, Rearrangements of the RAF kinase pathway in prostate cancer, gastric cancer and melanoma, *Nat Med* **16**: 793–798 (2010).

Panagopoulos, I., L. Gorunova, B. Bjerkehagen, I. Lobmaier, and S. Heim, Fusion of the TBL1XR1 and HMGA1 genes in splenic hemangioma with t(3;6)(q26;p21), *Int J Oncol* **48**: 1242–1250 (2016).

Panagopoulos, I., M. Isaksson, R. Billström, B. Strömbeck, F. Mitelman, and B. Johansson, Fusion of the NUP98 gene and the homeobox gene HOXC13 in acute myeloid leukemia with t(11;12)(p15;q13), *Genes Chromosomes Cancer* **36**: 107–112 (2003).

Panagopoulos, I., F. Mertens, R. Löfvenberg, and N. Mandahl, Fusion of the COL1A1 and USP6 genes in a benign bone tumor, *Cancer Genet Cytogenet* **180**: 70–73 (2008).

Panagopoulos, I., J. Thorsen, L. Gorunova, F. Micci, L. Haugom, B. Davidson, and S. Heim, RNA sequencing identifies fusion of the EWSR1 and YY1 genes in mesothelioma with t(14;22)(q32;q12), *Genes Chromosomes Cancer* **52**: 733–740 (2013).

Panarello, C., C. Rosanda, and C. Morerio, Cryptic translocation t(5;11)(q35;p15.5) with involvement of the NSD1 and NUP98 genes without 5q deletion in childhood acute myeloid leukemia, *Genes Chromosomes Cancer* **35**: 277–281 (2002).

Park, T.S., S.G. Lee, J. Song, K.A. Lee, J. Kim, J.R. Choi, S.T. Lee, R. Marschalek, and C. Meyer, CASP8AP2 is a novel partner gene of MLL rearrangement with t(6;11)(q15;q23) in acute myeloid leukemia, *Cancer Genet Cytogenet* **195**: 94–95 (2009).

Pérot, C., L. Boccon-Gibod, R. Bouvier, F. Doz, J.C. Fournet, P. Fréneaux, A. Vieillefond, and J. Couturier, Five new cases of juvenile renal cell carcinoma with translocations involving Xp11.2: a cytogenetic and morphologic study, *Cancer Genet Cytogenet* **143**: 93–99 (2003).

Pession, A., L. Lo Nigro, L. Montemurro, S. Serravalle, R. Fazzina, G. Izzi, G. Nucifora, R. Slany, and R. Tonelli, ArgBP2, encoding a negative regulator ABL. of, is fused to MLL in a case of infant M5 acute myeloid leukemia involving 4q35 and 11q23, *Leukemia* **20**: 1310–1313 (2006).

Petit, M.M., R. Mols, E.F. Schoenmakers, N. Mandahl, and W.J. Van de Ven, LPP, the preferred fusion partner gene of HMGIC in lipomas, is a novel member of the LIM protein gene family, *Genomics* **36**: 118–129 (1996).

Petit, M.M., E.F. Schoenmakers, C. Huysmans, J.M. Geurts, N. Mandahl, and W.J. Van de Ven, LHFP, a novel translocation partner gene of HMGIC in a lipoma, is a member of a new family of LHFP-like genes, *Genomics* **57**: 438–441 (1999).

Pflueger, D., S. Terry, A. Sboner, L. Habegger, R. Esgueva, P.C. Lin, M.A. Svensson, N. Kitabayashi, B.J. Moss, T.Y. MacDonald, X. Cao, T. Barrette, A.K. Tewari, M.S. Chee, A.M. Chinnaiyan, D.S. Rickman, F. Demichelis, M.B. Gerstein, and M.A. Rubin, Discovery of non-ETS gene fusions in human prostate cancer using next-generation RNA sequencing, *Genome Res* **21**: 56–67 (2011).

Poitras, J.L., P. Dal Cin, J.C. Aster, D.J. Deangelo, and C.C. Morton, Novel SSBP2-JAK2 fusion gene resulting from a t(5;9)(q14.1;p24.1) in pre-B acute lymphocytic leukemia, *Genes Chromosomes Cancer* **47**: 884–889 (2008).

Przybyl, J., R. Sciot, P. Rutkowski, J.A. Siedlecki, V. Vanspauwen, I. Samson, and M. Debiec-Rychter, Recurrent and novel SS18-SSX fusion transcripts in synovial sarcoma: description of three new cases, *Tumor Biol* **33**: 2245–2253 (2012).

Put, N., K. Van Roosbroeck, I. Vande Broek, L. Michaux, and P. Vandenberghe, PDS5A, a novel translocation partner of MLL in acute myeloid leukemia, *Leuk Res* **36**: e87–89 (2012).

Queimado, L., C.S. Lopes, and A.M. Reis, WIF1, an inhibitor of the Wnt pathway, is rearranged in salivary gland tumors, *Genes Chromosomes Cancer* **46**: 215–225 (2007).

Reiter, A., C. Walz, A. Watmore, C. Schoch, I. Blau, B. Schlegelberger, U. Berger, N. Telford, S. Aruliah, J.A. Yin, D. Vanstraelen, H.F. Barker, P.C. Taylor, A. O'Driscoll, F. Benedetti, C. Rudolph, H.J. Kolb, A. Hochhaus,

R. Hehlmann, A. Chase, and N.C. Cross, The t(8;9)(p22;p24) is a recurrent abnormality in chronic and acute leukemia that fuses PCM1 to JAK2, *Cancer Res* **65**: 2662–2667 (2005).

Rimkunas, V.M., K.E. Crosby, D. Li, Y. Hu, M.E. Kelly, T.L. Gu, J.S. Mack, M.R. Silver, X. Zhou, and H. Haack, Analysis of receptor tyrosine kinase ROS1-positive tumors in non-small cell lung cancer: identification of a FIG-ROS1 fusion, *Clin Cancer Res* **18**: 4449–4457 (2012).

Robinson, B.W., N.K. Cheung, C.P. Kolaris, S.C. Jhanwar, J.K. Choi, N. Osheroff, and C.A. Felix, Prospective tracing of MLL-FRYL clone with low MEIS1 expression from emergence during neuroblastoma treatment to diagnosis of myelodysplastic syndrome, *Blood* **111**: 3802–3812 (2008).

Robinson, D.R., S. Kalyana-Sundaram, Y.M. Wu, S. Shankar, X. Cao, B. Ateeq, I.A. Asangani, M. Iyer, C.A. Maher, C.S. Grasso, R.J. Lonigro, M. Quist, J. Siddiqui, R. Mehra, X. Jing, T.J. Giordano, M.S. Sabel, C.G. Kleer, N. Palanisamy, R. Natrajan, M.B. Lambros, J.S. Reis-Filho, C. Kumar-Sinha, and A.M. Chinnaiyan, Functionally recurrent rearrangements of the MAST kinase and Notch gene families in breast cancer, *Nat Med* **17**: 1646–1651 (2011).

Robinson, D.R., Y.M. Wu, S. Kalyana-Sundaram, X. Cao, R.J. Lonigro, Y.S. Sung, C.L. Chen, L. Zhang, R. Wang, F. Su, M.K. Iyer, S. Roychowdhury, J. Siddiqui, K.J. Pienta, L.P. Kunju, M. Talpaz, J.M. Mosquera, S. Singer, S.M. Schuetze, C.R. Antonescu, and A.M. Chinnaiyan, Identification of recurrent NAB2-STAT6 gene fusions in solitary fibrous tumor by integrative sequencing, *Nat Genet* **45**: 180–185 (2013).

Rogalla, P., I. Lemke, B. Kazmierczak, and J. Bullerdiek, An identical HMGIC-LPP fusion transcript is consistently expressed in pulmonary chondroid hamartomas with t(3;12)(q27–28;q14–15), *Genes Chromosomes Cancer* **29**: 363–366 (2000).

Saborowski, A., M. Saborowski, M.A. Davare, B.J. Druker, D.S. Klimstra, and S.W. Lowe, Mouse model of intrahepatic cholangiocarcinoma validates FIG-ROS as a potent fusion oncogene and therapeutic target, *Proc Natl Acad Sci USA* **110**: 19513–19518 (2013).

Saito, T., M. Nagai, and M. Ladanyi, SYT-SSX1 and SYT-SSX2 interfere with repression of E-cadherin by snail and slug: a potential mechanism for aberrant mesenchymal to epithelial transition in human synovial sarcoma, *Cancer Res* **66**: 6919–6927 (2006).

Saito, T.. The SYT-SSX fusion protein and histological epithelial differentiation in synovial sarcoma: relationship with extracellular matrix remodeling. *Int J Clin Exp Pathol* **6**: 2272–2279 (2013).

Salzman, J., R.J. Marinelli, P.L. Wang, A.E. Green, J.S. Nielsen, B.H. Nelson, C.W. Drescher, and P.O. Brown, ESRRA-C11orf20 is a recurrent gene fusion in serous ovarian carcinoma, *PLoS Biol* **9**: e1001156 (2011).

Scheele, J.S., M. Kolanczyk, M. Gantert, T. Zemojtel, A. Dorn, D.B. Sykes, D.C. Möbest, M.P. Kamps, and D. Räpple, The Spt-Ada-Gcn5-acetyltransferase complex interaction motif of E2a is essential for a subset of transcriptional and oncogenic properties of E2a-Pbx1, *Leuk Lymphoma* **50**: 816–828 (2009).

Seshagiri, S., E.W. Stawiski, S. Durinck, Z. Modrusan, E.E. Storm, C.B. Conboy, S. Chaudhuri, Y. Guan, V. Janakiraman, B.S. Jaiswal, J. Guillory, C. Ha, G.J. Dijkgraaf, J. Stinson, F. Gnad, M.A. Huntley, J.D. Degenhardt, P.M. Haverty, R. Bourgon, W. Wang, H. Koeppen, R. Gentleman, T.K. Starr, Z. Zhang, D.A. Largaespada, T.D. Wu, and F.J. de Sauvage, Recurrent R-spondin fusions in colon cancer, *Nature* **488**: 660–664 (2012).

Shiba, N., H. Ichikawa, T. Taki, M.J. Park, A. Jo, S. Mitani, T. Kobayashi, A. Shimada, M. Sotomatsu, H. Arakawa, S. Adachi, A. Tawa, K. Horibe, M. Tsuchida, R. Hanada, I. Tsukimoto, and Y. Hayashi, NUP98-NSD1 gene fusion and its related gene expression signature are strongly associated with a poor prognosis in pediatric acute myeloid leukemia, *Genes Chromosomes Cancer* **52**: 683–693 (2013).

Shinmura, K., T. Kahyo, H. Kato, H. Igarashi, S. Matsuura, S. Nakamura, K. Kurachi, T. Nakamura, H. Ogawa, K. Funai, M. Tanahashi, H. Niwa, and H. Sugimura, RSPO fusion transcripts in colorectal cancer in Japanese population, *Mol Biol Rep* **41**: 5375–5384 (2014).

Sidhar, S.K., J. Clark, S. Gill, R. Hamoudi, A.J. Crew, R. Gwilliam, M. Ross, W.M. Linehan, S. Birdsall, J. Shipley, and C.S. Cooper, The t(X;1)(p11.2;q21.2) translocation in papillary renal cell carcinoma fuses a novel gene PRCC to the TFE3 transcription factor gene, *Hum Mol Genet* **5**: 1333–1338 (1996).

Sjögren, H., B. Wedell, J.M. Meis-Kindblom, L.G. Kindblom, and G. Stenman, Fusion of the NH2-terminal domain of the basic helix-loop-helix protein TCF12 to TEC in extraskeletal myxoid chondrosarcoma with translocation t(9;15)(q22;q21), *Cancer Res* **60**: 6832–6835 (2000).

Skalsky, Y.M., P.M. Ajuh, C. Parker, A.I. Lamond, G. Goodwin, and C.S. Cooper, PRCC, the commonest TFE3 fusion partner in papillary renal carcinoma is associated with pre-mRNA splicing factors, *Oncogene* **20**: 178–187 (2001).

Smith, S., B.R. Reeves, L. Wong, and C. Fisher, A consistent chromosome translocation in synovial sarcoma, *Cancer Genet Cytogenet* **26**: 179–180 (1987).

Specht, K., L. Zhang, Y.S. Sung, M. Nucci, S. Dry, S. Vaiyapuri, G.H. Richter, C.D. Fletcher, and C.R. Antonescu, Novel BCOR-MAML3 and ZC3H7B-BCOR gene fusions in undifferentiated small blue round cell sarcomas, *Am J Surg Pathol* **40**: 433–442 (2016).

Stephens, P.J., D.J. McBride, M.L. Lin, I. Varela, E.D. Pleasance, J.T. Simpson, L.A. Stebbings, C. Leroy, S. Edkins, L.J. Mudie, C.D. Greenman, M. Jia, C. Latimer, J.W. Teague, K.W. Lau, J. Burton, M.A. Quail, H. Swerdlow, C. Churcher, R. Natrajan, A.M. Sieuwerts, J.W. Martens, D.P. Silver, A. Langerød, H.E. Russnes, J.A. Foekens, J.S. Reis-Filho, L. van 't Veer, A.L. Richardson, A.L. Børresen-Dale, P.J. Campbell, P.A. Futreal, and M.R. Stratton, Complex landscapes of somatic rearrangement in human breast cancer genomes, *Nature* **462**: 1005–1010 (2009).

Storlazzi, C.T., F. Mertens, N. Mandahl, D. Gisselsson, M. Isaksson, P. Gustafson, H.A. Domanski, and I. Panagopoulos, A novel fusion gene, SS18L1/SSX1, in synovialsarcoma, *Genes Chromosomes Cancer* **37**: 195–200 (2003).

Storm, E.E., S. Durinck, F. de Sousa e Melo, J. Tremayne, N. Kljavin, C. Tan, X. Ye, C. Chiu, T. Pham, J.A. Hongo, T. Bainbridge, R. Firestein, E. Blackwood, C. Metcalfe, E.W. Stawiski, R.L. Yauch, Y. Wu, and F.J. de Sauvage, Targeting PTPRK-RSPO3 colon tumours promotes differentiation and loss of stem-cell function, *Nature* **529**: 97–100 (2016).

Sugita, S., Y. Arai, A. Tonooka, N. Hama, Y. Totoki, T. Fujii, T. Aoyama, H. Asanuma, T. Tsukahara, M. Kaya, T. Shibata, and T. Hasegawa, A novel CIC-FOXO4 gene fusion in undifferentiated small round cell sarcoma: a genetically distinct variant of Ewing-like sarcoma, *Am J Surg Pathol* **38**: 1571–1576 (2014).

Sugita, S., Y. Arai, A. Tonooka, N. Hama, Y. Totoki, T. Fujii, T. Aoyama, H. Asanuma, T. Tsukahara, M. Kaya, T. Shibata, and T. Hasegawa, A novel CIC-FOXO4 gene fusion in undifferentiated small round cell sarcoma: a genetically distinct variant of Ewing-like sarcoma, *Am J Surg Pathol* **38**: 1571–1576 (2014).

Sumegi, J., J. Nishio, M. Nelson, R.W. Frayer, D. Perry, and J.A. Bridge, A novel t(4;22)(q31;q12) produces an EWSR1-SMARCA5 fusion in extraskeletal Ewing sarcoma/primitive neuroectodermal tumor, *Mod Pathol* **24**: 333–342 (2011).

Sun, Y., J. Perera, B.P. Rubin, and J. Huang, SYT-SSX1 (synovial sarcoma translocated) regulates PIASy ligase activity to cause overexpression of NCOA3 protein, *J Biol Chem* **286**: 18623–18632 (2011).

Szuhai, K., M. Ijszenga, D. de Jong, A. Karseladze, H.J. Tanke, and P.C. Hogendoorn, The NFATc2 gene is involved in a novel cloned translocation in a Ewing sarcoma variant that couples its function in immunology to oncology, *Clin Cancer Res* **15**: 2259–2268 (2009).

Takahashi, T., N. Nagai, H. Oda, K. Ohama, N. Kamada, and K. Miyagawa, Evidence for RAD51L1/HMGIC fusion in the pathogenesis of uterine leiomyoma, *Genes Chromosomes Cancer* **30**: 196–201 (2001).

Taki, T., M. Akiyama, S. Saito, R. Ono, M. Taniwaki, Y. Kato, Y. Yuza, Y. Eto, and Y. Hayashi, The MYO1F, unconventional myosin type 1F, gene is fused to MLL in infant acute monocytic leukemia with a complex translocation involving chromosomes 7, 11, 19 and 22, *Oncogene* **24**: 5191–5197 (2005).

Tardío, J.C., I. Machado, L. Navarro, F. Idrovo, J. Sanz-Ortega, A. Pellín, and A. Llombart-Bosch, Ewing-like sarcoma with CIC-DUX4 gene fusion in a patient with neurofibromatosis type 1. A hitherto unreported association, *Pathol Res Pract* **211**: 877–882 (2015).

Thaete, C., D. Brett, P. Monaghan, S. Whitehouse, G. Rennie, E. Rayner, C.S. Cooper, and G. Goodwin, Functional domains of the SYT and SYT-SSX synovial sarcoma translocation proteins and co-localization with the SNF protein BRM in the nucleus, *Hum Mol Genet* **8**: 585–591 (1999).

Thanasopoulou, A., A. Tzankov, and J. Schwaller, Potent co-operation between the NUP98-NSD1 fusion and the FLT3-ITD mutation in acute myeloid leukemia induction, *Haematologica* **99**: 1465–1471 (2014).

Tirado, C.A., D. Shabsovich, L. Yeh, S.T. Pullarkat, L. Yang, M. Kallen, and N. Rao, A (1;19) translocation involving TCF3-PBX1 fusion within the context of a hyperdiploid karyotype in adult B-ALL: a case report and review of the literature, *Biomark Res* **3**: 4 (2015).

Trautmann, M., E. Sievers, S. Aretz, D. Kindler, S. Michels, N. Friedrichs, M. Renner, J. Kirfel, S. Steiner, S. Huss, A. Koch, R. Penzel, O. Larsson, A. Kawai, S. Tanaka, H. Sonobe, A. Waha, P. Schirmacher, G. Mechtersheimer, E. Wardelmann, R. Büttner, and W. Hartmann, SS18-SSX fusion protein-induced Wnt/β-catenin signaling is a therapeutic target in synovial sarcoma, *Oncogene* **33**: 5006–5016 (2014).

Turc-Carel, C., P. Dal Cin, J. Limon, U. Rao, F.P. Li, J.M. Corson, R. Zimmerman, D.M. Parry, J.M. Cowan, and A.A. Sandberg, Involvement of chromosome X in primary cytogenetic change in human neoplasia: nonrandom translocation in synovial sarcoma, *Proc Natl Acad Sci USA* **84**: 1981–1985 (1987).

Udayakumar, A.M., T.S. Sundareshan, G. Mukherjee, S. Biswas, K.R. Rajan, and P.S. Prabhakaran, Submandibular synovial sarcoma with t(X;18) and synovial sarcoma of the toe with additional cytogenetic abnormalities: presentation of two cases and review of the literature, *Cancer Genet Cytogenet* **134**: 151–155 (2002).

Van Roosbroeck, K., L. Cox, T. Tousseyn, I. Lahortiga, O. Gielen, B. Cauwelier, P. De Paepe, G. Verhoef, P. Marynen, P. Vandenberghe, C. De Wolf-Peeters, J. Cools, and I. Wlodarska, JAK2 rearrangements, including the novel SEC31A-JAK2 fusion, are recurrent in classical Hodgkin lymphoma, *Blood* **117**: 4056–4064 (2011).

Voz, M.L., A.K. Aström, K. Kas, J. Mark, G. Stenman, and W.J. Van de Ven, The recurrent translocation t(5;8)(p13;q12) in pleomorphic adenomas results in upregulation of PLAG1 gene expression under control of the LIFR promoter, *Oncogene* **16**: 1409–1416 (1998).

Wang, G.G., L. Cai, M.P. Pasillas, and M.P. Kamps, NUP98-NSD1 links H3K36 methylation to Hox-A gene activation and leukaemogenesis, *Nat Cell Biol* **9**: 804–812 (2007).

Wang, L., R. Bhargava, T. Zheng, L. Wexler, M.H. Collins, D. Roulston, and M. Ladanyi, Undifferentiated small round cell sarcomas with rare EWS gene fusions: identification of a novel EWS-SP3 fusion and of additional cases with the EWS-ETV1 and EWS-FEV fusions, *J Mol Diagn* **9**: 498–509 (2007).

Wang, L., T. Motoi, R. Khanin, A. Olshen, F. Mertens, J. Bridge, P. Dal Cin, C.R. Antonescu, S. Singer, M. Hameed, J.V. Bovee, P.C. Hogendoorn, N. Socci, and M. Ladanyi, Identification of a novel, recurrent HEY1-NCOA2 fusion in mesenchymal chondrosarcoma based on a genome-wide screen of exon-level expression data, *Genes Chromosomes Cancer* **51**: 127–139 (2012).

Weterman, M.A., J.J. van Groningen, L. Tertoolen, and A.G. van Kessel, Impairment of MAD2B-PRCC interaction in mitotic checkpoint defective t(X;1)-positive renal cell carcinomas. *Proc Natl Acad Sci USA* **98**: 13808–13813 (2001).

Weterman, M.A., M. Wilbrink, and A. Geurts van Kessel, Fusion of the transcription factor TFE3 gene to a novel gene, PRCC, in t(X;1)(p11;q21)-positive papillary renal cell carcinomas, *Proc Natl Acad Sci USA* **93**: 15294–15298 (1996).

Wiesner, T., J. He, R. Yelensky, R. Esteve-Puig, T. Botton, I. Yeh, D. Lipson, G. Otto, K. Brennan, R. Murali, M. Garrido, V.A. Miller, J.S. Ross, M.F. Berger, A. Sparatta, G. Palmedo, L. Cerroni, K.J. Busam, H. Kutzner, M.T. Cronin, P.J. Stephens, and B.C. Bastian, Kinase fusions are frequent in Spitz tumours and spitzoid melanomas, *Nat Commun* **5**: 3116 (2014).

Xie, H., P.S. Rachakonda, B. Heidenreich, E. Nagore, A. Sucker, K. Hemminki, D. Schadendorf, and R. Kumar, Mapping of deletion breakpoints at the

CDKN2A locus in melanoma: detection of MTAP-ANRIL fusion transcripts, *Oncotarget* **7**: 16490–16504 (2016).

Yang, J.J., T.S. Park, S.T. Lee, J.Y. Seo, S.H. Oh, E.H. Cho, T. Burmeister, W.D. Ludwig, C. Meyer, R. Marschalek, H.J. Kim, and S.H. Kim, Molecular characterization and clinical course of MLL-ACTN4 rearrangement in therapy-related hematologic malignancies, *Haematologica* **99**: e49–e51 (2014).

Yano, M., S. Toyooka, K. Tsukuda, H. Dote, Y. Morimoto, N. Ohata, K. Ichimura, M. Aoe, H. Date, and N. Shimizu, SYT-SSX fusion genes in synovial sarcoma of the thorax, *Lung Cancer* **44**: 391–397 (2004).

Yoneda, Y., S. Ito, T. Kunisada, Y. Morimoto, H. Kanzaki, A. Yoshida, K. Shimizu, T. Ozaki, and M. Ouchida, Truncated SSX protein suppresses synovial sarcoma cell proliferation by inhibiting the localization of SS18-SSX fusion protein, *PLoS One* **8**: e77564 (2013).

Yoo, H.Y. P. Kim, W.S. Kim, S.H. Lee, S. Kim, S.Y. Kang, H.Y. Jang, J.E. Lee, J. Kim, S.J. Kim, Y.H. Ko, and S. Lee, Frequent CTLA4-CD28 gene fusion in diverse types of T cell lymphoma, *Haematologica* **101**: 757–763 (2016).

Yoon, J.K. and J.S. Lee, Cellular signaling and biological functions of R-spondins, *Cell Signal* **24**: 369–377 (2012).

Yoshida, H., M. Miyachi, K. Ouchi, Y. Kuwahara, K. Tsuchiya, T. Iehara, E. Konishi, A. Yanagisawa, and H. Hosoi, Identification of COL3A1 and RAB2A as novel translocation partner genes of PLAG1 in lipoblastoma, *Genes Chromosomes Cancer* **53**: 606–611 (2014).

Zhang, Y., X.Y. Mao, X. Liu, R.R. Song, D. Berney, Y.J. Lu, and G. Ren, High frequency of the SDK1: AMACR fusion transcript in Chinese prostate cancer, *Int J Clin Exp Med* **8**: 15127–15136 (2015).

21

Targeting Fusion Genes for Cancer Therapy

*Nand K. Roy, Devivasha Bordoloi, Ganesan Padmavathi and Ajaikumar B. Kunnumakkara**

INTRODUCTION

The fusion genes are of immense biological significance due to their specificity to cancer cells making them an excellent target for molecular therapy. The close association of the gene fusion and the tumor phenotype makes them ideal for various diagnostic and therapeutic purposes. It enables the sub classification of otherwise seemingly identical disease entities. Moreover, different fusion genes add key features required for risk stratification and increasing numbers of chimeric proteins encoded by the gene fusions serve as specific targets for treatment, resulting in the development of many therapies against fusion genes (Table 21.1)

*Author for correspondence: Ajaikumar B. Kunnumakkara, Cancer Biology Laboratory, Department of Biosciences and Bioengineering, Indian Institute of Technology Guwahati, Assam 781039, India. kunnumakkara@iitg.ernet.in

Table 21.1: Various compounds targeted against fusion oncogenes

Fusion Gene	Compound(s)	Cancer	Reference
BCR-ABL	CHMFL-ABL-053	CML	Liang *et al.* (2016)
BCR-ABL	CR-LAAO	CML	Burin *et al.* (2016)
BCR-ABL	EGCG-MP	CML	Jung *et al.* (2015)
BCR-ABL	CD-200	CML	Fang *et al.* (2015)
BCR-ABL	Pyrazolopyrimidines	CML	Liu *et al.* (2015)
BCR-ABL	PEITC	CML	Roy *et al.* (2015)
BCR-ABL	E35	CML	Li *et al.* (2015a)
BCR-ABL	Imatinib	CML	Payandeh *et al.* (2015)
BCR-ABL	ATRA	CML	Wang *et al.* (2014)
BCR-ABL	Imatinib and TG101348	CML	Okabe *et al.* (2014)
BCR-ABL	ATO and bortezomib	CML	Xu *et al.* (2014)
BCR-ABL	Thiotanib	CML	Fan *et al.* (2014)
BCR-ABL	TKI258	Leukemia	Eucker *et al.* (2014)
BCR-ABL	TKI258 and RAD001	Leukemia	Eucker *et al.* (2014)
BCR-ABL	DCC-2036	CML	Eide *et al.* (2011)
BCR-ABL	Bosutinib	ALL	Cortes *et al.* (2011a)
BCR-ABL	Imatinib	ALL	Soverini *et al.* (2011)
BCR-ABL	GNF2 and imatinib	CML	Zhang *et al.* (2010)
BCR-ABL	GNF2	CML	Hassan *et al.* (2010)
BCR-ABL	Ponatinib	ALL	O'Hare *et al.* (2009)
BCR-ABL	Imatinib	ALL	Hantschel *et al.* (2008)
BCR-ABL	Nilotinib	ALL	Hantschel *et al.* (2008)
BCR-ABL	Dasatinib	ALL	Hantschel *et al.* (2008)
BCR-ABL	Dasatinib	ALL	Rix *et al.* (2007)
BCR-ABL	Nilotinib	ALL	von Bubnoff *et al.* (2006)
BCR-ABL	GNF2	CML	Adrian *et al.* (2006)
BCR-ABL	AMN107	ALL	Weisberg *et al.* (2005)
BCR-ABL	BMS-354825	ALL	Shah *et al.* (2004)
BCR-ABL	TPA	Leukemia	Campbell *et al.* (1993)

(Continued)

Table 21.1: (*Continued*)

Fusion Gene	Compound(s)	Cancer	Reference
BRD4-NUT	OTX015/MK-8628	NMC	Stathis *et al.* (2016)
EML4-ALK	Crizotinib	NSCLC	Bayliss *et al.* (2016)
EML4-ALK	Crizotinib	NSCLC	Casaluce *et al.* (2013)
EML4-ALK	Crizotinib and TAE684	Lung cancer	Heuckmann *et al.* (2012)
EML4-ALK	NVP-TAE684	NSCLC	Katayama *et al.* (2011)
EML4-ALK	AP26113	NSCLC	Katayama *et al.* (2011)
EML4-ALK	17-AAG	NSCLC	Katayama *et al.* (2011)
ETV6-NTRK3	PKC412	—	Chi *et al.* (2012)
ETV6-NTRK3	SU6656	—	Jin *et al.* (2007)
EWS-ATF1	Romidepsin	Sarcoma	Liu *et al.* (2008)
KIAA1549-BRAF	Sorafenib, temsirolimus and bevacizumab	MSCN	Subbiah *et al.* (2014)
MLL-AF9	Dinaciclib	MLL	Baker *et al.* (2016)
NPM-ALK	Crizotinib	Lymphoma	Hamedani *et al.* (2014)
NPM-ALK	GC & rapamycin	Lymphoma	Gu et *al.* (2008)
NPM-ALK	Herbimycin A	Lymphoma	Turturro *et al.* (2002)
NPM-ALK	17-AAG	Lymphoma	Bonvini *et al.* (2002)
PAX5-PML	ATO	ALL	Kurahashi *et al.* (2011)
PAX8-PPARγ	Pioglitazone	TC	Dobson *et al.* (2011)
PCM1-JAK2	Ruxolitinib	CEL	Rumi *et al.* (2013)
PCM1-JAK2	Ruxolitinib	CEL	Lierman *et al.* (2012)
PML-RARA	ATRA	APL	Fang *et al.* (2015)
PML-RARA	ATRA	APL	Wei *et al.* (2015)
PML-RARA	Bortezomib	APL	Takenokuchi *et al.* (2015)
PML-RARA	ATRA and ATO	APL	Vitaliano-Prunier *et al.* (2014)
PML-RARA	ATRA and ATO	APL	Isakson *et al.* (2010)
PML-RARA	ATRA and ATO	APL	Bøe *et al.* (2010)

(*Continued*)

Table 21.1: (*Continued*)

Fusion Gene	Compound(s)	Cancer	Reference
PML-RARA	ATRA	APL	Kuyama *et al.* (2004)
RANBP2-ALK	Crizotinib	EIMS	Kimbara *et al.* (2014)
RANBP2-ALK	Crizotinib	AML	Maesako *et al.* (2014)
RANBP2-ALK	Crizotinib	Leukemia	Maesako *et al.* (2014)
RET-PTC	Vandetanib	Lung cancer	Suzuki *et al.* (2013)
RET-PTC	Lenvatinib (E7080)	TC	Okamoto *et al.* (2013)
SND1-BRAF	Trametinib	PACC	Chmielecki *et al.* (2014)
SYT-SSX	MS-275	Sarcoma	Liu *et al.* (2008)
TEL-PDGFβR	CGP57148	CMML	Tomasson *et al.* (1999)
TPM3-ALK	Herbimycin A	Lymphoma	Giuriato *et al.* (2007)

*EIMS: Epithelioid inflammatory myofibroblastic sarcoma; MSCN: Malignant spindle cell neoplasm; TC: Thyroid carcinoma.

(Annala *et al.*, 2013, Mertens *et al.*, 2015). This chapter deals with the various chemotherapeutics developed against fusion genes and their importance in cancer therapy.

Therapies for Fusion Genes

BCR/ABL is one of the most common genetic abnormalities detected in leukemia particularly in ALLs and CML (Ye *et al.*, 2014). Therefore, targeting the tyrosine kinase activity of BCR/ABL can prove to be an attractive therapeutic strategy to combat leukemia. Tyrosine kinase inhibitors (TKI) are mostly used to target BCR/ABL fusion gene. Depending on the molecular mechanism of TKIs, it can be classified into two types i.e. type 1 inhibitors and type 2 inhibitors. Type 1 has been found to target the active conformation of kinase domain that are active for catalysis because of even distribution of essential elements required for binding the ATP and substrate. On the other hand, type 2 was shown to target only the inactive conformation of the kinase domain. Generally, type 2 inhibitors are believed to be more specific compared to type 1 inhibitors since most kinases possess the similar active conformation (Hantschel *et al.*, 2012; Davis *et al.*, 2011). Imatinib is the first generation of TKIs which has revolutionized the targeted cancer therapy (Druker, 2008). Imatinib treatment in chronic phase led to durable remissions in majority of CML patients and resulted in better response in Ph+ ALL patients. However, various BCR/ABL mutations which include G250E, Q252H, Y253H/F and E255K/V in the Gly-rich loop; T315I; H395P/R in the activation loop, M244V, F317L, M351T, E355G and F359V in other regions of kinase domain were found to result in imatinib resistance significantly (Hochhaus *et al.*, 2002, 2009; Soverini *et al.*, 2011). To overcome the resistance developed, investigators have come up with second- and third-generation TKIs. Few of them were found to meet the regulatory approval criteria while others are undergoing clinical trials at present (Schiffer, 2010). Nilotinib, dasatinib and bosutinib are considered as second generation BCR/ABL TKIs. Dasatinib and nilotinib were shown to inhibit almost all frequently occurring imatinib resistance associated mutations where T315I mutation is the only exception. Compared to imatinib, second generation TKIs showed less spectrum of emerging resistance mutations, although differences in the comparative sensitivities for these two TKIs for particular mutations *in vitro* existed. However, their clinical significance is yet to be validated (Weisberg *et al.*, 2005; Shah *et al.*, 2004; von Bubnoff *et al.*, 2006; Burgess *et al.*, 2005; Laneuville *et al.*, 2010; Hantschel *et al.*, 2012). In spite of great similarity observed between nilotinib and dasatinib, they belong to different classes of inhibitors. Nilotinib is a type 2 inhibitor while dasatinib belongs to type 1 inhibitor category. Nilotinib interacts with an auxiliary binding pocket of Abl kinase domain that allows elevated lipophilic interactions and reduction in the number of hydrogen bonds with the target. Consequently, the binding interface has greater flexibility and can act against a broad spectrum of imatinib resistance mutations. Although nilotinib shows similar spectrum of targets as imatinib, it shows a greater affinity towards BCR/ABL. Dasatinib, on the contrary, targets many other types of tyrosine kinases, particularly Src, Tec, Csk and Eph families, in addition to quite a few Ser/Thr kinases besides ABL1/2, KIT, PDGFRA/B and DDR1/2 PDGFR (Rix *et al.*, 2007; Vajpai *et al.*, 2008; Weisberg *et al.*, 2005; Hantschel *et al.*, 2008). Bosutinib is another second-generation TKI approved by U.S. Food and

Drug Administration (FDA) for the treatment of all stages CML patients exhibiting intolerance or resistance to alternate therapies (FDA, 2012). This inhibitor belongs to type 1 inhibitor and is quite similar to dasatinib. Notably, bosutinib was unable to inhibit KIT and PDGFR. Besides targeting most of the imatinib resistant BCR/ABL mutants excluding T315I gatekeeper mutation, it was found to target Ser/Thr kinases, including mitogen-activated protein kinase family members (Puttini *et al.*, 2006; Remsing *et al.*, 2009). Since the second generation TKIs were unable to target T315I BCR/ABL mutant, the third generation TKIs have been developed. Ponatinib is one such third generation TKI which can target both wild-type and imatinib-resistant BCR/ABL mutants along with T315I, with equal efficacy. However, ponatinib shows medium range specificity as it can target other kinases such as SRC kinases and several RTKs like KIT, RET, PDGFR, VEGFR, DDR, EPH, TRK and FGFR family member. An ethinyl linkage present in ponatinib facilitates its binding to the kinase domain in spite of the existence of bulky isoleucine residue in T315I gatekeeper mutation, which otherwise was inaccessible to imatinib as well as second-generation BCR/ABL TKIs. It has similar features of methylphenyl and trifluormethylphenyl rings as nilotinib that occupy nearly identical positions in bounded state with ABL kinase domain (O'Hare *et al.*, 2009; Cortes *et al.*, 2011a, 2011b). DCC-2036 is another third generation TKI in which a carboxamide-substituted pyridine ring binds to the hinge region and a fluor-phenyl ring in order to avoid clashes with the gatekeeper residue. Moreover, the binding of DCC-2036 can displace the αC-helix and stabilize the inactive conformation of the kinase domain. The DCC-2036 also shows medium specificity and can target other kinases like SRC kinases and RTKs, especially FLT3, TIE2, MER, DDR2 and TRK, EPH, PDGFR family members. The *in vitro* analysis has shown that co-treatment of DCC-2036 with nilotinib or dasatinib abrogated the occurrence of drug-resistant colonies (Chan *et al.*, 2011; Eide *et al.*, 2011).

Although the currently available TKIs are promising therapeutic approaches, they are associated with the development of resistance, a major obstacle in cancer therapy. The frequent mutation of T315I gatekeeper residue as mentioned earlier is one of the main reasons behind the development of resistance. Though the third generation TKIs can overcome this resistance, they don't show high level of specificity. To overcome these issues, several approaches have been implemented such as the development of allosteric inhibitors that target the sites present outside the ATP-binding cleft. These allosteric inhibitors possess the ability to alter the kinase conformation or they can compete with the protein substrates directly (Radi *et al.*, 2013). The benefit non-ATP competitive kinase inhibitors provide is that they can be highly selective for a specific kinase as they target non-conserved kinase regulatory mechanisms (Deng *et al.*, 2010). GNF2 is one such allosteric inhibitor which has shown potency similar to imatinib. Different experimental methods showed that GNF2 binds to the myristate pocket of the kinase protein. GNF2 binds to the remote region from the ATP pocket which makes it an appealing candidate for inhibiting different BCR/ABL mutations. However, it was found to be ineffective against T315I gatekeeper mutation. This resistance was overthrown when its variant GNF5 was combined with nilotinib (Adrian *et al.*, 2006; Zhang *et al.*, 2010; Hassan *et al.*, 2010). Recently, many other inhibitors and their combinations such as imatinib and TG101348, arsenic trioxide (ATO) and bortezomib, ATRA, Thiotanib, TKI258, alone or in combination with RAD001, EGCG-monopalmitate (EGCG-MP), CD-200,CR-LAAO,18a (CHMFL-ABL-053), alkyne-containing pyrazolopyrimidines are being studied which showed some promising outcomes in treating patients carrying BCR/ABL fusion gene (Okabe *et al.*, 2014; Xu *et al.*, 2014; Wang *et al.*, 2014; Fan *et al.*, 2014; Eucker *et al.*, 2014; Hershkovitz-Rokah *et al.*, 2015; Jung *et al.*, 2015; Fang *et al.*, 2015; Liu *et al.*, 2015; Liang *et al.*, 2016; Burin *et al.*, 2016).

In addition to BCR-ABL fusion gene, other fusion genes such as PCM1-JAK2, RUNX1-EVI1, TEL-RUNX1, RUNX1-ETO, RANBP2-ALK, PML-RARA, AML1-ETO, etc. are also found to be implicated in case of leukemia. For targeting PML/RARA fusion gene, ATO and ATRA were used in different studies. In the year 2004, Kuyama *et al.* successfully treated tetraploid APL with double PML-RARA gene rearrangements by using ATRA. Similarly, in another study of randomized, controlled, multicentre, clinical trial on acute promyelocytic leukaemia (APL) patient harboring PML-RARA fusion gene, it was found that ATRA and ATO might be a plausible treatment option for low and high-risk APL patients. Moreover, another study reported that APL patient with iso(17q) as the only cytogenetic aberration and a cryptic PML-RARA transcript upon treatment with ATRA and ATO after unsuccessful response to chemotherapy attained complete remission (Kuyama *et al.*, 2004; Burnett *et al.*, 2015; Shepshelovich *et al.*, 2015). Studies have shown that administration of a tyrosine kinase inhibitor crizotinib in AML having RANBP2-ALK chromosomal rearrangement leads to the reduction in leukemia cell burden and restoration of normal hematopoiesis (Maesako *et al.*, 2014). In another study, Sasaki *et al.* (2008) investigated the effect of trichostatin A and valproic acid on leukemia cell lines carrying different fusion genes such as RUNX1-ETO, RUNX1-EVI1, TEL-RUNX1 and it was found to result in cell cycle arrest and induction of apoptosis (Sasaki *et al.*, 2008). Likewise, ruxolitinib- a Janus kinase inhibitor was found to exhibit great efficacy against transforming JAK2 fusion proteins *in vitro* and in t(8;9)(p22;p24)-*PCM1-JAK2*-positive chronic eosinophilic leukemia total cytogenetic remission was induced (Lierman *et al.*, 2012). This activity was further validated by a clinical study (Rumi *et al.*, 2013).

In case of lung cancer as well, several fusions involving genes such as *RET*, *ROS1*, *NTRK1*, *NRG1*, *FGFR1* and *FGFR3* have been identified (Solomon, 2015). In lung adenocarcinomas, kinesin family member 5B-Ret proto-oncogene (*KIF5B-RET*), *CCDC6-ROS1* and *FGFR2*-citron (*CIT*) are some of the fusion genes that have been reported so far (Parker BC, Zhang, 2013). While in lung squamous cell carcinoma, three fusions have been reported such as *FGFR3-TACC3* fusion, *FGFR3-KIAA1967* and *FGFR1-BCL2*-associated athanogene (*BAG4*) (Parker and Zhang, 2013). The ROS1 tyrosine kinase was known to be frequently involved in various chromosomal rearrangements and the resulting fusion oncogenes were found to occur in approx. 1–2% of NSCLC patients (Solomon, 2015). Eventually, around 11 gene fusions of *ROS1* have been identified thus far including *CD74-ROS1*, *SDC4-ROS1*, *EZR-ROS1* and *SLC34A2-ROS1*. Further, all these fusion genes were shown to have the ROS1 kinase domain which results in the overexpression of ROS1 tyrosine kinase (Solomon, 2015). In NSCLC, ALK fusion has also been found to be expressed and the fusion partners of ALK were found to be echinoderm microtubule-associated protein-like

4 (EML4), TRK-fused gene (TFG), kinesin family member 5B, kinesin light chain 1 (KLC1), protein tyrosine phosphatase and non-receptor type3 and huntingtin interacting protein 1 (HIP1) (Choi *et al.*, 2014). The EML4-ALK fusion oncogene has been recognized as a novel molecular target for the treatment of NSCLCs (Parker and Zhang, 2013; Mano, 2015; Miyanaga *et al.*, 2013; Shaw *et al.*, 2009). An inversion in chromosome 2 mediates the fusion of these two genes thereby upregulating the ALK tyrosine kinase activity. The drugs such as crizotinib, ceritinib, and alectinib have been found to target kinase activity of ALK (Mano, 2015; Casaluce *et al.*, 2013; Mok, 2011; Sasaki *et al.*, 2010). In another study, on treatment with crizotinib, a marked downregulation in the phosphorylation of ALK and its downstream signaling was observed (Isozaki *et al.*, 2014; Parker and Zhang, 2013). Crizotinib (PF-02341066) has been noted to suppress ALK and hepatocyte growth factor receptor (c-MET) and is found to be ATP-competitive. The drug has been found beneficial in the treatment of EML4-ALK positive advanced NSCLC pre-treated patients (Casaluce *et al.*, 2013; Gröschel *et al.*, 2013; Sasaki *et al.*, 2010). Another fusion gene CCDC6-RET has been found to be actively expressed in LC-2/ad cells of lung adenocarcinoma. The decrease in the expression of RET tyrosine kinase and phosphorylation of ERK1/2 was observed on application of siRNA that targets the RET 3′ region. Vandetanib, an inhibitor of RET, was shown to decrease the cell proliferation and oveexpression of AKT and ERK1/2 (Suzuki *et al.*, 2013). The combination therapy of ALK kinase inhibitors (crizotinib, TAE684) and the HSP90 inhibitors have been found to reduce tumor growth in EML4-ALK positive tumor (Heuckmann *et al.*, 2012). Histone deacetylase inhibitor romidepsin (depsipeptide, FK228) is found to target SS18-SSX and SYT-SSX in different *in vitro* and *in vivo* sarcoma models. It was found that this inhibitor led to the suppression of cancer cell growth and its invasion to surrounding tissues and also induced apoptosis (Ito *et al.*, 2005; Su *et al.*, 2012). In another study, growth inhibition and differentiation effects of the histone deacetylase inhibitors MS-275 and romidepsin (FK228 depsipeptide) were evaluated on EWS-ATF1 positive sarcoma cells. It was observed that their treatment increased the expression of SOX9, MYOD1 and PPARG and decreased the expression of EWS-ATF1 fusion gene

suggesting the possible therapeutic potential of HDAC inhibitors against sarcoma (Liu *et al.*, 2008).

TARGETING FUSION GENES BY RNAi

The finding of RNA interference (RNAi) in mammalian cells in the year 2002 was considered as the "breakthrough of the year" and had raised the expectations of gene therapy. RNAi is a natural host defense mechanism associated with degradation of target mRNA transcripts in a sequence-specific manner and their protein products. The specificity of RNAi makes it a perfectly appropriate tool for targeted therapies against different fusion oncogenes that contain unique sequences. The inhibition of growth and progression of cancer cells by RNAi is a great challenge; despite that it can have some potential impact. In the recent period, researchers have taken keen interest in developing RNAi technology as a laboratory tool for the downregulation of the expression of a gene of interest. Furthermore, RNAi technology holds immense potential for gene therapy of particular cancer cells by the specific inhibition of a cancer-associated target (Lage, 2005; Cheng and Sakamoto, 2004; Bakalova, 2007). One of the early reports of application of RNAi in killing of BCR/ABL positive cells comes from the work of Wilda *et al.* in the year 2002 where they found that the administration of dsRNA specific for BCR/ABL gene led to the induction of apoptosis. However, combination of M-BCR/ABL-dsRNA with the FDA approved TKI imatinib (STI 571) did not exert any synergistic effect on the apoptotic induction. Nevertheless, these data have definitely provided important clues for RNA interference gene-therapeutic approaches for killing tumor cells having specific genetic abnormalities (Wilda *et al.*, 2002). The potential of RNAi was also proved in Ewing's sarcoma. It was observed that RNAi mediated suppression of EWS-FLI1 resulted in increased differentiation and chemosensitivity. Hence, RNAi holds immense potential as an adjuvant to chemotherapy (Kovar *et al.*, 2003). In 2008, in a study on the inhibitory effect of RNAi on the expression of AML1-ETO gene in Kasumi-1 cells, it was shown that AML1-ETO specific siRNA mediated suppression of AML1-ETO fusion protein results in the G1 cell cycle arrest and inhibition of proliferation of the leukemic cells (Wei *et al.*, 2008). In case of BCR/ABL fusion gene, RNAi was also suggested as an important therapeutic option. Lentivirus-mediated RNAi was successfully demonstrated to induce gene silencing in a dose-dependent fashion in BCR-ABL+ cells which indicated its therapeutic usefulness in primary hematopoietic cells (Scherr *et al.*, 2005). Similarly, in another study, a marked inhibition of the overexpressed BCR/ABL leading to elevated apoptosis of CML cells was obtained after *in vivo* application of targeted non-virally delivered synthetic BCR/ABL siRNA in a recurrent philadelphia chromosome positive CML patient with imatinib resistance Y253F mutation (Koldehoff and Elmaagacli, 2009). The RNAi-mediated therapy can also help in sensitizing the cancer cells against conventional chemotherapeutics. Furthermore, Wohlbold and colleagues have shown that RNAi can selectively inhibit BCR/ABL-dependent cell growth. Moreover, siRNA directed against BCR/ABL caused enhanced sensitivity to imatinib in BCR/ABL-overexpressing cells (Wohlbold *et al.*, 2003). In line with this report, siRNA homologous for different regions of BCR/ABL such as p190 and p210 showed synergism with imatinib mesylate and 17-allylamino-17-demetoxygeldanamycin in killing the BCR/ABL positive cells selectively in both *in vitro* and *in vivo* conditions (Futami *et al.*, 2008; Zhu *et al.*, 2012). In a recent study, a marked inhibition of the overexpressed BCR/ABL oncogene was observed after application of siRNA which caused elevated apoptosis of CML cells. Also, *in vivo* siRNA application was found to be well tolerated with no clinical adverse events (Koldehoff, 2015).

CONCLUSION

Genomic aberrations such as gene mutation, amplification, translocation, deletion and inversion are important hallmarks of cancer which led to the formation of fusion genes. These genes have significant role in the development of cancer. Furthermore, it has been observed that there exists a strong correlation between recurrent gene fusions and cancer types, and their detection has been used for finding different tumor types. Therefore, identification of fusion genes has enormous potential in the development of different therapeutic approaches. However, more studies are required in this area to find out novel, safe and affordable drugs for targeting fusion genes.

CONFLICT OF INTEREST

The authors express no conflict of interest.

REFERENCES

Adrián, F.J., Q. Ding, T. Sim, A. Velentza, C. Sloan, Y. Liu, G. Zhang, W. Hur, S. Ding, P. Manley, and J. Mestan, Allosteric inhibitors of Bcr-abl–dependent cell proliferation, *Nature Chemical Biology* **2**(2): 95–102 (2006).

Annala, M.J., B.C. Parker, W. Zhang, and M. Nykter, Fusion genes and their discovery using high throughput sequencing, *Cancer Letters* **340**(2): 192–200 (2013).

Bakalova, R., RNA interference — About the reality to be exploited in cancer therapy, *Methods Find Exp Clin Pharmacol* **29**(6): 417–421 (2007).

Baker, A., G.P. Gregory, I. Verbrugge, L. Kats, J.J. Hilton, E. Vidacs, E.M. Lee, R.B. Lock, J. Zuber, J. Shortt, and R.W. Johnstone, The CDK9 inhibitor Dinaciclib exerts potent apoptotic and antitumor effects in preclinical models of MLL-rearranged Acute Myeloid Leukemia, *Cancer Res* **76**(5): 1158–1169 (2016).

Bayliss, R., J. Choi, D.A. Fennell, A.M. Fry, and M.W. Richards, Molecular mechanisms that underpin EML4-ALK driven cancers and their response to targeted drugs, *Cell Mol Life Sci* **73**(6): 1209–1224 (2016).

Bøe, S.O. and A. Simonsen, Autophagic degradation of an oncoprotein, *Autophagy* **6**(7): 964–965. doi: 10.4161/auto.6.7.13066.

Bonvini, P., T. Gastaldi, B. Falini, and A. Rosolen, Nucleophosmin-anaplastic lymphoma kinase (NPM-ALK), a novel Hsp90-client tyrosine kinase: down-regulation of NPM-ALK expression and tyrosine phosphorylation in ALK(+) CD30(+) lymphoma cells by the Hsp90 antagonist 17-allylamino, 17-demethoxygeldanamycin, *Cancer Res* **62**(5): 1559–1566 (2002).

Burgess, M.R., B.J. Skaggs, N.P. Shah, F.Y. Lee, and C.L. Sawyers, Comparative analysis of two clinically active BCR-ABL kinase inhibitors reveals the role of conformation-specific binding in resistance, *Proceedings of the National Academy of Sciences of the United States of America*, **102**(9): 3395–3400 (2005).

Burin, S.M., S. Ghisla, A.T. Ouchida, A.F. Aissa, M.G. Coelho, T.R. Costa, A.P. Marsola, B. Pinto-Simões, L.M. Antunes, C. Curti, and S.V. Sampaio, CR-LAAO antileukemic effect against Bcr-Abl+ cells is mediated by apoptosis and hydrogen peroxide, *International Journal of Biological Macromolecules* **86**: 309–320 (2016).

Burnett, A.K., N.H. Russell, R.K. Hills, D. Bowen, J. Kell, S. Knapper, Y.G. Morgan, J. Lok, A. Grech, G. Jones, and A. Khwaja, Arsenic trioxide and all-trans retinoic acid treatment for acute promyelocytic leukaemia in all risk groups (AML17): results of a randomized, controlled, phase 3 trial, *The Lancet Oncology* **16**(13): 1295–1305 (2015).

Campbell, M.L., D. Lu, J.Q. Guo, and R.B. Arlinghaus, Inhibition of phosphorylation of p160 BCR within p210 BCR-ABL complexes during early stages of phorbol ester-induced differentiation of K562 cells, *Cell Growth Differ* **4**: 581–588 (1993).

Casaluce, F., A. Sgambato, P. Maione, A. Rossi, C. Ferrara, A. Napolitano, G. Palazzolo, F. Ciardiello, and C. Gridelli, ALK inhibitors: a new targeted therapy in the treatment of advanced NSCLC, *Target Oncol* **8**(1): 55–67 (2013).

Chan, W.W., S.C. Wise, M.D. Kaufman, Y.M. Ahn, C.L. Ensinger, T. Haack, M.M. Hood, J. Jones, J.W. Lord, W.P. Lu, and D. Miller, Conformational control inhibition of the BCR-ABL1 tyrosine kinase, including the gatekeeper T315I mutant, by the switch-control inhibitor DCC-2036, *Cancer cell* **19**(4): 556–568 (2011).

Charest, A., K. Lane, K. McMahon, J. Park, E. Preisinger, H. Conroy, and D. Housman, Fusion of FIG to the receptor tyrosine kinase ROS in a glioblastoma with an interstitial del (6)(q21q21), *Genes, Chromosomes and Cancer* **37**(1): 58–71 (2003).

Cheng, J.C., and K.M. Sakamoto, The emerging role of RNA interference in the design of novel therapeutics in oncology, *Cell Cycle* **3**(11): 1398–1401 (2004).

Chi, H.T., B.T. Ly, Y. Kano, A. Tojo, T. Watanabe, and Y. Sato, ETV6-NTRK3 as a therapeutic target of small molecule inhibitor PKC412, *Biochem Biophys Res Commun* **429**(1–2): 87–92 (2012).

Chmielecki, J., K.E. Hutchinson, G.M. Frampton, Z.R. Chalmers, A. Johnson, C. Shi, J. Elvin, S.M. Ali, J.S. Ross, O. Basturk, S. Balasubramanian, D. Lipson, R. Yelensky, W. Pao, V.A. Miller, D.S. Klimstra, and P.J. Stephens, Comprehensive genomic profiling of pancreatic acinar cell carcinomas identifies recurrent RAF fusions and frequent inactivation of DNA repair genes, *Cancer Discov* **4**(12): 1398–1405 (2014).

Choi, Y.L., M.E. Lira, M. Hong, R.N. Kim, S.J. Choi, J.Y. Song, K. Pandy, D.L. Mann, J.A. Stahl, H.E. Peckham, Z. Zheng, J. Han, M. Mao, and

J. Kim, A novel fusion of TPR and ALK in lung adenocarcinoma, *J Thorac Oncol* **9**(4): 563–566 (2014).

Cortes, J.E., D.W. Kim, J. Pinilla-Ibarz, Le P.D. Coutre, C. Chuah, F.E. Nicolini, R. Paquette, J.F. Apperley, J.F. DiPersio, H.J. Khoury, and D. Rea, Initial findings from the PACE trial: a pivotal phase 2 study of ponatinib in patients with CML and Ph+ ALL resistant or intolerant to dasatinib or nilotinib, or with the T315I mutation, *Blood* **118**(21): 109 (2011a).

Cortes, J.E., H.M. Kantarjian, T.H. Brümmendorf, D.W. Kim, A.G. Turkina, Z.X. Shen, R. Pasquini, H.J. Khoury, S. Arkin, A. Volkert, and N. Besson, Safety and efficacy of bosutinib (SKI-606) in chronic phase Philadelphia chromosome–positive chronic myeloid leukemia patients with resistance or intolerance to imatinib, *Blood* **118**(17): 4567–4576 (2011b).

Davis, M.I., J.P. Hunt, S. Herrgard, P. Ciceri, L.M. Wodicka, G. Pallares, M. Hocker, D.K. Treiber, and P.P. Zarrinkar, Comprehensive analysis of kinase inhibitor selectivity, *Nature biotechnology* **29**(11): 1046–1051 (2011).

Deng, X., B. Okram, Q. Ding, J. Zhang, Y. Choi, F.J. Adrián, A. Wojciechowski, G. Zhang, J. Che, B. Bursulaya, and S.W. Cowan-Jacob, Expanding the diversity of allosteric bcr-abl inhibitors. *Journal of Medicinal Chemistry*, **53**(19): 6934–6946 (2010).

Dobson, M.E., E. Diallo-Krou, V. Grachtchouk, J. Yu, L.A. Colby, J.E. Wilkinson, T.J. Giordano, and R.J. Koenig, Pioglitazone induces a proadipogenic antitumor response in mice with PAX8-PPARgamma fusion protein thyroid carcinoma, *Endocrinology* **152**(11): 4455–4465 (2011).

Druker, B.J., Translation of the Philadelphia chromosome into therapy for CML, *Blood* **112**(13): 4808–4817.

Eide, C.A., L.T. Adrian, J.W. Tyner, Mac M. Partlin, D.J. Anderson, S.C. Wise, B.D. Smith, P.A. Petillo, D.L. Flynn, M.W. Deininger, and T. O'Hare, The ABL switch control inhibitor DCC-2036 is active against the chronic myeloid leukemia mutant BCR-ABLT315I and exhibits a narrow resistance profile, *Cancer Research* **71**(9): 3189–3195 (2011).

Eucker, J., C. Zang, Y. Zhou, X. Li, P. Habbel, C. Neumann, C. Scholz, and H. Liu, The multi-tyrosine kinase inhibitor TKI258, alone or in combination with RAD001, is effective for treatment of human leukemia with BCR-ABL translocation *in vitro*, *Anticancer Res* **34**(9): 4909–4914 (2014).

Fan, J., X. Dong, W. Zhang, X. Zeng, Y. Li, Y. Sun, S. Wang, Z. Wang, H. Gao, W. Zhao, and D. Ju, Tyrosine kinase inhibitor Thiotanib targets Bcr-Abl and induces apoptosis and autophagy in human chronic myeloid leukemia cells, *Appl Microbiol Biotechnol* **98**(23): 9763–9775 (2014).

Fang, Z., K.H. Jung, H.H. Yan, S.J. Kim, M.K. Son, M. Rumman, H. Lee, K.W. Kim, H.D. Yoo, and S.S. Hong, CD-200 induces apoptosis and inhibits Bcr-Abl signaling in imatinib-resistant chronic myeloid leukemia with T315I mutation, *Int J Oncol* **47**(1): 253–261 (2015).

FDA approved drug products. (Cited 2012 Sep 19). Available from: http://www.fda.gov/

Futami, M., T. Hatano, Y. Soda, S. Kobayashi, M. Miyagishi, and A. Tojo, RNAi-mediated silencing of p190Bcr-Abl inactivates Stat5 and cooperates with imatinib mesylate and 17-allylamino-17-demetoxygeldanamycin in selective killing of p190Bcr-Abl-expressing leukemia cells, *Leukemia* **22**(6): 1131–1138 (2008).

Giuriato, S., N. Faumont, E. Bousquet, M. Foisseau, A. Bibonne, M. Moreau, Al T. Saati, D.W. Felsher, G. Delsol, and F. Meggetto, Development of a conditional bioluminescent transplant model for TPM3-ALK-induced tumorigenesis as a tool to validate ALK-dependent cancer targeted therapy, *Cancer Biol Ther* **6**(8): 1318–1323 (2007).

Gröschel, A., A. Warth, and N. Reinmuth, (Crizotinib — molecular therapy for lung cancer), *Pneumologie* **67**(4): 205–208 (2013).

Gu, L., J. Gao, Q. Li, Y.P. Zhu, C.S. Jia, R.Y. Fu, Y. Chen, Q.K. Liao, and Z. Ma, Rapamycin reverses NPM-ALK-induced glucocorticoid resistance in lymphoid tumor cells by inhibiting mTOR signaling pathway, enhancing G1 cell cycle arrest and apoptosis, *Leukemia* **22**(11): 2091–2096 (2008).

Hamedani, F.S., M. Cinar, Z. Mo, M.A. Cervania, H.M. Amin, and S. Alkan, Crizotinib (PF-2341066) induces apoptosis due to downregulation of pSTAT3 and BCL-2 family proteins in NPM-ALK(+) anaplastic large cell lymphoma, *Leuk Res* **38**(4): 503–508 (2014).

Hantschel, O., F. Grebien, G. Superti-Furga, The growing arsenal of ATP-competitive and allosteric inhibitors of BCR–ABL, *Cancer Research* **72**(19): 4890–4895 (2012).

Hantschel, O., U. Rix, and G. Superti-Furga, Target spectrum of the BCR-ABL inhibitors imatinib, nilotinib and dasatinib, *Leukemia & Lymphoma* **49**(4): 615–619 (2008).

Hassan, A.Q., S.V. Sharma, and M. Warmuth, Allosteric inhibition of BCR-ABL, *Cell Cycle* **9**(18): 3734–3738 (2010).

Hershkovitz-Rokah, O., S. Modai, M. Pasmanik-Chor, A. Toren, N. Shomron, P. Raanani, O. Shpilberg, and G. Granot, Restoration of miR-424 suppresses BCR-ABL activity and sensitizes CML cells to imatinib treatment, *Cancer Lett* **360**(2): 245–256 (2015).

Heuckmann, J.M., H. Balke-Want, F. Malchers, M. Peifer, M.L. Sos, M. Koker, L. Meder, C.M. Lovly, L.C. Heukamp, W. Pao, R. Küppers, and R.K. Thomas, Differential protein stability and ALK inhibitor sensitivity of EML4-ALK fusion variants, *Clin Cancer Res* **18**(17): 4682–4690 (2012).

Hiroyuki, M.A., The EML4-ALK oncogene: targeting an essential growth driver in human cancer. Proceedings of the Japan Academy, *Series B, Physical and Biological Sciences* **91**(5): 193 (2015).

Hochhaus, A., S. Kreil, A.S. Corbin, La P. Rosee, M.C. Muller, T. Lahaye, B. Hanfstein, C. Schoch, N.C. Cross, U. Berger, and H. Gschaidmeier, Molecular and chromosomal mechanisms of resistance to imatinib (STI571) therapy, *Leukemia* **16**(11): 2190–2196 (2002).

Hochhaus, A., S.G. O'brien, F. Guilhot, B.J. Druker, S. Branford, L. Foroni, J.M. Goldman, M.C. Müller, J.P. Radich, M. Rudoltz, and M. Mone, Six-year follow-up of patients receiving imatinib for the first-line treatment of chronic myeloid leukemia, *Leukemia* **23**(6): 1054–1061 (2009).

Isakson, P., M. Bjørås, S.O. Bøe, and A. Simonsen, Autophagy contributes to therapy-induced degradation of the PML/RARA oncoprotein, *Blood* **116**(13): 2324–2331. doi: 10.1182/blood-2010-01-261040.

Isozaki, H., M. Yasugi, N. Takigawa, K. Hotta, E. Ichihara, A. Taniguchi, S. Toyooka, S. Hashida, T. Sendo, M. Tanimoto, and K. Kiura, A new human lung adenocarcinoma cell line harboring the EML4-ALK fusion gene, *Jpn J Clin Oncol* **44**(10): 963–968 (2014).

Ito, T., M. Ouchida, Y. Morimoto, A. Yoshida, Y. Jitsumori, T. Ozaki, H. Sonobe, H. Inoue, and K. Shimizu, Significant growth suppression of synovial sarcomas by the histone deacetylase inhibitor FK228 *in vitro* and *in vivo*, *Cancer Letters* **224**(2): 311–319 (2005).

Jin, W., C. Yun, A. Hobbie, M.J. Martin, P.H. Sorensen, and S.J. Kim, Cellular transformation and activation of the phosphoinositide-3-kinase-Akt cascade by the ETV6-NTRK3 chimeric tyrosine kinase requires c-Src, *Cancer Res* **67**(7): 3192–3200 (2007).

Jung, J.H., M. Yun, E.J. Choo, S.H. Kim, M.S. Jeong, D.B. Jung, H. Lee, E.O. Kim, N. Kato, B. Kim, S.K. Srivastava, K. Kaihatsu, and S.H. Kim, A derivative of epigallocatechin-3-gallate induces apoptosis via SHP-1-mediated suppression of BCR-ABL and STAT3 signalling in chronic myelogenous leukaemia, *Br J Pharmacol* **172**(14): 3565–3578 (2015).

Katayama, R., T.M. Khan, C. Benes, E. Lifshits, H. Ebi, V.M. Rivera, W.C. Shakespeare, A.J. Iafrate, J.A. Engelman, and A.T. Shaw, Therapeutic strategies to overcome crizotinib resistance in non-small cell lung cancers harboring the fusion oncogene EML4-ALK, *Proc Natl Acad Sci USA* **108**(18): 7535–7540 (2011).

Kimbara, S., K. Takeda, H. Fukushima, T. Inoue, H. Okada, Y. Shibata, U. Katsushima, A. Tsuya, S. Tokunaga, H. Daga, T. Okuno, and T. Inoue, A case report of epithelioid inflammatory myofibroblastic sarcoma with RANBP2-ALK fusion gene treated with the ALK inhibitor, crizotinib, *Jpn J Clin Oncol* **44**(9): 868–871 (2014).

Koldehoff, M. and A.H. Elmaagacli, Therapeutic targeting of gene expression by siRNAs directed against BCR-ABL transcripts in a patient with imatinib-resistant chronic myeloid leukemia. siRNA and miRNA Gene Silencing: From Bench to Bedside, pp. 1–6 (2009).

Koldehoff, M., Targeting bcr-abl transcripts with siRNAs in an imatinib-resistant chronic myeloid leukemia patient: challenges and future directions. RNA Interference: Challenges and Therapeutic Opportunities, pp. 277–292 (2015).

Kovar, H., J. Ban, and S. Pospisilova, Potentials for RNAi in sarcoma research and therapy: Ewing's sarcoma as a model, *Semin Cancer Biol* **13**(4): 275–281 (2003).

Kurahashi, S., F. Hayakawa, Y. Miyata, T. Yasuda, Y. Minami, S. Tsuzuki, A. Abe, and T. Naoe, PAX5-PML acts as a dual dominant-negative form of both PAX5 and PML, *Oncogene* **30**(15): 1822–1830. doi: 10.1038/onc.2010.554.

Kuyama, J., Y. Tsumori, K. Aoyama, S. Kosugi, H. Take, and T. Matsuyama, Tetraploid acute promyelocytic leukemia with double PML/RARA gene rearrangements successfully treated with all-trans retinoic acid, *Int J Hematol* **79**(4): 405–406 (2004).

Lage, H., Potential applications of RNA interference technology in the treatment of cancer, *Future Oncol* **1**(1): 103–113 (2005).

Laneuville, P., C. DiLea, O.Q. Yin, R.C. Woodman, J. Mestan, and P.W. Manley, Comparative *in vitro* cellular data alone are insufficient to predict clinical responses and guide the choice of BCR-ABL inhibitor for treating imatinib-resistant chronic myeloid leukemia, *Journal of Clinical Oncology* **28**(11): e169–171 (2010).

Leow, P.C., C.S. Ku, R. Soo, and R. Soong, Technological Advances in the Detection of Novel Fusion Genes, eLS (2001).

Liang, X., X. Liu, B. Wang, F. Zou, A. Wang, S. Qi, C. Chen, Z. Zhao, W. Wang, Z. Qi, F. Lv, Z. Hu, L. Wang, S. Zhang, Q. Liu, and J. Liu, Discovery of 2-((3-Amino-4-methylphenyl)amino)-N-(2-methyl-5-(3-(trifluoromethyl) benzamido)phe nyl)-4-(methylamino)pyrimidine-5-carboxamide (CHMFL-ABL-053) as a Potent, Selective, and Orally Available BCR-ABL/SRC/p38

Kinase Inhibitor for Chronic Myeloid Leukemia, *J Med Chem* **59**(5): 1984–2004 (2016).

Lierman, E., D. Selleslag, S. Smits, J. Billiet, and P. Vandenberghe, Ruxolitinib inhibits transforming JAK2 fusion proteins *in vitro* and induces complete cytogenetic remission in t(8;9)(p22;p24)/PCM1-JAK2-positive chronic eosinophilic leukemia, *Blood* **120**(7): 1529–1531 (2012)

Liu X, A. Kung, B. Malinoski, G.K. Prakash, and C. Zhang, Development of Alkyne-Containing Pyrazolopyrimidines To Overcome Drug Resistance of Bcr-Abl Kinase, *J Med Chem* **58**(23): 9228–9237 (2015).

Liu, S., H. Cheng, W. Kwan, J.M. Lubieniecka, and T.O. Nielsen, Histone deacetylase inhibitors induce growth arrest, apoptosis, and differentiation in clear cell sarcoma models, *Molecular cancer therapeutics* **7**(6): 1751–1761 (2008).

M White, N., Y.F. Feng and A.C. Maher, Recurrent rearrangements in prostate cancer: causes and therapeutic potential, *Current drug targets* 14(4): 450–459 (2013).

Maesako, Y., A. Okumura, K. Takeoka, C. Kishimori, K. Izumi, Y. Kamoda, F. Iioka, T. Akasaka, and H. Ohno, Reduction of leukemia cell burden and restoration of normal hematopoiesis at 3 months of crizotinib treatment in RAN-binding protein 2 (RANBP2)-anaplastic lymphoma kinase (ALK) acute myeloid leukemia, *Leukemia* **28**(9): 1935–1937 (2014).

Mano, H., The EML4-ALK oncogene: targeting an essential growth driver in human cancer, *Proc Jpn Acad Ser B Phys Biol Sci* **91**(5): 193–201 (2015).

Mertens, F., B. Johansson, T. Fioretos, and F. Mitelman, The emerging complexity of gene fusions in cancer, *Nature Reviews Cancer* **15**(6): 371–381 (2015).

Mitelman, F., B. Johansson, and F. Mertens, The impact of translocations and gene fusions on cancer causation, *Nature Reviews Cancer* **7**(4): 233–245 (2007).

Miyanaga, A., K. Shimizu, R. Noro, M. Seike, K. Kitamura, S. Kosaihira, Y. Minegishi, T. Shukuya, A. Yoshimura, M. Kawamoto, S. Tsuchiya, K. Hagiwara, M. Soda, K. Takeuchi, N. Yamamoto, H. Mano, Y. Ishikawa, and A. Gemma, Activity of EGFR-tyrosine kinase and ALK inhibitors for EML4-ALK-rearranged non-small-cell lung cancer harbored coexisting EGFR mutation, *BMC Cancer* **13**: 262 (2013).

NewsEvents/Newsroom/PressAnnouncements/ucm318160.htm.

Nicorici, D., M. Satalan, H. Edgren, S. Kangaspeska, A. Murumagi, O. Kallioniemi, S. Virtanen, and O. Kilkku, FusionCatcher-a tool for finding somatic fusion genes in paired-end RNA-sequencing data, *BioRxiv* 011650 (2014).

O'Hare, T., W.C. Shakespeare, X. Zhu, C.A. Eide, V.M. Rivera, F. Wang, L.T. Adrian, T. Zhou, W.S. Huang, Q. Xu, and C.A. Metcalf, AP24534, a pan-BCR-ABL inhibitor for chronic myeloid leukemia, potently inhibits the T315I mutant and overcomes mutation-based resistance, *Cancer Cell* **16**(5): 401–412 (2009).

Okabe, S., T. Tauchi, S. Katagiri, Y. Tanaka, and K. Ohyashiki, Combination of the ABL kinase inhibitor imatinib with the Janus kinase 2 inhibitor TG101348 for targeting residual BCR-ABL-positive cells, *J Hematol Oncol* **7**: 37 (2014).

Okamoto, K., K. Kodama, K. Takase, N.H. Sugi, Y. Yamamoto, M. Iwata, and A. Tsuruoka, Antitumor activities of the targeted multi-tyrosine kinase inhibitor lenvatinib (E7080) against RET gene fusion-driven tumor models, *Cancer Lett* **340**(1): 97–103 (2013).

Payandeh, M., M. Sadeghi, and E. Sadeghi, Treatment and Survival in Patients with chronic myeloid leukemia in a chronic phase in West Iran, *Asian Pac J Cancer Prev* **16**(17): 7555–7559 (2015).

Pierotti, M.A., P. Vigneri, and I. Bongarzone, Rearrangements of RET and NTRK1 tyrosine kinase receptors in papillary thyroid carcinomas. InGenes and Environment in Cancer 1998 (pp. 237–247). Springer Berlin Heidelberg.

Puttini, M., A.M. Coluccia, F. Boschelli, A. Franceschino, L. Tornaghi, S. Ahmed, S. Redaelli, R. Piazza, V. Magistroni, F. Andreoni, and L. Scapozza, *In vitro* and *in vivo* activity of SKI-606, a novel Abl/Src inhibitor, against imatinib resistant BCR-ABL+ neoplastic cells, *Blood* **108**(11): 2176 (2006).

Radi, M., S. Schenone, and M. Botta, Allosteric inhibitors of Bcr-Abl: towards novel myristate-pocket binders, *Current Pharmaceutical Biotechnology* **14**(5): 477–487 (2013).

Rix, U., O. Hantschel, G. Dürnberger, L.L. Rix, M. Planyavsky, N.V. Fernbach, I. Kaupe, K.L. Bennett, P. Valent, J. Colinge, and T. Köcher, Chemical proteomic profiles of the BCR-ABL inhibitors imatinib, nilotinib, and dasatinib reveal novel kinase and nonkinase targets, *Blood* **110**(12): 4055–4063 (2007).

Roy, M., R. Sarkar, A. Mukherjee, and S. Mukherjee, Inhibition of crosstalk between Bcr-Abl and PKC signaling by PEITC, augments imatinib sensitivity in chronic myelogenous leukemia cells, *Chem Biol Interact* **242**: 195–201 (2015).

Rumi, E., J.D. Milosevic, I. Casetti, I. Dambruoso, D. Pietra, E. Boveri, M. Boni, P. Bernasconi, F. Passamonti, R. Kralovics, and M. Cazzola, Efficacy of ruxolitinib in chronic eosinophilic leukemia associated with a PCM1-JAK2 fusion gene, *J Clin Oncol* **31**(17): e269–e271 (2013).

Sasaki, K., T. Yamagata, and K. Mitani, Histone deacetylase inhibitors trichostatin A and valproic acid circumvent apoptosis in human leukemic cells expressing the RUNX1 chimera, *Cancer Science* **99**: 414–422 (2008).

Sasaki, T., S.J. Rodig, L.R. Chirieac, and P.A. Jänne, The biology and treatment of EML4-ALK non-small cell lung cancer, *Eur J Cancer* **46**(10): 1773–1780 (2010).

Scherr, M., K. Battmer, B. Schultheis, A. Ganser, and M. Eder, Stable RNA interference (RNAi) as an option for anti-bcr-abl therapy, *Gene Ther* **12**(1): 12–21 (2005).

Schiffer, C.A., CML: how low can you go?. *Blood* **116**(19): 3686–3687 (2010).

Shah, N.P., C. Tran, F.Y. Lee, P. Chen, D. Norris, and C.L. Sawyers, Overriding imatinib resistance with a novel ABL kinase inhibitor, *Science* **305**(5682): 399–401 (2004).

Shaw, A.T., B.Y. Yeap, M. Mino-Kenudson, S.R. Digumarthy, D.B. Costa, R.S. Heist, B. Solomon, H. Stubbs, S. Admane, U. McDermott, J. Settleman, S. Kobayashi, E.J. Mark, S.J. Rodig, L.R. Chirieac, E.L. Kwak, T.J. Lynch, and A.J. Iafrate, Clinical features and outcome of patients with non-small-cell lung cancer who harbor EML4-ALK, *J Clin Oncol* **27**(26): 4247–4253 (2009).

Shepshelovich, D., N. Oniashvili, D. Parnes, A. Klein, E. Muchtar, J. Yeshaya, A. Aviram, E. Rabizadeh, and P. Raanani, Acute promyelocytic leukemia with isochromosome 17q and cryptic PML-RARA successfully treated with all-trans retinoic acid and arsenic trioxide, *Cancer Genet* **208**(11): 575–579 (2015).

Soda, M., Y.L. Choi, M. Enomoto, S. Takada, Y. Yamashita, S. Ishikawa, S.I. Fujiwara, H. Watanabe, K. Kurashina, H. Hatanaka, and M. Bando, Identification of the transforming EML4–ALK fusion gene in non-small-cell lung cancer, *Nature* **448**(7153): 561–566 (2007).

Solomon, B., Validating ROS1 rearrangements as a therapeutic target in non-small-cell lung cancer, *J Clin Oncol* **33**(9): 972–974 (2015).

Soverini, S., A. Hochhaus, F.E. Nicolini, F. Gruber, T. Lange, G. Saglio, F. Pane, M.C. Müller, T. Ernst, G. Rosti, and K. Porkka, BCR-ABL kinase domain mutation analysis in chronic myeloid leukemia patients treated with tyrosine kinase inhibitors: recommendations from an expert panel on behalf of European LeukemiaNet, *Blood* **118**(5): 1208–1215 (2011).

Stathis, A., E. Zucca, M. Bekradda, C. Gomez-Roca, J.P. Delord, T. de La Motte Rouge, E. Uro-Coste, F. de Braud, G. Pelosi, and C.A. French, Clinical

Response of carcinomas harboring the BRD4-NUT oncoprotein to the targeted bromodomain inhibitor OTX015/MK-8628, *Cancer Discov* **6**(5): 492–500 (2016).

Su, L., A.V. Sampaio, K.B. Jones, M. Pacheco, A. Goytain, S. Lin, N. Poulin, L. Yi, F.M. Rossi, J. Kast, and M.R. Capecchi, Deconstruction of the SS18-SSX fusion oncoprotein complex: insights into disease etiology and therapeutics, *Cancer Cell* **21**(3): 333–347 (2012).

Subbiah, V., S.N. Westin, K. Wang, D. Araujo, W.L. Wang, V.A. Miller, J.S. Ross, P.J. Stephens, G.A. Palmer, and S.M. Ali, Targeted therapy by combined inhibition of the RAF and mTOR kinases in malignant spindle cell neoplasm harboring the KIAA1549-BRAF fusion protein, *J Hematol Oncol* **7**: 8 (2014).

Suzuki, M., H. Makinoshima, S. Matsumoto, A. Suzuki, S. Mimaki, K. Matsushima, K. Yoh, K. Goto, Y. Suzuki, G. Ishii, A. Ochiai, K. Tsuta, T. Shibata, T. Kohno, H. Esumi, and K. Tsuchihara, Identification of a lung adenocarcinoma cell line with CCDC6-RET fusion gene and the effect of RET inhibitors *in vitro* and *in vivo*, *Cancer Sci* **104**(7): 896–903 (2013).

Takenokuchi, M., K. Miyamoto, K. Saigo, and T. Taniguchi, Bortezomib Causes ER Stress-related Death of Acute Promyelocytic Leukemia Cells Through Excessive Accumulation of PML-RARA, *Anticancer Res* **35**(6): 3307–3316 (2015).

Tomasson, M.H., I.R. Williams, R. Hasserjian, C. Udomsakdi, S.M. McGrath, J. Schwaller, B. Druker, and D.G. Gilliland, TEL/PDGFbetaR induces hematologic malignancies in mice that respond to a specific tyrosine kinase inhibitor, *Blood* **93**(5): 1707–1714 (1999).

Turturro, F., M.D. Arnold, A.Y. Frist, and K. Pulford, Model of inhibition of the NPM-ALK kinase activity by herbimycin A, *Clin Cancer Res* **8**(1): 240–245 (2002).

Vajpai, N., A. Strauss, G. Fendrich, S.W. Cowan-Jacob, P.W. Manley, S. Grzesiek, and W. Jahnke, Solution conformations and dynamics of ABL kinase-inhibitor complexes determined by NMR substantiate the different binding modes of imatinib/nilotinib and dasatinib, *Journal of Biological Chemistry* **283**(26): 18292–18302 (2008).

Vitaliano-Prunier, A., J. Halftermeyer, J. Ablain, A. de Reynies, L. Peres, M. Le Bras, D. Metzger, and H. de Thé, Clearance of PML/RARA-bound promoters suffice to initiate APL differentiation, *Blood* **124**(25): 3772–3780 (2014).

von Bubnoff, N., P.W. Manley, J. Mestan, J. Sanger, C. Peschel, and J. Duyster, Bcr-Abl resistance screening predicts a limited spectrum of point mutations to be associated with clinical resistance to the Abl kinase inhibitor nilotinib (AMN107), *Blood* **108**(4): 1328–1333 (2006).

Wang, Z., Z. Liu, X. Wu, S. Chu, J. Wang, H. Yuan, M. Roth, Y.C. Yuan, R. Bhatia, and W. Chen, ATRA-induced cellular differentiation and CD38 expression inhibits acquisition of BCR-ABL mutations for CML acquired resistance, *PLoS Genet* **10**(6): e1004414 (2014).

Wei, J., S. Li, C. Wang, Y.W. Qin, X.X. Ma, K.C. Xie, S.K. Yan, Y.R. Gao, and Q. Cai, (Inhibitory effect of Rnai on AML1 -ETO fusion gene expression in leukemia cells), *Zhonghua Xue Ye Xue Za Zhi* **29**(9): 607–610 (2008).

Wei, S., S. Kozono, L. Kats, M. Nechama, W. Li, J. Guarnerio, M. Luo, M.H. You, Y. Yao, A. Kondo, H. Hu, G. Bozkurt, N.J. Moerke, S. Cao, M. Reschke, C.H. Chen, E.M. Rego, F. Lo-Coco, L.C. Cantley, T.H. Lee, H. Wu, Y. Zhang, P.P. Pandolfi, X.Z. Zhou, and K.P. Lu, Active Pin1 is a key target of all-trans retinoic acid in acute promyelocytic leukemia and breast cancer, *Nat Med* **21**(5): 457–466 (2015).

Weisberg, E., P.W. Manley, W. Breitenstein, J. Brüggen, S.W. Cowan-Jacob, A. Ray, B. Huntly, D. Fabbro, G. Fendrich, E. Hall-Meyers, and A.L. Kung, Characterization of AMN107, a selective inhibitor of native and mutant Bcr-Abl, *Cancer cell* **7**(2): 129–141 (2005).

Wilda, M., U. Fuchs, W. Wössmann, and A. Borkhardt, Killing of leukemic cells with a BCR/ABL fusion gene by RNA interference (RNAi), *Oncogene* **21**(37): 5716–5724 (2002).

Wohlbold, L., H. van der Kuip, C. Miething, H.P. Vornlocher, C. Knabbe, J. Duyster, and W.E. Aulitzky, Inhibition of bcr-abl gene expression by small interfering RNA sensitizes for imatinib mesylate (STI571), *Blood* **102**(6): 2236–2239 (2003).

Xu, W., W. Wei, Q. Yu, C. Wu, C. Ye, Y. Wu, and H. Yan, Arsenic trioxide and bortezomib interact synergistically to induce apoptosis in chronic myelogenous leukemia cells resistant to imatinib mesylate through Bcr/Abl-dependent mechanisms, *Mol Med Rep* **10**(3): 1519–1524 (2014).

Ye, Y.X., J. Zhou, Y.H. Zhou, Y. Zhou, X.B. Song, J. Wang, L. Lin, B.W. Ying, and X.J. Lu, Clinical significance of BCR-ABL fusion gene subtypes in chronic myelogenous and acute lymphoblastic leukemias, *Asian Pac J Cancer Prev* **15**(22): 9961–9966 (2014).

Zhang, J., F.J. Adrián, W. Jahnke, S.W. Cowan-Jacob, A.G. Li, R.E. Iacob, T. Sim, J. Powers, C. Dierks, F. Sun, and G.R. Guo, Targeting Bcr–Abl by combining allosteric with ATP-binding-site inhibitors, *Nature* **463**(7280): 501–506 (2010).

Zhu, Y.F., Y.Z. Wang, and F.Y. Meng, Stable interference on P210(bcr/abl) gene expression by lentiviral vector-delivered shRNA *in vitro* and *in vivo*, *Zhongguo Shi Yan Xue Ye Xue Za Zhi* **20**(5): 1090–1094 (2012).

Index

O

P

Q

T